Fundamentals of
U.S. Health Care

Principles and Perspectives

Charles E. Yesalis • Harry D. Holt • Robert M. Politzer

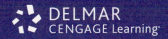
DELMAR
CENGAGE Learning·

Australia • Brazil • Japan • Korea • Mexico • Singapore • Spain • United Kingdom • United States

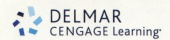
DELMAR
CENGAGE Learning®

**Fundamentals of U. S. Health Care:
Principles and Perspectives**
Charles Yesalis, Harry Holt, Robert Politzer

Vice President, Careers & Computing:
Dave Garza

Director of Learning Solutions:
Matthew Kane

Senior Acquisitions Editor: Tari Broderick

Managing Editor: Marah Bellegarde

Product Manager: Natalie Pashoukos

Editorial Assistant: Nicole Manikas

Vice President, Marketing: Jennifer Baker

Marketing Director: Wendy Mapstone

Senior Marketing Manager:
Michelle McTighe

Marketing Coordinator: Scott Chrysler

Production Director: Andrew Crouth

Senior Content Project Manager:
Kenneth McGrath

Senior Art Director: Jack Pendleton

Media Editor: William Overocker

For product information and technology assistance, contact us at
Cengage Learning Customer & Sales Support, 1-800-354-9706

For permission to use material from this text or product,
submit all requests online at **www.cengage.com/permissions**.
Further permissions questions can be e-mailed to
permissionrequest@cengage.com

Library of Congress Control Number: 2011943672

ISBN-13: 978-1-4283-1735-2

ISBN-10: 1-4283-1735-X

Delmar
5 Maxwell Drive
Clifton Park, NY 12065-2919
USA

Cengage Learning is a leading provider of customized learning solutions with office locations around the globe, including Singapore, the United Kingdom, Australia, Mexico, Brazil, and Japan. Locate your local office at: **international.cengage.com/region**

Cengage Learning products are represented in Canada by Nelson Education, Ltd.

To learn more about Delmar, visit **www.cengage.com/delmar**

Purchase any of our products at your local college store or at our preferred online store **www.cengagebrain.com**

Printed in Canada
1 2 3 4 5 6 7 16 15 14 13 12

Table of Contents

Preface

▪ Introduction

The U.S. health care system is complex and often confusing. Whether you are a health care provider or a patient, an administrator or an informal caregiver, you may have found it difficult and frustrating to navigate through the various parts of the health care system. The purpose of this text, *Fundamentals of U.S. Health Care: Principles and Perspectives*, is to provide a roadmap to guide you through the health care system—describing it component by component and explaining the interrelationships among these components, thereby making it easier to understand as a whole.

▪ Instructional Approach

Our framework for writing this text is to offer objective, fair, and balanced perspectives on the U.S. health care system. Our aim is to present both sides of any issue when addressing controversial topics. We made every attempt to withhold our biases as authors and focused on presenting all positions, clearly and simply. Once informed, the readers then can decide for themselves which position they support. Our goal is to allow the readers to be the final judge, as they are charged with making the crucial decisions in the modern health care world.

This text focuses on the fundamental problems of the U.S. health care system and strives to provide clear objective coverage of the salient issues. We do not explore fads, but attend to the factors that have been decisive in the past and will remain so in the future. Fundamental concerns such as cost, access, quality, financing, health workforce, and public health represent key chapters. Throughout the text we provide vignettes, or case studies, which permit students to apply these topics or problems to real-life situations. It should be noted that although entire chapters are devoted to subjects such as cost, financing, access, and quality, these issues can also be found in other chapters throughout the text. This approach is purposeful, to allow the reader to recognize how these topics interact with each other within the whole health care system.

▪ Organization of This Text

The text is divided into 16 chapters. Chapter 1, Introduction: The Big Picture, provides an overview of some of the key issues and problems facing the health care system today, as well as many of the trends that have occurred over time. Chapter 2, Health Status, explores how we measure the performance of the health care system on the health of the population. Chapter 3, Health Services in Perspective takes health status a step further to address whether the United States receives high-quality care commensurate with the amount of investment. Chapter 4, Organization of Health

Services, provides a description of the various settings in which health providers and patients interact. Chapter 5, Health Manpower, presents a comprehensive discussion of the various types of health providers in the health workforce, their training, certification, and care they provide. Chapter 6, Public Health, takes a macro approach to health care delivery, using the entire population as the focus of health care impact. Chapter 7, Long-Term Care, delves into a growing and vital component of health care delivery for populations with special and unique needs. Chapter 8, Medicare and Medicaid, tackles the complex organization and financing of the largest insurance products in the world, designed to assist the elderly and the poor, respectively. Chapter 9, Health Care Facilities, covers the organization of the largest segment of the health care system, the delivery of inpatient services in hospitals, surgical centers, and nursing homes. Chapter 10, Costs of Health Care Services, switches gears and addresses the most limiting aspect of health care delivery and the barriers to improvement in quality and access. Chapter 11, Health Care Financing, is a sister chapter of costs, and explains the manner in which public and private funds are used to cover the costs and pay for the delivery of health care. Chapter 12, Managed Care, addresses a fundamental delivery model used to insure patients, deliver health care services, and pay clinicians for their services while controlling costs and maintaining quality. Chapter 13, Utilization of Health Services, discusses the theories that predict the patterns of use (or nonuse) of services by patients. Chapter 14, Quality, similarly describes the factors that determine how well care is delivered and how patient health is improved. Chapter 15, Health Planning and Regulation, addresses another macro approach to health care delivery, the task of providing essential services to populations to protect and improve the health of all. Finally, Chapter 16, National Health Policy, attempts to place the reader in the driver seat of the health care system by addressing the most pressing issues facing national health policy makers today.

Instructional Features

There are several features of this text that distinguish it from all others and usher learning into the twenty-first century. Each chapter stresses opposing perspectives on selected issues along with an objective treatment of all others. For instance, in the sections entitled Your Opinion Matters (YOM), the authors have designed the content to provide a balanced approach to the fundamental issues facing the industry. In addition, each chapter begins with Learning Objectives to inform the reader of the main points that will be presented in each chapter, along with a list of Key Terms. Vignettes, or case studies, are presented in each chapter to highlight and apply the main messages. Discussion questions are offered at the end of each YOM and Vignette, along with critical thinking, thought-provoking Review Questions at the end of each chapter. A Glossary of Terms is presented at the end of the text for students to quickly access the meanings of unfamiliar words and acronyms. We selected this format in an attempt to preclude advocating an agenda or one perspective. We present the information so that students can decide for themselves and form their own opinions regarding controversial topics. Our desire is that students interpret the facts on their own and continue to hone their critical and analytical thinking skills to apply them in their future professional careers.

Text material is presented in full-color, graphically where appropriate, utilizing many visual aids. We want the audience to be excited and intrigued when reading this text and eager to learn more about the health care system. Pie charts, histograms, illustrations, and graphs are used to provide a perspective and context for each issue. Graphic representations are used to convey the role and significance of health care spending in the national budget. Pie charts are used to illustrate how such national spending is allocated. A visual presentation of the content facilitates greater understanding by readers of all learning types.

▪ Ancillary Materials

▪ Instructor Companion Site (ISBN: 978-1-4283-1736-9)

The Instructor Companion Site is a robust tool designed to meet your instructional needs. A must-have for all instructors, this comprehensive site contains the following components:

Instructor's Manual

The Instructor's Manual provides a wealth of additional resources to maximize the value of the student's learning experience and provide assistance to the instructor. An overview of the Your Opinion Matters features from the textbook are included along with instructor talking points to facilitate group discussions and debates as classroom exercises. Vignette overviews with suggested solutions to the discussion questions are also provided. Answers to the Review Questions contained within the textbook have been included. The Review Questions are designed to assess the students' accomplishments of the chapter Learning Objectives and may be useful as a homework assignment or simply as a self-assessment tool for the student.

PowerPoint® Presentations

The text is complemented with over 600 full-color slides that can be edited by the instructor to include their personal approach to delivering the material.

Computerized Test Bank in ExamView®

The question bank includes 800 test questions that are multiple choice, matching, or fill in the blanks. Users can add their own questions. The software allows the user to create tests in less than five minutes, with the ability to print them out in a variety of layouts. It also has electronic "take-home testing" and Internet-based testing capabilities.

In addition to these resources, the Instructor Companion Site houses a sample course syllabus.

▪ WebTUTOR™ on Blackboard (ISBN: 978-1-4283-1738-3)
▪ WebTUTOR™ on WebCT (ISBN: 978-1-4283-1737-6)

Designed to complement the textbook, WebTUTOR™ is a content-rich, Web-based teaching and learning aid that reinforces and clarifies complex concepts. The Blackboard™ platform also provides rich communication tools to instructors and students, including a course calendar, chat, email, and threaded discussions.

▪ Goals for the Future

Through the next decade, the U.S. health care system will face two opposing but inevitable forces, limited resources to provide care and a growing aging patient population that will demand more care. These unstoppable forces must be addressed by policy makers and payers and consumers of health care services. Clinicians will be providing care to a healthier aging population with an increased life expectancy and radically different expectations. At the same time, the U.S. government and the nation's employers will wrestle with demands for universal access, universal insurance, and world class care for our society.

Reducing medical errors and increasing quality of care are critical issues that must be addressed by administrators and clinicians. The authors' goal is that those who use this text will be motivated to confront these difficult issues head on and will become leaders in shaping the health care system of the future. Ultimately, our goal is to improve the health care of our fellow human beings, and enable administrators and clinicians to deliver the highest quality, most effective health care in the world.

▪ About the Data

With the advent of high-powered technology used by many of the data sources cited in this text, like the Bureau of the Census, Centers for Medicare and Medicaid Services, and the Centers for Disease Control and Prevention's National Center for Health Statistics, long-term trends are updated annually with great regularity. This process is faster than any reasonable course a manuscript must take to reach publication. As such, the authors have provided the Web sites for data updates for each of the trends depicted in the text to assure that faculty and students can obtain the latest data points if necessary. It should be mentioned, however, that providing the very latest data points was never a purpose of our authorship. As lifelong students of the health care system, we have come to understand that such trends do not "turn on a dime." Data points with extremely large denominators do not change dramatically from one year to the next, but take decades to develop. The authors' intention was to provide extensive trend data on important health care issues and problems and then offer the readers the tools necessary to first understand the meaning of the trends and, second, to find the latest data points to update if necessary. We hope the text meets this objective.

▪ About the Authors

Students and instructors should not hesitate to contact the authors at their respective email addresses below.

▪ Dr. Charles E. Yesalis

Dr. Yesalis has served on the faculties of the Johns Hopkins School of Hygiene and Public Health, the University of Iowa College of Medicine, and the Pennsylvania State University. He is currently an Emeritus Professor at Pennsylvania State University.

For the past 28 years, much of Dr. Yesalis' research has been devoted to the nonmedical use of anabolic-androgenic steroids (AS) and other performance-enhancing drugs and dietary supplements. In 1988, he directed the first national study of AS use among adolescents and was the first to present evidence of psychological dependence on AS. In addition, he has studied the incidence of AS use among elite power lifters, collegiate athletes, and professional football players. In 1993, using nationwide data, he demonstrated the association between AS use and violent behavior as well as an association with the use of other illicit drugs and alcohol. He also presented an estimate of lifetime AS use in the U.S. population (over 1 million). In 1998, he wrote *The Steroids Game*, which focuses on prevention, education, and intervention regarding AS use by adolescents. He is the editor of a medical reference text, *Anabolic Steroids in Sport and Exercise* (2nd ed.) and coeditor of *Performance Enhancing Substances in Sport and Exercise*.

On six occasions he has been asked to testify before the U.S. Congress on legislation related to the control of AS and growth hormone abuse. Dr. Yesalis has been a consultant to, among others, the U.S. Office of National Drug Control Policy, the U.S. Senate and House of Representatives, the Drug Enforcement Administration, the Centers for Disease Control and Prevention, the Food and Drug Administration, Center on Addiction and Substance Abuse: National Commission on Sports and Substance Abuse, the NFL Players Association, the U.S. Olympic Committee, the National Collegiate Athletic Association, and the National Strength and Conditioning Association.

Dr. Yesalis completed his Bachelor of Science from the University of Michigan and Masters in Public Health from the University of Michigan, School of Public Health, and earned his doctor of science degree from the then Johns Hopkins School of Hygiene and Public Health. (Cey2@psu.edu)

▪ Dr. Harry D. Holt

Dr. Holt's scholarship efforts focus on hospitals and health system performance. His research explores relevant factors including organizational characteristics, management strategy, quality, local market structure, strategic alliances, and characteristics of executive leadership teams. Dr. Holt began his career at the Cleveland Clinic, working to expand patient services in satellite facilities throughout Ohio. While working in the health care industry, he provided consulting and legal services to hospitals, health systems, and health insurance companies, and clients located in the Americas.

Harry Holt recently graduated from the Pennsylvania State University with a PhD in Health Policy and Administration in the health care management and organization track. He earned a Bachelor of Arts degree from Indiana University of Pennsylvania in Economics and Political Science. He earned a Juris Doctorate, with a concentration in health law, and a Masters of Business Administration, with a concentration in health systems management, from Case Western Reserve University. While in law school, he served as an associated editor of *Health Matrix*, an internationally subscribed journal that provides law review articles focusing on the most recent developments in health law. He is admitted to practice law in the state of Ohio and is a member of the American College of Health Care Executives, the Academy of Management, and Academy of Health. (hdh118@psu.edu)

Dr. Robert M. Politzer

Dr. Politzer's career spanned 27 years in the U.S. Public Health Service, Health Resources and Services Administration, Department of Health and Human Services. He served as Senior Policy Advisor to the Bureau Director and Director of the Office of Data Evaluation Analysis and Research in the Bureau of Primary Health Care. Prior to those positions, Dr. Politzer served as Associate Director for Primary Care Policy and Special Assistant to the Director, Bureau of Health Professions. He was also Chief, Workforce Analysis and Research Branch of the Bureau of Health Professions' Office of Research and Planning. Dr. Politzer also served in several capacities within the National Health Service Corps.

During his distinguished career, Dr. Politzer received many honors, among them the highest honors within the department. In addition, Dr. Politzer has coauthored numerous articles that have appeared in such noteworthy journals as the *Journal of the American Medical Association, Health Affairs, American Journal of Preventive Medicine, Medical Care, American Journal of Public Health, Journal of Public Health Policy, Health Services Research*, and the *Milbank Memorial Quarterly*.

Since 2006, Dr. Politzer has served as Senior Health Policy Consultant for Management Solutions Consulting Group, advising on the analytic agenda for the nation's health centers. After retiring in 2005, Dr. Politzer entered full time into private practice as a Certified Addictions Specialist, a part-time activity since 1983. In 1978, he founded and directed the Johns Hopkins Center for Pathological Gambling, a pilot outpatient and inpatient treatment program funded by the state of Maryland. He was asked by then-Governor William Donald Schaefer to serve as co-chair of the Maryland Task Force on Gambling Addiction that released its seminal report in 1990.

Prior to his federal service, Dr. Politzer served on the faculty of the then Johns Hopkins School of Hygiene and Public Health as the Director of Primary Care Education Evaluation. Also as faculty, he established the Center for Pathological Gambling.

Dr. Politzer received his B.A. degree in mathematics and his M.S. degree in biostatistics from the University of Vermont. He received his doctor of science degree in health services research from the then Johns Hopkins School of Hygiene and Public Health. Dr. Politzer also received a certification as a Certified Addictions Specialist from the American Academy of Health Care Providers in the Addictive Disorders. (Robert.politzer@gmail.com)

Acknowledgments

There are many people and institutions who have helped us gather the information and data for this endeavor. However, we would like to thank the institutions that trained us in this subject matter, including the then Johns Hopkins School of Hygiene and Public Health; the University of Michigan, School of Public Health; the University of Vermont, College of Medicine; the U.S. Public Health Service; and the Department of Health Policy and Administration at Pennsylvania State University. We especially want to thank Cengage Publishing and its subsidiaries for recognizing the importance of this subject matter, the quality of the draft text, and the timeliness of its publication.

The authors also thank our respective families for displaying the patience of Job during the writing, editing, and finalizing of the text.

We are specifically grateful for the expertise and contribution of Dr. Andrea S. Yesalis. She provided a wealth of knowledge and insights into the issues of long-term care and is the primary author of Chapter 7, Long-Term Care. She also provided editorial support and guidance for these respective areas throughout the text.

Dr. Holt would like to thank his loving parents, Jerry and Olive Holt, who provided him with much encouragement and support throughout the process of writing this book. Both have been unequaled role models who have always encouraged him to strive for excellence in everything he does. He would also like to thank his sister, Lynn, and his brothers, Stephen and Samuel Holt, all of with whom he shares many cherished childhood memories.

■ Author Signatures

Dr. Charles E. Yesalis
Cey2@psu.edu

Dr. Harry D. Holt
hdh118@psu.edu

Dr. Robert M. Politzer
Robert.politzer@gmail.com

Reviewers

Lavonna Blair Lewis, Ph.D., MPH

USC SPPD
Los Angeles, CA

James R. Ciesla, Ph.D.

Northern Illinois University
DeKalb, IL

Phillip Decker, Ph.D., MBA

University of Houston at Clear Lake
Houston, TX

Dorothy Gargis Foote, Ph.D., FNP-BC, GNP-BC

University of Alabama in Huntsville
Huntsville, AL

Pam Hildebrandt

Cornell University
Ithaca, NY

Maria A. Kronenburg, MBA, Ph.D.

Troy University – Global Campus – Atlantic Region
Norfolk, VA

Michael Markowski, Ph.D.

Pennsylvania State University
Downingtown, PA

Susan Radius, Ph.D.

Towson University
Towson, MD

Ramani Ranagavajhula, Ph.D., M.D.

San Jose State University
San Jose, CA

Dr. John Sellers

Lincoln Memorial University
Knoxville, TN

Vicki Zeman, MA, RHIA

The College of St. Scholastica
Duluth, MN

Introduction: The Big Picture

Key Terms

access

allopathic medicine

alternative medicine

biologically based practices

community- or population-based health care

complementary medicine

cost

emergency care

energy medicine

health

health care system

health education

homeopathy

informal medicine

long-term care

manipulative and body-based practices

mind–body medicine

Continued

Learning Objectives

- Describe an overview of the U.S. health care system, including the relationships among quality, cost, and access; stakeholders; and types of health care services.

- Discuss key medical care and health care designations and definitions.

- Identify and discuss the principle problems in the U.S. health care system.

- Describe the major forces that have shaped the delivery of health care services, and cite examples of each.

▪ What Is Health and Health Care?

The most commonly used definition of **health** is the one posited by the World Health Organization (WHO) and recorded in the organization's 1946 constitution. WHO defines *health* as "a state of complete physical, mental and social well-being and not merely the absence of disease or infirmity" (WHO, 1946).

Health status is determined by many factors that lead to the outcome of better or worse health. The four major components contributing to health status are heredity or genetics, the environment, lifestyle, and the organization and delivery of health care services. All of these factors interact to determine an individual's health status. Heredity refers to the genetic makeup and its impact on health status. For example, Caucasians may be more susceptible to skin cancer or breast cancer, whereas blacks may be more susceptible to sickle cell anemia. Some diseases such as heart disease and colon cancer have a strong hereditary link, whereby parents or grandparents with the disease determine that offspring are predisposed to them as well. Other diseases such as Huntington's disease, a degenerative nerve disorder, have a more specific genetic link because a faulty gene inherited from one or both parents causes the disease.

Our environment affects our health status because we interact with it every day. It may prevent or promote disease. The environment has physical, social, and economic components. The physical environment includes radon and ozone levels, as well as air and water quality. If the air we breathe or the water we drink is polluted, the likelihood of illness increases. If we live near a factory that is polluting the air and water, our health may be altered. Prolonged exposure to radon gas can actually cause death.

The social environment includes our social institutions and government regulations that affect health through laws, for example, by prohibiting smoking in restaurants or increasing access to health care through Medicare. The economic component refers to the wealth of a nation and how much money can be spent on the search for new and more effective treatments for disease, or personal wealth that enables patients to secure health care services.

Our lifestyle or individual behavior is another determinant of health status. Lifestyle includes such activities as drinking and driving, smoking or taking drugs, practicing safe sex, exercising, and eating a low-fat diet, all of which can influence health negatively or positively. In his book *Who Shall Live?* the noted health economist Victor Fuchs (1974) wrote, "The greatest current potential for improving the health of the American people is to be found in what they do and don't do to and for themselves."

Organization and delivery of health care services, hereafter called the **health care system**, refers to a complex set of arrangements in our society that mediate between the human being and our vulnerability to disease. The three goals of a health care system are to treat the sick, prevent disease, and set goals for maintenance and promotion of health. Determining the balance among these often-competing goals has been

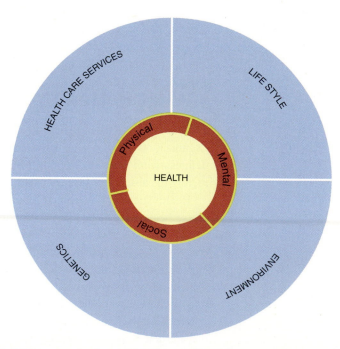

Figure 1–1 The organization and delivery of health care services.
Source: Adapted from H. Blum. (1981). Planning for Health, *2nd ed. New York: Human Sciences Press, p. 3.*

a dilemma for the United States health care delivery system, which has traditionally invested in the provision of personal health care services, such as treating sick people, at the expense of public health services that focus on heath promotion and disease prevention. In fact, we spend approximately 97 percent of our health care dollars on curative health care services as opposed to preventive care. In 1988, the Centers for Disease Control and Prevention (CDC) estimated that we spent only 3 percent of our health care dollars on prevention (CDC, 1992). By 2005, that percentage had declined to 2.32 percent (Beitsch et al., 2006). Absent a substantial emphasis on prevention, health care generally can only have a minimal impact on health status. By focusing our health care dollars more on prevention, the U.S. health care system might better address many of the problems caused by lifestyle choices that place Americans at a higher risk for disease. Figure 1–1 illustrates the relationships among the various inputs to health from the environment, lifestyle, health care services, and genetics. Although it is true that all of these components affect our health and well-being, lifestyle has the greatest influence.

▪ The "Iron Triangle" of Health Care

The pillars of a health care system are access, cost, and quality, as shown in Figure 1–2. **Access** is the potential or ability to use health care services. **Cost** is the price of health care services. **Quality** refers to how good or bad the health care services are at the time of delivery. Each of these factors can be described at the micro level, such as between the individual patient and provider, and at the macro, or system, level.

Changes in funding or infrastructure in one vector of the triangle will produce changes in the other sectors. The "iron triangle" operates like a balloon. Pressure on one side of the balloon forces the other sides to expand. For example, in 2008, the United States spent approximately *$2.3 trillion* on health care, yet it is estimated that *46.3 million* people living in the United States in 2007 did not have any form of health insurance (Centers for Medicare and Medicaid Services [CMS], 2010; U.S. Census Bureau, 2009). If the government mandated that everyone had some form of insurance, thereby reducing the price of care for the patient at the time of service, then access to the health care system would increase. However, costs to society would increase as well. The uninsured who previously were unable to purchase care could now use health care services more frequently by filling formerly unmet health care needs. In addition, insurance does stimulate the insured to use more health care services than they need.

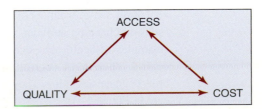

Figure 1–2 The "iron triangle" of cost, access, and quality—altering one will likely alter the others.

© Cengage Learning 2013

If health insurance were mandated for everyone, quality of care would improve for the millions of uninsured Americans who gained access to the health care system. However, as a nation we are concerned that spending additional funds on health care means fewer resources for other priorities. These increased health care expenditures would likely lead to cost containment policies and restrictions on use, which could result in decreasing the quality of care for some. History has shown that increasing access to care for the previously underserved can actually decrease access to care for others because of increased waiting times.

You will note that this discussion includes terms such as "may" and "likely." We can predict the effects of government intervention on the health care system to some degree, based on previous experiences. However, government intervention can and often does have unintended consequences, which may manifest in unpredictable changes in the relationships among these factors. For sure, however, changing any of these factors will affect the others.

▪ Types of Health Care Services

As stated above, most of the U.S. health care dollars are spent on health care treatment of acute and chronic diseases. Because our system is designed to heal one individual at a time, it is an illness-driven system of medicine rather than a comprehensive health care system.

There are two types of health care services available in our system: personal and community- or population-based services. **Personal health care services** focus on the provider and patient relationship. For example, a personal health service is delivered when patients visit their family doctors. Because 97 percent of our health care dollars are allotted to personal care, our spending reveals the importance of personal health care services within our current system.

Community-, or population-based, health care services are provided to prevent disease for large groups of people living together in a community, city, or county. For example, sanitation strategies such as developing proper sewage and waste disposal mechanisms, ensuring water quality and air quality, requiring childhood vaccinations, and offering screening programs are all community-based health care measures. Local or state public health departments provide most of these services.

▪ Types of Care

The care that patients receive falls somewhere on a continuum ranging from health education and prevention to long-term care. **Health education** and **preventive care** focus on changing attitudes and behaviors to prevent or lessen the impact of disease. Examples of health education and prevention include immunizations, hypertension control, cholesterol control, smoking cessation, exercise, stress management, and breast cancer screening. They fall under population-based care and clinical preventive care in Figure 1–3.

Primary care is often referred to as "first contact" care, such as that received from the family doctor, hospital outpatient department, community health center, or university health service. Primary care is delivered by clinicians in general practice

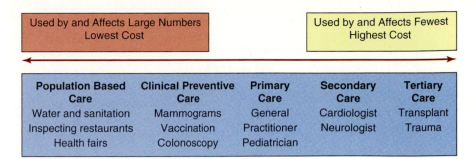

Figure 1–3 Continuum of health care services, community-based to personal.
© *Cengage Learning 2013*

and the medical specialties of family practice, obstetrics and gynecology, pediatrics, and general internal medicine. Primary care clinicians are generalists and treat a wide range of health care problems. **Secondary care** is typically provided in community hospitals, outpatient testing centers, and specialists' offices. Some examples of secondary care include referral to specialist, surgical consults, and magnetic resonance imaging (MRI) and computerized axial tomography (CAT) scanning. Specialists include cardiologists, neurologists, radiologists, and gastroenterologists, just to name a few. Some insurance plans may require that patients obtain a referral from their primary care providers before they can see a specialist. Some specialists will not accept appointments unless patients have been referred by a primary care provider. Since secondary care is more costly than primary care, this referral hierarchy assures insurance companies that secondary care is necessary and affirms that patients need the specialist physicians' expertise.

Tertiary care, or "super" specialty care, is often delivered at large medical centers, referral hospitals, and teaching hospitals. Tertiary care hospitals do provide almost all levels of service, including primary and secondary care. They also perform complex medical procedures such as transplants, open-heart surgery, neurosurgery, and advanced cancer treatment, and are likely to have intensive care and critical care units such as neonatal intensive care, cardiac intensive care, and burn units. Most large metropolitan areas have at least one tertiary care facility. Examples of tertiary care centers throughout the country include Cleveland Clinic (Cleveland, Ohio), Mayo Clinic, (Rochester, Minnesota), Johns Hopkins University Hospital (Baltimore, Maryland), Mount Sinai Medical Center (New York, New York), and University of California Los Angeles Hospital (Los Angeles, California). Although much of care delivered today is shifting from inpatient to outpatient settings, tertiary care facilities have adapted by providing services in both settings.

Population-based health care services, such as health education and preventive services, reach or affect the health of many individuals, whereas tertiary care services are utilized by and affect a much smaller percentage of our population. Sanitation services benefit everyone who lives in an area where the services are provided. Although over 80 percent of the population in the United States incurs at least one doctor visit in any given year (National Center for Health Statistics [NCHS], 2010), only a slight majority of those visits are in a primary care setting (50.4%), with fewer at the secondary or tertiary levels (NCHS, 2010). About 6 to 7 percent of Americans, on average, are admitted to a secondary care facility in a year (Bernstein et al., 2003).

However, a disproportionate amount of the health care dollar is spent on secondary and tertiary care. So much of our health care dollar covers services that are received by so few people. These personal health care costs leave very little to spend on preventive care (3%).

Emergency care can be provided at the scene of an accident, en route to the hospital, or at the hospital emergency department. The main purpose of emergency care is to stabilize the patient until arrival at a hospital trauma center or emergency room. Emergency care can include transport by fixed-wing aircraft, helicopters, boats, or even snowmobiles equipped to provide emergency care such as basic and advanced life support. Emergency care providers can include physicians, nurse practitioners, nurses and emergency medical technicians (EMTs). Approximately 43 percent of inpatient admissions originate in the emergency department (ED), and they have the potential of generating substantial revenue for hospitals if the patients are well insured (Merrill & Elixhauser, 2005). However, if the patients are poor and have little or no insurance for their health care, emergency departments can be a financial drain on the hospital.

Long-term care focuses upon the treatment of chronic illnesses and disability. Demand for long-term care services has increased in recent years and will become even more critical as our population ages and people live longer. Long-term care is generally less expensive and less intensive than acute hospital care. Long-term care services include nursing homes, home health care, assisted living facilities, and hospice care.

Long-term care, including physical and occupational therapy, is becoming more important as life expectancy increases, patients suffer from more debilitating diseases, and patients desire to retain as much personal independence and daily functioning as possible. **Rehabilitative care** is an example of the increasing demands placed on the health care system and the increasing importance of physical medicine. With each generation, there appear to be increasing demands for health care technology and decreasing tolerance of illness. Thus, with each new generation the expectations of the health care system, or access to high-quality care, increase.

Finally, health education and prevention are aimed at producing changes in behavior. However, humans are creatures of habit; many of the unhealthy behaviors are enjoyable in the short run, and changing these behaviors frequently requires significant discipline and hard work. Health education programs and information are designed to educate the public and individuals about health issues and diseases. Preventive medicine offers services that aim to stop the onset of disease. Through health education and preventive health services, healthy changes in lifestyle can produce significant societal health benefits. Nevertheless, the health system devotes relatively few resources to preventive health, and Americans often ignore health education. For example, smoking is the single greatest *preventable* cause of death, followed by healthy diet and exercise. The National Cancer Institute (NCI) estimated that in the years 2000–2004, an average of 443,000 people in the United States died each year from diseases caused by smoking (NCI, 2010), and 350,000–400,000 died yearly from diseases caused by obesity (Mokdad et al., 2005; Mokdad et al., 2004). Examples of preventive care are listed in Table 1–1.

Stopping people from smoking would seem to have many positive health-related consequences; however, at the societal level, some of the consequences may be negative. For instance, the farming and tobacco industries would lose business and income; the funds raised by the cigarette tax would vanish; the number of people who reach the age at which they can collect Social Security would increase, thus further taxing

Table 1–1: Types of Preventive Care		
Immunizations	Prenatal care visits	Exercise
Hypertension control	Pap smears	Smoking cessation
Cholesterol control	Mammography	Stress relief

© *Cengage Learning 2013*

the system; and scientists involved in research on the health consequences of tobacco (the single largest research endeavor) may lose their funding sources. Thus, the economy would have to adjust to account for these changes.

In addition, efforts to counter the health effects of smoking frequently emphasize treatment as opposed to prevention. The decision to invest in smoking cessation strategies should be based on a cost-effectiveness analysis that compares the improved outcomes of prevention versus treatment of smoking-related diseases. There are preventive health services that have a dramatic impact on the health of individuals and populations at relatively low cost, such as prenatal care, whereas others are not as cost-effective, such as annual physical exams. If the cost-effectiveness of the preventive health strategy is low, should society make the investment in that strategy and balance its expenditures on treatment of diseases?

■ Types of Medicine

There are several types of medicine and alternative healing that are practiced in the United States, with some important distinctions. Traditional medicine is practiced by physicians, both allopathic and osteopathic. Complementary and alternative medicine is practiced by clinicians, including chiropractors, acupuncturists, homeopaths, naturopaths, and faith healers.

■ Traditional or Conventional Medicine

Providers who have received a Doctor of Medicine (MD) degree practice **allopathic medicine**. Allopathic medicine is conventional or traditional scientific medicine. Doctors trained in allopathic medicine use drugs, devices, and surgery to treat diseases to produce alterations in the paths of diseases. Providers who have received a Doctor of Osteopathy (DO) degree practice **osteopathic medicine**. Osteopathic physicians are trained to use drugs, devices, and surgery like MDs, but, traditionally, they have focused on treating the person holistically rather than focusing on symptoms or diseases. In osteopathic medicine, *holistic* means that structure influences function; if there is a problem in one part of the body's structure, function in that area, and possibly in other areas, may be affected. Thus, part of a DO's training includes combining manual musculoskeletal manipulation with other medical treatment. This system of hands-on techniques helps alleviate pain, restores motion, supports the body's natural functions, and influences the body's structure to help it function more efficiently. Another integral tenet of osteopathic medicine is the body's innate ability to heal itself. Many of the manipulative techniques used in osteopathic medicine are aimed at reducing or eliminating the impediments to proper structure and function so the self-healing mechanism can assume its role in restoring a person to health.

By current standards, there is very little, if any, difference between osteopathic and allopathic medical practice. However, chiropractors, who are trained differently and are not osteopathic doctors, use physical manipulation for treatment of some (or many) diseases.

■ Complementary and Alternative Medicine (CAM)

Complementary and **alternative medicine** uses alternative therapies in place of conventional medicine. Although some scientific evidence has been produced to demonstrate the effectiveness of some alternative therapies, most of the practices that constitute complementary and alternative medicine still have not been proven as effective and/or safe. The National Institutes of Health (NIH), National Center for Complementary and Alternative Medicine (NCCAM), classifies CAM into five domains: whole medical systems, mind–body medicine, biologically based practices, manipulative and body-based practices, and energy medicine. **Homeopathy** and **naturopathy** are examples of whole medical systems. Homeopathy is the use of "very low doses of drugs that produce patient signs or symptoms" as a means of curing them. For example, a homeopath may try to relieve nausea by administering a small amount of *Psychotria ipecacuanha*, the plant used to make ipecac, which induces vomiting (National Center for Homeopathy, 2007). Naturopathy uses all-natural treatments such as herbal medicine, massage, acupuncture, manual manipulation, hydrotherapy, and aromatherapy. Naturopaths believe that natural treatments can help the human body to heal itself.

Mind–body medicine is designed to "enhance the mind's capacity to affect bodily function and symptoms" (NCCAM, 2007). These interventions include support groups such as Alcoholics Anonymous or cancer support groups, meditation, faith medicine (healing practices, such as prayer, that appeal to a supernatural power), and creative therapies such as art.

Biologically based practices involve the use of natural substances such as herbs, vitamins, and supplements to improve health or prevent disease. Examples include taking Ginkgo biloba to improve memory or zinc or vitamin C to prevent a cold.

Manipulative and body-based practices include chiropractic and massage therapy. Chiropractic doctors treat problems with the musculoskeletal and nervous system, largely using spinal manipulation or "chiropractic adjustment." Chiropractors may also prescribe exercises used in physical therapy or counsel patients on nutrition, diet, and exercise (American Chiropractic Association, 2007).

Finally, **energy medicine** involves the use of energy (biofield therapy) and electromagnetic fields (bioelectromagnetic-based therapy) to affect health. The National Center for Complementary and Alternative Medicine divides the practice of energy medicine into two categories: veritable and putative, the former confined to energy systems whose existence has been confirmed and proven by scientific investigation like electromagnetism, and the latter based on theorized energy forms for which scientific investigation has not confirmed the existence, like biofield energy (NCCAM, 2007).

Yet another classification of medicine is one that we practice and receive more regularly than either traditional or complementary and alternative medicine. **Informal medicine** is practiced when family and friends influence our health and medical-seeking behavior. For example, comments such as "You don't look well. You should take some vitamin C," or "You should see a doctor" are examples of informal medicine.

■ Major Stakeholders in the U.S. Health Care System

A stakeholder is an individual or group that has an investment or personal interest in something. Stakeholders can either lose or gain from their investment or interest. By their very name, stakeholders have a great investment in outcomes in which their interest lies. In health care, any changes in the macro system affect the stakeholders. These stakeholders therefore attempt to influence the health care system and create changes that will be beneficial for them. The interaction between stakeholders affects the "iron triangle" of access, cost, and quality.

The following are major stakeholders in the health care industry: providers (e.g., physicians, nurses, hospitals, chiropractors), consumers (patients), insurers (e.g., health maintenance organizations [HMOs], preferred provider organizations [PPOs], BlueCross/Blue Shield, Prudential), businesses (employers), and government (regulation, Medicaid/Medicare). Providers and consumers are the frontline participants in the health care system, because most health care contacts are made between doctors and other providers and patients. Insurers, or third-party payers, pay hospitals and physicians and other providers for patient care. Individuals and/or employers pay premiums to the insurers to cover health care costs for themselves or their employees. Hence, businesses or employers also act as insurers for their employees. The federal and state governments also act as insurers through Medicare, funded and administered at the federal level, and Medicaid, which is a federal-state matching program. Medicare and Medicaid are government-run financing programs that provide insurance primarily for the elderly and poor, respectively. In addition to acting as an insurer, the government also acts as a provider in the Department of Defense, Department of Veteran Affairs, Bureau of Prisons, and other federal and state hospitals and clinics. The federal government regulates health care providers by requiring licenses and is a major funding source for health-related research.

■ Illness and Disease, the Sick Role

The following definitions provide a useful background to understand the differences among illness, disease, and sickness. Illness is a subjective notion that focuses on how patients feel. Disease is an objective designation or diagnosis made by a medical or health professional.

Sickness, or the sick role, is relative and relates closely to social position, which includes age, occupation, marital status, and education. Therefore, any definition of illness varies with social role.

According to Parsons (1951) there are four components of the sick role:

1. Individuals are not held responsible for their disease.

2. Individuals are exempt from normal social responsibilities and role obligations.

3. The state of illness is undesirable, and patients want to recover.

4. Sick people are obligated to seek help from health care experts.

When someone we know is ill, we generally recognize that it is not a desirable state of being, and we do not blame the person for getting sick; more often than not, we feel sorry for him or her. Often, when people are sick, they also are excused from going to school and work, or doing normal housework or other duties. Finally, because people do not want to be sick and want to recover, we expect them to seek help from a health care professional. Today, all ills cannot necessarily be treated by a visit to a doctor, but a person's work or school may require a doctor's "note" before granting an excused absence.

The perception of illness will vary with a person's societal or individual role. As a result, the same illness will affect individual lives differently. Several factors explain why individuals perceive illnesses differently. First, a person's occupation will influence his or her perception. For instance, back pain may cause only slight discomfort for an executive, but it will prevent a construction worker from obtaining employment. Second, a patient's marital status determines obligations to his or her spouse and children. Therefore, illness will be a significant factor in the person's ability to fulfill those obligations. If one spouse has primary responsibility for taking care of the children, the other spouse may have to help more when that person is sick. Third, a person's education level will affect his or her perception of illness. More educated persons may view changes in their body as requiring medical attention because they may know of the benefits of early detection and treatment. They may also be informed about the benefits of preventive care and the dangers of allowing a condition to go untreated for a period of time. Fourth, the passage of time influences our perception of illness. Many illnesses today were not considered illnesses 50 years ago, like mental illness and alcoholism. Fifth, a person's age will elicit different responses to the same illness. For example, an elderly person may assume that arthritis or loss of mobility is a natural condition due to age and endure the symptoms, whereas a younger person may find the condition an impediment to earning a living and demand exhaustive treatment.

Sixth, our religion influences the way we perceive illness. Believers who are members of the Church of Christian Scientists and Jehovah's Witnesses possess unique beliefs about seeking care from health care professionals and receiving blood products, respectively. Seventh, our ethnic heritage also influences our response to disease and illness. For example, Hispanic women often do not use screening services for breast or cervical cancer because they are afraid of the disease and would prefer not to know whether they have it (Austin et al., 2002).

Medicalization of Social Problems

Vignette

Anna lives with her boyfriend of 9 months. She does not work and is dependent on him for shelter and food. One night, she is driven by her boyfriend to her local emergency room and tells the intake nurse that she fainted and hit her head. Anna does not have any insurance, but the hospital is a part of the state university system. After several hours of waiting, she is taken back to a room, and her boyfriend joins them. Mary is a nurse who has worked in the ED for 1 month. Previously, she worked in critical care but wanted a change that would be exciting. In one month, she has seen numerous problems from gunshot wounds to stabbings, to car accident trauma, to the run-of-the-mill conditions that are treated in every emergency room. Mary enters Anna's room and asks her to recount what happened. As Anna is telling her story, Mary notices that Anna has a black eye that is healing. She then asks Anna about the black eye. Anna states that it occurred while doing yard work. Mary looks at Anna's address again and notices that she lives in an apartment. Mary suspects that Anna is a victim of domestic violence. With the boyfriend in the room, Mary does not want to question Anna further. She tells Anna that the doctor will be right with her. The doctor then examines Anna and has the same suspicions. He sends Anna for an X-ray and asks the boyfriend to wait in the waiting room. Mary and the doctor discuss the issue while Anna is getting an X-ray. They decide that Mary will talk with Anna once she returns. When Anna returns, Mary tells her that she believes Anna is being abused by her boyfriend, and Anna denies it. Mary tries to convince Anna that if she is being abused, she should get out of the situation and press charges. Anna continues to deny the accusation. There is a social worker in the ER who handles cases of suspected child abuse and a police officer who is stationed there for the employees' and patients' protection. Mary wonders whether she should contact either of these people on Anna's behalf.

1. What should Mary do?

2. Does Mary have a moral responsibility as well as a professional responsibility to report the incident of suspected abuse to the social worker as well as to the appropriate authorities?

3. Is it the responsibility of healthcare clinicians to intervene in cases of domestic spousal or child abuse or to merely treat the patients that may be injured from such cases?

Historically, medicine in the United States focused on the technical aspects of treating traditional diseases. In the minds of some, this emphasis on traditional disease ignored the role that social problems play in the health of the community. Nevertheless, over the past several decades there has been a move to medicalize social problems and add them to the responsibilities of the health care system, as evidenced by the WHO definition of health presented at the beginning of this chapter. Some advocates of this strategy have attempted, at least partially, to redirect such social issues as gun violence, domestic violence, literacy, and substance abuse to the responsibility of the health care delivery system (see Table 1–2 for more examples).

For example, it is recommended that hospitals and physician offices create informed consent forms, which describe medical procedures and their risks and benefits, at the

Table 1–2: **Common Social Problems Targeted by Health Care**		
Poverty	Substance abuse	Unemployment
Illiteracy	Racism	Violent crime
Health habits and diet	Spouse abuse	Injury caused by guns

© *Cengage Learning 2013*

sixth-grade reading level. However, health care administrators and providers often find it difficult to translate complex medical procedures into shorter, less complex language. By federal law, health care organizations that receive federal funding, including Medicare, Medicaid, or SCHIP reimbursement, must provide language translation for patients with limited English proficiency (Office for Civil Rights, Department of Health and Human Services [DHHS], 2001).

There are additional social problems that laws and policies have not yet included in treatment but which may arise in the future. For example, health care providers are required to report suspected child abuse to child welfare agencies, but should they also be required to report suspected spousal abuse, as in the case of Anna in the story above? To whom would it be reported? The American Public Health Association (APHA) supports gun control in an effort to reduce firearm-related injuries, but does this position conflict with a person's Second Amendment rights? (This issue is debated in the next Your Opinion Matters section.) In general, medical schools do not train doctors to deal with these types of problems. Furthermore, although adding health services directed at these issues does increase access to care and likely increases the quality of care, it also increases costs.

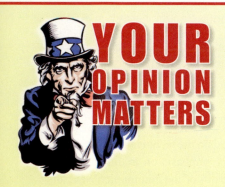

Should the Health Care System Be Responsible for Treating Social Problems?

Yes

We have a health care system, not just a medical care system. Health includes social and psychological health as well as physical health. For example, if child abuse is suspected or a person seeks treatment for a gunshot wound, health care providers are required to notify authorities. This stipulation protects the abused and can prevent future crime. For this purpose, providers should have to contact the authorities in all cases of suspected abuse or assault, even when the victim is an adult. It is in the patients' and public's interest to prevent abuse and crimes when possible.

Another social problem that must be addressed by health care providers is literacy. We have the responsibility to ensure that people get all the treatment they need and that all patients are treated with respect. All patients must provide informed consent for treatment. If a patient cannot understand the language that the doctor speaks or read the informed consent form, then he or she cannot truly provide informed consent. By law, health care providers have to provide translators for people who do not speak English and informed consent forms written in other languages. Because not all English speakers can read English well, most forms are written at no higher than an eighth-grade reading level. Not providing these services and accommodations would be unethical because we would be treating people without their knowing what was being done to them, thus violating the tenet of respect for persons.

To treat the whole person, we have to be prepared to handle people's entire needs: medical, social, psychological, and spiritual. This philosophy may require that social workers, translators, psychologists, and pastors be on staff in addition to doctors, to fully ensure patients' health.

No

The U.S. health care system is truly a medical care or illness-driven system. Doctors are not trained to deal with a host of social issues that confront them, and therefore may not handle them well. Social services exist to help people with social problems and should be used in conjunction with the medical care system. Doctors contact social services when child abuse is suspected, but it would create a huge burden on the system if providers were required to do so for every person who walked through the emergency room doors and appeared to be assaulted or abused.

For translation and literacy issues, people who do not speak English should bring someone with them to translate. It should not be the burden of the hospital to pay for these services for all possible languages. When the federal government mandates these ancillary services, it increases the cost of health care, which in turn leads to higher premiums and higher taxes for Americans. These requirements should be the responsibility of the individual in a free society and not the burden of government.

You decide:

1. What role should the health care system play in addressing social issues?

2. Can the health care system effectively engage in the holistic assessment and treatment of patients to address such issues as lack of employment, domestic abuse, and spiritual needs?

3. Where does the health care system draw the line between treating a condition or episode of care and dedicating resources to address other societal issues?

4. What are the unintended consequences of diagnosing societal issues as medical conditions?

5. Does the health care system have sufficient resources to treat patients holistically or should clinicians concentrate on the physical "disease"?

Principle Problems of the U.S. Health Care System

There are many problems with our health care system, including rising costs of health care, access barriers for the uninsured, the Medicare/Medicaid deficit, and the war against terrorism. All current problems affect access, cost, and quality and the dynamic interaction among them. A list of the principal problems discussed in this chapter is provided in Table 1–3.

First, many people believe that the *United States is spending too much money and too great a percentage of its scarce resources on health care.* The United States spends more than any other country in the world in total actual dollars ($2.49 trillion in 2009), percent of the gross domestic product (GDP; 17.6% in 2009), and per capita ($8,160 in 2009). In fact, the increase in 2009 over the previous year was the largest percent increase since 1960 (CMS 2011). At the same time, the United States is one of only two developed countries that do not have some form of universal coverage, national health insurance, or national health system. It is estimated that 50.7 million people living in the United States in 2009 did not have insurance (U.S. Census Bureau, 2010). Although our spending levels have increased over time, we have not achieved a proportional decrease in mortality or disability/restricted activity days or a proportional increase in life expectancy. Additionally, as costs increase, citizens demand more insurance coverage, mostly from employers. This response in turn leads to insensitivity to price on the part of consumers, higher demand for health care, and higher health care costs.

Figure 1–4 illustrates the rising health care expenditures in billions from 1960 through 2009. Health care expenditures have grown between 4.4 and 9.1 percent each year from 2000–2009 (CMS, 2011). The increases in health care spending are also reflected in the higher percentage of GDP spent on health care. The GDP is the market value of all of the goods and services produced in the United States in a given year. Historically, except 1997–1998, the amount of money spent on health care as a percentage of our GDP has increased every year, with the second highest increase occurring between 2004 and 2005 and the highest between 2008 and 2009 (see Figure 1–4). Simultaneously, the number of uninsured people living in America has increased over time. It

Table 1–3: Principal Problems of the U.S. Health Care System

Many of the arguments in the health care industry focus on the following issues:

- We are spending too much on health care services, not too little.

- We are spending too little on health care services, not too much.

- The rise in costs has been uncontrollable by any interventions tried to date.

- The distribution of health services is highly variable throughout the population.

- Much that could be done to prevent disease and promote health, using available knowledge and techniques, is not done.

- Many health care needs are under-met (e.g., not enough home health care for the infirm elderly), while others are over-met (e.g., too many hospital beds).

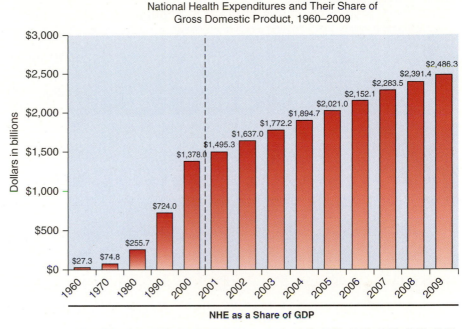

Figure 1–4 National health expenditures, 1960–2009.

Source: Centers for Medicare and Medicaid Services (CMS) (2011). National Health Expenditures: 2009. Highlights: Retrieved December 2011 from https://www.cms.gov/NationalHealthExpendData/25_ NHE_Fact_Sheet.asp

is estimated that there were over 50 million uninsured people living in America in 2009. This number has increased from 38.8 million in 1999 (see Table 1–4) (U.S. Census Bureau, 2010). As a percentage of the U.S. population, however, the number of uninsured has remained fairly stable, fluctuating from 13.7 percent (2000) to 16.7 percent (2009). Some believe that we should redistribute the existing dollars that we spend on health care to provide universal access to care through health insurance. Others point out that health care, like housing or food, is not a right guaranteed under the Constitution.

Still others argue *we are spending too little*, not too much on health care. Despite spending *17.6 percent* of the GDP on health care in 2009, many argue that we need to spend more money to expand access to care and develop better technology and methods for treating illness. If we spent more on health care, then we could give everyone the same level of quality of care that those with the best health insurance currently receive. Still others argue that resources that we spend elsewhere (e.g., the United Nations, aid to foreign countries, or the War on Terror) would be better spent on health care.

Yet *the rise in health care costs and expenditures has been uncontrollable* by any intervention tried to date. The increase in expenditure growth slowed in the 1990s because of a lower *overall* (i.e., for the entire U.S. economy) inflation rate, but it is increasing at rates last seen in the early 1990s. Managed care had some modest success in slowing the rise in costs and expenditures in the 1990s, but the success was not sustained. The three major factors driving rising health care costs and expenditures are *an aging population, a growth in technology, and an increase in demand for and expectations of health care*. We have little or no control over these aspects of the health care system.

Table 1–4: Insurance Status of the U.S. Population, 1999–2009							
Year	U.S. Population (in millions)	Number Uninsured (in millions)	%	Number Privately Insured* (in millions)	%	Number Publicly Insured** (in millions)	%
1999	276,804	38,767	14.0	200,721	72.5	67,683	24.5
2000	279,517	38,426	13.7	202,794	72.6	69,037	24.7
2001	282,082	39,760	14.1	201,695	71.5	71,295	25.3
2002	285,933	42,019	14.7	200,891	70.3	73,624	25.7
2003	288,280	43,404	15.1	199,871	69.3	76,755	26.6
2004	291,166	43,498	14.9	200,924	69.0	79,486	27.3
2005	293,834	44,815	15.3	201,167	68.5	80,213	27.3
2006	296,824	46,995	15.8	201,695	67.9	80,270	27.0
2007	299,106	45,657	15.3	201,991	67.5	83,031	27.8
2008	301,483	46,340	15.4	200,721	66.7	87,411	29.0
2009	304,280	50,674	16.7	194,545	63.9	93,167	30.6

*Employment-based and direct purchase

**Medicaid, Medicare, and military health care

Source: *U.S. Bureau of the Census (2010 September) Income, Poverty, and Health Insurance Coverage in the United States: 2009. Department of Commerce Washington D.C.*

The distribution of health services varies across the U.S. population. This inequality includes the disparity between the poor and the rich, rural settings versus urban areas, and others. The U.S. health care system is described by its critics as a "two-tiered" system, where different levels of access to care and different levels of quality care exist based on the demographic and socioeconomic characteristics of the individual. Health care disparities are a growing area of health services research.

Much that could be done to prevent disease and promote health, using knowledge and technology, is not done. As a society, we have not been very successful at encouraging individuals to exercise, change their diets, stop smoking (especially among the young), or adopt behaviors that could dramatically alter the burden of disease. Finally, many health care needs are under-met (not enough home health care for the elderly), whereas others are over-met (too many acute care hospital beds).

▪ The Culture War—Polarization of the Nation

The United States is composed of individuals with differing values and opinions that often guide thoughts and decisions and heavily influence how people feel about different social issues, including the provision and regulation of health care. There is a philosophical divide between those who favor government involvement in our lives and those who view it as intrusion. Those who believe strongly in egalitarianism and government programs to improve the common good are often at odds with those who believe that personal responsibility and freedom will lead to the common good. There are also moral struggles in our society over entitlements and welfare, abortion, stem cell research, gun ownership, homosexuality, and many other issues, some of which are fought in the health policy arena.

Secularists, people who believe that religion should not play a role in the public and governments' decisions, are at the polar opposite from those who believe in traditional religion and its influence in their lives and decisions. This polarization of opinions of the roles of government and religion in society has often been called the "culture war," and it affects U.S. health care policy in a number of ways: the interpretation of the Constitution and the rights granted to U.S. citizens (right to health or health care); the role of health care in the economy and the level of regulation needed; the battle between personal freedom and property rights versus government ownership and control; and the role of the federal government versus the role of state governments in creating policy.

Citizens of the United States have no constitutional right to health care or health insurance. This edict has charged a battle between the camps that espouse a moral obligation versus those who claim there is a constitutional obligation to provide health care. Those who believe we only have a moral obligation to provide health care believe that everyone deserves health care treatment but that they must pay for it directly (out of pocket) or indirectly (insurance), with charity care provided for those who truly cannot afford care. Those who believe we have a constitutional obligation espouse that the government should pay for everyone's health care, using tax dollars. However, the Constitution does not contain the word "health." It does contain a clause in the preamble to "promote the general welfare." This broad phrase leads many Americans to believe that health care is a right or should be a right. To some extent, our nation does grant a right to health care. The Emergency Medical Treatment and Active Labor Act of 1986 (EMTALA) mandates that hospitals with Emergency Departments that participate in Medicare evaluate any patient who seeks care, regardless of the patient's ability or willingness to pay, and that they treat or stabilize anyone who is found to have an emergency medical condition. This act means that any person who goes to an emergency room will be seen by a health care professional.

In addition to disagreement over whether citizens have a right to health care, there is also disagreement regarding the appropriate role of government in the marketplace (competition vs. regulation). The United States has a private–public health care system where we struggle to maintain the free-market system while simultaneously ensuring the welfare of our citizens. Determining the appropriate amount of government regulation or involvement in the health care system is what is referred to as the *health care tug-of-war* (Figure 1–5). What criteria should determine when the government should intervene in the private marketplace? Should health care be a right specified in the Constitution? We debate these questions in the next Your Opinion Matters section.

No regulation
"Laissez-Faire"　　　　　　　　　　　　Current U.S. regulation　　　　　　　　　Total regulation

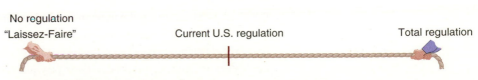

Figure 1–5 Health care tug-of-war.
© Cengage Learning 2013

The government's involvement in the market exists along a continuum (see Figure 1–5). At the far left, limited government regulation in the system allows businesses to freely compete. This type of system, a system with limited or no regulations, is described by the term *laissez-faire*, or "hands off." At the far right, complete regulation could be characterized by government owning and running the entire health care system and mandating all components from the types of services provided to the prices that clinicians could charge or how much salary clinicians could earn. Examples of a fully regulated system are the National Health Service in Great Britain, the French health care system or the health care system of the People's Republic of China. According to a study of the cost components of health care, approximately 14.5 percent of the dollars spent on actual use of medical and health care services ($339.2 billion of $1.34 trillion in personal health expenditures in 2002) in the United States is spent on regulation (Conover, 2004), and only $170 billion of benefit is derived from that government regulation.

It is important to recognize that the health care system is a key component of the U.S. economy. Action taken by government that produces significant changes in the health care system (e.g., cutting jobs, closing hospitals, or expanding health care entitlement programs such as Medicare) ripple throughout the entire economy. For example, the expansion of Medicare to cover prescription drugs in 2003 created a demand for pharmacists to provide medication therapy management in addition to dispensing medications and providing advice. It also created hundreds of fee-for-service prescription drug plans and Medicare Advantage-Prescription Drug plans. This legislation could lead to positive changes in the economy such as increased training for pharmacists, a need for more pharmacy techs as the pharmacists' duties change, and an increase in the number of people employed by the health insurance industry. However, if the Medicare prescription drug program follows the same pattern as Medicare Parts A and B, it will also lead to higher prices for prescription drugs, which will necessitate an increase in taxation and an increase in the national debt. Higher taxes mean that people have less money to spend on other things, and the national debt adversely affects inflation and the stock market. The health care industry is one of the largest industries in the United States; health care provided 14.3 million jobs for wage and salary workers; 10 of the 20 fastest-growing occupations are health care related (Bureau of Labor Statistics, 2010). Program expansions such as the Medicare prescription drug plans and the proposed State Children's Health Insurance Program (SCHIP) expansions will lead to a greater percentage of our GDP devoted to health care, which means that other sectors of the economy may not fare as well unless the overall GDP grows proportionally to the growth in health care spending, which has not happened in recent memory.

In the United States, there is often an inherent struggle between personal freedom and property rights on the one hand and the community good on the other. Virtually all government actions can be measured against values of personal freedom and property rights. For example, the government must take "property" (income) from citizens, in the form of taxes, to fund Medicare and Medicaid. To what extent is it right for the government to pay for some people's care with others' money? The answer depends upon your own personal values and opinions. Personal freedoms in health care include the ability of patients to choose their providers and the ability of providers to own their own hospitals. Depending on how it is structured, a national insurance system could limit a person's choice of provider (as in the case of the proposed 1993 Health

Security Act). Federal law prohibits providers from referring Medicare and Medicaid patients for health care services (e.g., lab, X-ray) to a health care facility in which they or their immediate family members are owners. This regulation is an attempt by the government to limit the number of unnecessary tests and procedures, thereby saving the taxpayers money, yet it curtails a physician's ability to invest in other health care organizations or to refer patients where they wish.

Finally, there is a struggle over the role of the federal government versus the role of the state government. The roles played by these two different levels of government are dynamic and differ by political ideology. Some believe that to have equitable access to care, the federal government must provide health care or health insurance to all Americans. Others believe that different states have different needs and different priorities, so it should be up to the citizens of each state to determine whether the state should require health insurance and how much. The 10th Amendment to the United States Constitution states, "The powers not delegated to the Federal government by the Constitution, are reserved to the States respectively, or to the people." However, the federal government has enacted many laws and created many programs that have given it power beyond what is explicitly stated in the Constitution; the 10th Amendment has not in the past prevented greater government involvement in the health care system.

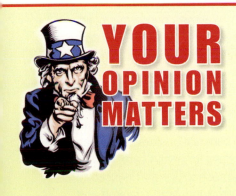

YOUR OPINION MATTERS

Should We Have a Right to Health Care in the United States?

Yes

Not all rights are specified in the Constitution—only minimal rights that the founding fathers sought to protect at the time. In our nation, and internationally, individuals and countries have recognized that human rights and civil rights exist along with liberty rights. Human and civil rights have evolved from liberty rights and continue to evolve as society changes. These rights include the right to vote, the right to education, the rights of disabled persons to education, and the right to health care.

The right to vote has evolved over time. When the Constitution was ratified in 1789, only property-holding white men over the age of 21 were permitted to vote. Other barriers such as religious tests, racial restrictions, literacy tests, and poll taxes were implemented and then abolished over time. Women in 1920 and adults between 18 and 21 in 1971 were also given the right to vote. This right took almost 200 years to fully evolve.

So it is with health care. Franklin Delano Roosevelt first proposed a recognized right to health care in his Economic Bill of Rights (never enacted). Among the economic rights President Roosevelt proposed was "The right to adequate medical care and the opportunity to achieve and enjoy good health . . ."

(Continued)

(Roosevelt, 1944). The Universal Declaration of Human Rights, developed by the United Nations with U.S. guidance, was adopted in 1948 (although not ratified by the United States) and includes a right to health care. Almost all other industrialized nations have established a right to health care and provided systems for universal access to health care in their nations. As founding nation and member of the United Nations, the United States should do the same. No one should be deprived of basic necessities such as food, housing, and health care.

No

There is no explicit right to health care in the United States Constitution. According to our founding fathers, our type of government cannot give you a right to anything; you either have that right or you do not. Regarding the rights of life, liberty, property and the pursuit of happiness, the government cannot take your life, imprison you, or take your property without a trial. You have the right to life, but the government doesn't give you food or clothing or housing, all of which are necessities of life. Similarly, we have the right to pursue health. It is our responsibility to maintain our health by engaging in healthy behaviors, going to the doctor, and by other means. Conversely, we also have the right to be destructive toward our own health. We can choose to smoke, drink excessively, or eat poorly and not exercise. It is the government's duty to protect those choices. As part of the right to pursue health, we can choose to purchase health care services. The government cannot stop anyone from obtaining health care, and in the case of emergencies, no one can be turned away, regardless of ability to pay. People who don't have insurance may be able to get charity care or go to community health centers or make financial arrangements with health care providers. But health care is a business, a service that is provided by trained professionals. When we pay for health care, we pay the salaries of those who work in health care, the technology that is used to diagnose and treat us, the training of health care providers, and research and development of new treatments. Fewer people would have jobs in health care if we didn't pay for health care privately and let the government pay for it all. Moreover, when government does for individuals what individuals should do for themselves, it creates a dependent class, which only widens socioeconomic inequalities and inhibits some people from pursuing the American dream.

You decide:

1. Why does the right to health care fall into the category of the right to vote, free speech, speedy trail, and assembly?

2. Is the right to health care more important than all of the rights in the United States Constitution, since those rights cannot be exercised without being healthy?

3. Did the writers of the Constitution embed the right to health care in the phrase, "life, liberty, and the pursuit of happiness"?

▪ Environmental Change and Restructuring

The health care system has changed dramatically over the last century. The major changes are listed in Table 1–5. The health care environment today is very different than it was in the early to mid-1900s, having experienced a great deal of restructuring. For example, the system shifted from a fee-for-service system (i.e., a billing system in which a health care provider charges a payer a set amount for a specific service) to a prospective payment system (i.e., a system for reimbursing providers using a predetermined, fixed fee or payment per diagnosis or unit of time). Prospective payment for Medicare was introduced in the 1980s as an attempt to reduce health care costs, and as a result this payment form rippled throughout the health care system. When the government implemented the DRG (diagnosis-related group) system in 1983, it changed the way hospitals were paid and eventually led to a number of hospital closures. To supplement the reduced payments from Medicare, hospitals began to charge privately insured patients more. This rebalance led insurance companies to increase premiums, which eventually resulted in many employers shifting their insurance plans from fee-for-service plans to managed care.

The U.S. health care system has evolved from a system of general practitioners to highly specialized medicine, where physicians obtain expertise in multiple discrete subdisciplines. Managed care in the 1990s used cost containment as a vehicle to revert to general medicine or primary care; however, medical education encourages specialization, so the health care system did not change overall. Some additional physicians may have entered primary care specialties, and departments of family and preventive medicine were created in many medical schools, but the specialty subdisciplines remained far more popular.

Managed care also produced a shift from private practice to corporate medicine in the 1990s. The percentage of physicians who became employees increased during this

Table 1–5: Environmental Change and Restructuring of the U.S. Health Care System	
From	**To**
Fee for service	Prospective payment
Mainline medicine	Multiple discrete subdisciplines
Private practice	Corporate medicine
Direct payer	Third-party payer
Inpatient	Outpatient
Intervention	Prevention
Medical model	Sociomedical model
Length of life	Quality of life
Absolute trust in physicians	Trust in several or no authorities
Confidence in institutions	No sense of obligation to institutions

© Cengage Learning 2013

time. If physicians did not join managed care plans as employees, they often became employees of hospitals and group practices. Rather than establish their own independent practices, many physicians preferred to join established practices or become employees of hospitals, group practices, and managed care organizations. The high cost of medical education and the costs associated with opening a practice make it extremely difficult for most medical school graduates to become solo practitioners.

Reimbursement for care has also produced changes in services, from a focus on inpatient to outpatient services. Hospital outpatient revenues now equal inpatient revenues for the first time ever. Since the introduction of health insurance and then Medicare and Medicaid, our system has changed from a direct pay at time of use of services to one where a third party pays (i.e., third-party payers refer to insurance companies, managed care companies, Medicare, and Medicaid). This shift in method of payment for services produced an increase in the cost of health care, which led to the prospective payment changes described above, which then led to a shift to less costly outpatient care.

Additionally, U.S. health care has tried to shift some of the focus on intervention to prevention. The public dialogue has increasingly included prevention strategies, and medical schools are training more clinicians in preventive care, but we are still an intervention—or illness—oriented system. We have not "put our money where our mouth is." We still spend 97 percent of our health care dollars on intervention. In addition, we are trying to shift the focus of care from length of life to quality of life. Hospice, home health care, and other services now exist to help patients receive treatment at home rather than the hospital and to help them die peacefully, with dignity and without pain. This change should have a positive impact on the cost of care if patients are shifting from costly inpatient care to care in the home. This shift represents a redirection of the health system from a predominantly medical model to a sociomedical model. In the sociomedical model, patients are viewed not only as biological organisms but also as social beings with role responsibilities. Hospice and home health care provide social services as well as health care services.

United States citizens are becoming better-educated consumers. Thus, our perception of physicians has also changed from one of absolute trust in one family physician to skeptical trust in several physicians or no trust at all. Similarly, patients' confidence in or loyalty to hospitals and other health facilities has changed to one of no obligation to any specific institution. This absence of loyalty has evolved in part from managed care and other changes in insurance coverage.

▪ Public Image of Health Care Entities

Our perceptions of doctors, hospitals, and insurers are vastly different as well. Today, unlike 20 or 30 years ago, the public is wary of physicians. Increasingly, patients question the knowledge and integrity of their physicians. For example, a survey at the end of the twentieth century was conducted with the following results, shown in Table 1–6.

Despite the lack of trust in physicians in general, patients tend to trust their own physicians. Moreover, people still do trust hospitals. When asked, if a company had a serious safety problem with one of its products or services, would the consumer "trust it to do the right thing or not?" 70 percent said that they would trust hospitals to do the right thing, a higher percentage than any other type of company (Harris Interactive,

Table 1–6: Public Opinion on Health Care Issues, 1997

Statement	Percent Agreed	Percent Disagreed
Doctors are usually up to date on new medical advances.	66%	26%
Most doctors take genuine interest in their patients.	63%	34%
Doctors explain things well to patients.	49%	48%
Doctors spend enough time with patients.	35%	61%
Doctors don't care as much about people as they used to.	53%	42%
Doctors do not involve patients enough in deciding on treatment.	57%	37%

Source: Harris Interactive. (1999). Public attitude toward 13 major industries. The Harris Poll, No. 28, April 1999.

1999). In 2007, the Harris Poll asked whether specific industries do a good or bad job in servicing their customers. Hospitals were ranked fourth overall, with 78 percent saying they did a good job and 20 percent answering that they did a bad job. They were rated higher than any other health care industry component. However, managed care, health insurance companies, and pharmaceutical companies all fare very poorly in public opinion, receiving low rankings and negative scores (Harris Interactive, 2007). Managed care and health insurance companies rank just above tobacco and oil companies in "doing a good job." However, as with physicians, most people are happy with their individual health insurance plans. In 2004, 67 percent of people surveyed gave their insurance plan an "A" or "B" ranking, and 76 percent would recommend their plan to a relative or friend (Harris Interactive, 2004). This poll result is a common example of Americans having a poor opinion of the U.S. health care system overall while being pleased with their own care.

■ The Authors' Intentions

The U.S. health care system has evolved over the past century, the product of a free society that struggles with the role of government and its obligations to take care of those in its midst who are less fortunate. Historically, policy makers and health care academicians have looked to the creation and expansion of government entitlement programs, both federal and state, to solve the nation's health and health care delivery problems, neglecting other viable solutions or strategies, which has resulted in segments of the population who are overly dependent on these programs, soaring health care costs, and exploding national debt.

By no means do these authors suggest that solutions are at hand. Rather, improvements are likely to be incremental and the product of dialogue among the interested parties with their various perspectives and interpretations of available data. The intent of this composite is to provide the debaters and discussants with a fair and balanced, solid foundation of knowledge of the various components of the health care delivery system so that such talks can ensue. Never before in the nation's history has such a compendium been needed as we observe the most polarized, acrimonious discourse on the subject. It is our desire, by presenting the spectrum of opinion and data, that factions in the debate can listen to and not just hear opposing positions. This kind of preparation can lead to productive negotiations that are vitally necessary to maintain what is wonderful about our current system while ameliorating its shortcomings.

There are several key issues to consider when evaluating the health care system:

- Do we have a moral obligation versus a constitutional obligation to provide health care to our fellow citizens?

- What is the appropriate role of government in the health care industry?

- How should the roles and responsibilities in the delivery of health care be divided between the federal and state governments?

- What should be the government's effect on the U.S. economy?

- The health care system is a major part of the U.S. economy; therefore, how should this component be regulated and managed?

So as the saying goes: "Hang on to your seats, folks, it's going to be a bumpy ride!"

▪ Summary

In this chapter we discussed the definition of health. The World Health Organization (WHO) defines health as "a state of complete physical, mental and social well-being and not merely the absence of disease or infirmity." Our health is predominately influenced by heredity or genetics, the environment, lifestyle, and the organization and delivery of health care services. The "iron triangle" of health care includes access, cost, and quality. Access is the potential or ability to use health care services. Cost is the price of health care services. Quality refers to how good or bad the health care services are at the time of delivery.

There are several types of care that consumers are able to access. They include health education and prevention, primary care, secondary care, tertiary care, emergency care, and long-term care. We also discussed the differences and similarities between allopathic medicine, osteopathic medicine, and complementary and alternative medicine. Although some scientific evidence has been produced to demonstrate the effectiveness of some alternative therapies, most of the practices that constitute complementary and alternative medicine still have not been proven as effective and/or safe.

The major stakeholders in the United States health care system include providers, consumers, insurers, businesses, and government. Each group plays an important role in the health care industry, with several of the groups playing two or three roles. For instance, the state and federal governments act as insurer, consumer, and provider of health care services. Employers both consume health care services and reimburse providers when they are self-insured. Each group is affected by the many problems with our health care system. All current problems affect access, cost, and quality and the dynamic interaction among them.

The United States health care system has many problems, including rising costs of health care, access barriers for the uninsured, the Medicare and Medicaid funding burden, high cost of pharmaceuticals, shortage of physicians and nurses, and medical errors.

Within this context, our goal in this book is to provide an objective, fact-based approach to understanding the health care industry. We desire to provide readers with a core set of analytical skills that will enable them to assess health care issues. These skills should be based on a thorough understanding of the health care industry and the key factors that impact cost, access, and quality across time.

▪ Review Questions

1. List and describe the four inputs to health and how these factors influence a person's health. What factor has the largest impact? What factor has the smallest impact?

2. Explain the "iron triangle" and how these factors are interrelated.

3. What are the differences between personal health care and community or population-based services? Give three examples of each.

4. Describe the different types of care and give two examples of each.

5. What are the differences between traditional medicine and complementary and alternative medicine? Give examples of each type of medicine.

6. What are the elements of Parson's sick role?

7. Explain the principal problems of the U.S. health care system.

8. Discuss the elements of the culture war in the U.S. health care system.

9. Discuss the major changes in the U.S. health care system over the last century.

▪ Additional Resources

World Health Organization (WHO) http://www.who.org

Centers for Disease Control and Prevention (CDC) http://www.cdc.gov

American Medical Association (AMA) http://www.ama-assn.org

American Osteopathic Association (AOA) http://www.osteopathic.org

National Center for Complementary and Alternative Medicine (NCCAM) http://nccam.nih.gov

United States Constitution: http://www.usconstitution.net/const.html

Universal Declaration of Human Rights (UDHR) (not ratified by the United States): http://www.un.org/en/documents/udhr/index.shtml

References

American Chiropractic Association. (2007). What is chiropractic? Available at http://www.acatoday.com/level2_css.cfm?T1ID=13&T2ID=61.

Austin, L.T., Amhad, F., McNallly, M., Stewart, D. (May/June 2002). Breast and Cervical Cancer Screening in Hispanic Women: A Literature Review using the Health Belief Model. *Women's Health Issues* 12(3): 122–128.

Beitsch, L. M., Brooks, R.G., Menachemi, N., & Libbey, P.M. (2006). Public health at center stage: New roles, old props. *Health Affairs, 25*(4): 911–922.

Blum, H. (1981). *Planning for Health*, 2nd ed. New York: Human Sciences Press.

Bureau of Labor Statistics, U.S. Department of Labor. (2010). *Career guide to industries 2010–11*. Washington, DC: Office of Occupational Statistics and Employment Projections. Available at http://www.bls.gov/oco/cg/cgs035.htm.

Centers for Medicare and Medicaid Services (CMS) (2011). National Health Expenditures: 2009. Highlights. Retrieved December 15, 2011 from https://www.cms.gov/NationalHealthExpendData/25_NHE_Fact_Sheet.asp.

Centers for Disease Control and Prevention (CDC). (1992). Effectiveness in disease and injury prevention estimated national spending on prevention—United States, 1988. *Morbidity and Mortality Weekly Review, 41*(29):529–531. Available at http://www.cdc.gov/mmwr/preview/mmwrhtml/00017286.htm.

Centers for Disease Control and Prevention (CDC). (2011). *Health United States 2010*. Hyattsville, MD: National Center for Health Statistics.

Conover, C. J. (2004). Health care regulation: A $169 billion hidden tax. *Policy Analysis, 527*, Cato Institute.

Fuchs, Victor. (1974). *Who shall live? Health, economics and social choice*. New York: Basic Books.

Harris Interactive. (1999). Public attitude toward 13 major industries. The Harris Poll, No. 28, April 1999.

Harris Interactive. (2004). Satisfaction with own health insurance remarkably stable. The Harris Poll, No. 31, March 29, 2004. Available at http://www.harrisinteractive.com/news/allnewsbydate.asp?NewsID=781.

Harris Interactive. (2007). Some substantial changes in how Americans view different industries. The Harris Poll, No. 79, August 8, 2007. Available at http://www.harrisinteractive.com/harris_poll/index.asp?PID=795.

Kaiser Family Foundation. (2009). Trends in health care costs and spending. March. Available at http://www.kff.org/insurance/upload/7692_02.pdf.

Merrill C. T., & Elixhauser A. (2005). *Hospitalization in the United States, 2002: HCUP fact book no. 6*. AHRQ Publication No. 05-0056, June 2005. Rockville, MD: Agency for Healthcare Research and Quality. Available at http://www.archive.ahrq.gov/data/hcup/factbk6/.

Mokdad, A. H., Marks, J. S., Stroup, D. F, & Gerberding J. L. (2005). Correction: Actual causes of death in the United States, 2000. *Journal of the American Medical Association*, 293:1918–19.

Mokdad, A. H., Marks, J. S., Stroup, D. F., & Gerberding, J. L. (2004). Actual causes of death in the United States, 2000. *Journal of the American Medical Association, 291*:1238–45.

National Center for Complementary and Alternative Medicine, National Institutes of Health. (2007). CAMBasics: What is CAM? NCCAM Report no. D437. Available at http://nccam.nih.gov/health/whatiscam/.

National Center for Health Statistics (NCHS), Centers for Disease Control and Prevention (CDC). (2010). NCHS fast stats: Ambulatory care use/physician visits, 2007. Available at http://www.cdc.gov/nchs/fastats/docvisit.htm.

National Cancer Institute (NCI). (2010). Tobacco statistics snapshot. Retrieved November 12, 2011, from http://www.cancer.gov/cancertopics/tobacco/statisticssnapshot.

National Center for Homeopathy. (2007). What is homeopathy? Available at http://www.homeopathic.org/whatis.htm.

Office for Civil Rights, Department of Health and Human Services (DHHS) (2001). Policy guidance: Title VI prohibition against national origin discrimination as it affects persons with limited English proficiency. Retrieved December 27, 2011 from http://www.acf.hhs.gov/programs/ocs/ssbg/procedures/memo1.html.

Parsons, Talcott. (1951). *The social system*. New York: Free Press.

Roosevelt, F. D. (1944). Economic bill of rights: Excerpt from January 11, 1944, message to Congress on the State of the Union. Retrieved August 8, 2005, from http://www.worldpolicy.org/globalrights/econrights/fdr-econbill.html (website no longer available).

U.S. Census Bureau. (2009). Health insurance coverage: 2008: Highlights. Available at http:www.census.gov/hhes/www/hlthins/data/historical/index.html.

U.S. Census Bureau. (2010). Income, poverty and health insurance coverage in the United States: 2009. September. Washington, DC: U.S. Dept. of Commerce.

World Health Organization. (1946). Constitution. Available at http://whqlibdoc.who.int/hist/official_records/constitution.pdf.

Key Terms

activities of daily living (ADLs)

compressed morbidity

disability-adjusted life expectancy

health status

incidence

infant mortality rate (IMR)

instrumental activities of daily living (IDLs)

life expectancy

living

morbidity rate

mortality rate

prevalence

quality-adjusted life years

years of healthy life

Learning Objectives

- Define health.

- Identify basic measures of health status, and explain how they are measured.

- Describe the challenges in measuring health status.

- Explain the major reasons for measuring health status.

- Describe the WHO method for comparing countries' health care systems.

- Describe the major causes of death and the major underlying causes of death.

- Describe the impact of smoking on health status.

- Describe the roles of age, sex, race, and poverty on health status.

- Define and discuss health disparities.

■ Definitions of Health

We introduced the first chapter with the most widely accepted definition of health: *"a state of complete physical, mental and social well-being and not merely the absence of disease or infirmity (WHO, 1946)."* There are many other definitions, but most are similar to the WHO definition in that they encompass more than just the absence of physical or mental disease but the presence of wellness. Definitions of health vary across time and cultures. Health includes the ability to contribute to society (cultural functioning) and maintain function in social roles. In addition, health reflects the ability to respond to changes in environment (physical and social) and maintain physical and psychological well-being. For example, physical relocation from one state to another or a change of jobs is often associated with anxiety, stress, and uncertainty. Healthy people adapt well to these major life changes, while others may have problems with depression or even physical illness as a result of stressful events.

Measuring Health Status

Health status is the level of health of a person, group, or nation. We can measure a person's health status in many ways. Physiological measures of health such as blood pressure, white blood cell count, and temperature can be used to diagnose signs of physical illness. Psychological measures such as the Center for Epidemiological Studies Depression Scale (CES-D) can be used to diagnose whether a person has a mental disorder, such as depression. Humans are also very good at measuring their own level of health. Health care–related surveys often ask how respondents perceive their physical and psychological well-being. Studies show that respondents are usually accurate in determining whether their health is excellent, very good, good, fair, or poor (Miilunpalo et al., 1997).

We can use similar measures for determining a group or nation's health status. By aggregating the causes of death for all of the members, we can compare rates of death by cause. Similarly, we can aggregate diagnoses to examine the incidence and prevalence of specific diseases (e.g., heart disease, cancer, stroke, AIDS). **Incidence** measures the number of new cases of a disease over a period of time. **Prevalence** measures the number of total cases of a disease (existing and new) over a period of time. Healthier groups or nations should have fewer cases for a given standardized group (such as per 1,000 or 100,000 people). National health status is often measured by calculating the infant mortality rate, life expectancy, disability-adjusted life expectancy, or years of healthy life. The **infant mortality rate (IMR)** is the rate of infant deaths (from live birth to 1 year) per 1,000 live births. **Life expectancy** is the average number of years people in a given population live. **Disability-adjusted life expectancy** and **years of healthy life** are calculated by subtracting the total number of sick and disabled days and years from the average life expectancy. These measures are used to determine the percentage of a person's or group's life that is spent in good health and to compare the disease and disability burdens of different groups. We will discuss the use of these measures in comparisons in the Your Opinion Matters section.

Measures of Health

A few measures of health have been introduced and defined. However, there are many ways to measure health status, using both traditional and newer measures. Over the past hundred years, there have been several measures routinely employed. Traditional measures include mortality rates, morbidity rates, disability measures, and self-rated health status.

Mortality Rates

A **mortality rate** is one of the earliest "formal" measures of health and is still one of the most commonly used measures of health. It calculates the incidence of death per year per 1,000 or 100,000 people. Generally, female mortality rates are lower than male mortality rates, while the poor have higher death rates than the non-poor, and older people have higher death rates than younger people. Mortality rates can be adjusted for age, sex, race, and other characteristics of the population to make the rates comparable across these factors.

Infant Mortality Rate

Infant mortality rate (IMR) is defined as the number of infants that die within the first year of life per 1,000 live births (i.e., an infant that took at least one breath). The United States ranks relatively low on this measure compared to other countries (the US rate was 28th in 2006). For example, Japan had a 2.6 per thousand live birth infant mortality rate compared to the United States rate of 6.7 deaths per 1,000 live births in 2006 (the rate for 2007 was 6.75, with whites having a 5.64 rate and blacks, a 13.24 rate) (CDC, 2010). The United States spends more per capita on health care than other countries, and we have more sophisticated health care technology than other countries, but still our infant mortality rate is relatively high.

One explanation for the higher infant mortality rate in the United States is that the nation's poor lack access to early prenatal care compared to those with higher incomes, and large-scale public health interventions directed at reducing infant mortality among the poor are not nearly as aggressive as those in other countries. At the same time, other countries may measure their infant mortality rates differently from the United States, excluding lower birth weight and/or shorter gestation births or deaths that occur within the first 24 hours after birth. However, researchers at the Centers for Disease Control and Prevention do not believe that variation in data collection is the main reason for the low ranking of the United States (MacDorman & Mathews, 2009). Nevertheless, the black–white disparity, where the black rate is nearly three times that of whites, explains in part why the U.S. infant mortality rate is relatively higher. This disparity is reflected in low birth weight rates, a contributing factor in infant mortality. It should be mentioned that infant mortality for all racial groups has decreased over time at much the same rate. Health care technology has improved our ability to keep premature and low birth weight babies alive. In addition, expectant mothers are obtaining prenatal care earlier and are more likely to avoid high-risk behaviors. However, early entrance into prenatal care and avoidance of high-risk behaviors like smoking are not comparable across income groups. Medicaid, the federal-state insurance program for the poor and near poor has facilitated access to prenatal care and delivery. Still, blacks and American Indians have higher infant mortality than whites. However, Hispanics in the United States, who also have high rates of poverty, have infant mortality and low birth weight rates comparable to whites. Although poverty is a major contributing factor to higher rates, a combination of lack of access to prenatal care and personal behaviors, as well as inherent discrimination within the U.S. health care system all contribute to infant mortality disparities.

■ Morbidity or Illness Rates

Examples of measures of morbidity include diagnoses of diseases, signs, symptoms, and clinical and laboratory abnormalities. **Morbidity rates** measure the number of people in a population who have a disease at one point in time per 100,000 people. Incidence and prevalence of diseases such as heart disease, cancer, and diabetes are often tracked over time to determine whether population health is improving or worsening. Clinical abnormalities such as high blood pressure (hypertension) and laboratory abnormalities such as hemoglobin A1C (diabetes) are measures used to diagnose morbidity. In general, the poor have higher morbidity rates than the non-poor, while women have higher morbidity (but lower mortality) rates than men, and older people higher morbidity rates than younger people.

▪ Disability

Disability can also be measured in a variety of ways including limitations in activities, burden of chronic diseases, and role interference such as school-loss or work-loss days. **Activities of daily living (ADLs)** and **instrumental activities of daily living (IADLs)** are common measures of limitations in activities. ADLs measure a person's ability to perform basic personal care tasks such as walking, bathing, dressing, toileting, and feeding oneself. IADLs measure ability to accomplish more independent tasks such as cleaning, shopping, managing finances, preparing meals, and using the telephone. There is a direct relationship between limitations in ADLs and IADLs and level of health status. A person with multiple limitations of ADLs will most likely not be able to live independently, whereas a person who only has limitations in one or a few IADLs may be able to live independently with help from family and social support services. In general, the poor have higher rates of disability than the non-poor, older people have higher disability rates than younger people, and women have higher disability rates than men.

▪ Perceived Health Status

Perceived health status is measured by asking how a person would rate their health status relative to others of their own age. Surveys often ask, "Compared to others your age, would you describe your health as excellent, very good, good, fair, or poor." Those with low incomes and minorities rate their health as fair or poor at a much higher rate than those with higher incomes and who are white.

▪ Other Measures of Health

Newer measures of health status incorporate social and quality aspects of **living** in the definition of health. These measures include medicalization of social problems, community health indicators, years of healthy life, also called quality-adjusted life years, and disability-adjusted life years.

Medicalization of Social Problems

The medicalization of social problems significantly expands our definition of health status. Examples of measures that influence health status are juvenile violent crime arrests, single-parent families, teen suicides, births to unmarried women, number or percentage of children on welfare or in poverty, and prevalence of drug and alcohol abuse. Community health indicators include measures of infertility, proportion of the population living alone, percentage of children who are immunized, marriage and divorce rates, unemployment rates, and smoking rates.

These measures add a new dimension to measuring health that transcend the measures of death, disease, and disability by assessing the impact of social environment and lifestyle on health status.

Years of Healthy Life

Years of healthy life (or healthy life years) and quality-adjusted life years (QALY) assess the percentage of life span that is healthy (free of significant disease or disability). It measures both quantity and quality of a person's healthy life. Healthy life years are calculated by measuring the number of people in certain health states at each age. Measures may differ depending on what elements are included in the calculations of nonhealthy life, but generally encompass morbidities, self-rated health status, functional impairment, and limitations in activities. The healthy life concept fits with the life goal held by many, described as **compressed morbidity**—that is to live a long and healthy life and then become acutely sick toward the end and die quickly.

Quality-adjusted life years are often used in cost-effectiveness calculations to determine whether a health care treatment provides a sufficient improvement in health for the amount of money that it costs. One quality-adjusted life year equals 1 year of perfect health. QALYs measure health states but also may assess health utility by asking people to rate their preferences for specific, hypothetical health states. Perfect health equals 1, death = 0 and some states, which people may deem worse than death, can take on negative values. Different treatments may have different values of QALYs, for example, a treatment that yields 0.25 QALYs for 4 years (¼ of the year is a full "quality" year and ¾ is less than full quality) may be preferable to a treatment that yields 0.50 QALYs for 1 year (only ½ of 1 year at full quality). The first treatment gives the patient a full quality-adjusted life year over time, whereas the second only gives ½ of a year of quality-adjusted life. Depending on the cost of the treatment, it may be deemed as cost-effective or not cost-effective. The decision maker, whether a person, business, insurer, or government, must set a threshold of what cost is considered too high per QALY. In the United States, the consensus is that a treatment is cost-effective if it costs less than $50,000 per QALY. In the example above, treatment 1 would be cost-effective if it cost less than $50,000 and treatment 2 would be cost-effective if it cost less than $25,000.

▪ Major Challenges in Measuring Health Status

There are several major challenges in measuring health status. First, it may be difficult to identify and measure all aspects of health status. Mortality data are collected from death certificates and are easy to measure. Functional status, activities of daily living, and other measures are usually estimated from large, nationally representative surveys, but are still subjective, self-reported limitations. It is also necessary to use a variety of scales and measures. No one measure is sufficient, yet it is also difficult to determine the relative importance of each measure. How the measures are weighted influences our interpretation of relative health status. As with developing QALYs, researchers use standard techniques to weight health states, but these adjustments have problems as well. Further, each component may have several dimensions, especially when measuring functional impairment, activities of daily living, or years of healthy life. Health status will depend on the duration of the illness or impairment (i.e., is it an isolated incident or chronic problem, a temporary disability or a permanent condition), the intensity or pain level, the severity of the illness or impairment, and other quality of life issues such as the impact of illness on the patient and those around him or her.

One challenge in particular in calculating quality-of-life estimates is that answers based on hypothetical health states may not reflect what a person will actually believe if he or she is ever in that state. For example, a person may believe that losing both legs would reduce his quality of life by 50 percent, but if that unlikely event happened, he might find that his quality of life was either better or worse than he expected. Opinions could also change over time as a person adjusts to the condition. QALYs also do not take into account externalities, both positive and negative. Externalities are treatments that may have a beneficial or negative impact on more people than just the one receiving the treatment. For example, those who are vaccinated for a communicable disease exert a positive externality on those who are not because the un-immunized cannot contract the disease from the immunized. That benefit to the un-immunized would not be captured in a QALY measurement. Finally, the value of a QALY or the cost-effectiveness of a QALY may differ depending on who is placing value on a person's life, whether it is the patient, the family, a physician, an insurer, or a government system. A child may be hesitant to take her elderly mother off life support, even if others may value the quality of life at zero or even a negative (worse than death) value.

▪ Why Measure Health Status?

Measuring health status is more than just an academic exercise. Determining the best way to measure and compare health status serves many purposes. First, insurance companies try to use previous indicators of health status to determine the health care costs of their applicant pool. The more accurately that the insurance company can measure health status, the better able they will be to set appropriate premiums, ones that will cover all costs of care and administration, and preserve a company profit without charging premiums that are too costly. We also use measures of health status to compare the effectiveness of various medical care devices and services. For example, clinical trials for drugs and medical devices must examine mortality, morbidities, side effects, and adverse events associated with the drug or device compared to a placebo or treatment without the device. Research has been conducted to determine whether HMOs have different mortality rates than fee-for-service insurance policies and if diagnosis-related groups (DRGs) led to poorer outcomes than what was experienced in the period prior to prospective payment (Draper et al., 1990; Kahn, Keeler, et al., 1990; Kahn, Rogers, et al., 1990; Maciejewski et al., 2001; Mukamel, Zwanziger, & Tomaszewski, 2001). Measuring health status can also help public and private health care providers detect unmet need and identify high-risk populations to determine how to plan and market services.

Health status measures and rankings are often used to support arguments for and against universal health care and health insurance systems. Researchers and organizations often use population-level health status measures to compare the health of the U.S. population (the only industrialized nation without universal coverage) to those in other countries with universal health care or health insurance systems. If we compare measures such as life expectancy, disability-adjusted life expectancy, and infant

Table 2–1: Life Expectancy from Birth in the United States and Selected Other Countries by Sex, 2006

Country	Men	Women	Country	Men	Women
Australia	79	84	Mexico	72	77
Austria	77	83	Netherlands	78	82
Canada	78	83	New Zealand	78	82
China	72	75	Norway	78	83
Cuba	76	80	Russian Federation	60	73
Denmark	76	81	Spain	78	84
France	77	84	Sweden	79	83
Germany	77	82	Switzerland	79	84
Italy	78	84	United Kingdom	77	81
Japan	79	86	United States	75	80

Source: World Health Organization. (2009). Statistical Information System, Core Health Indicators, Accessed January 2, 2012 from http://www.who.int/whosis/database/core/core_select.cfm.

Table 2–2: Healthy Life Expectancy from Birth in the United States and Selected Other Countries by Sex, 2003

Country	HALE Men	HALE Women	Country	HALE Men	HALE Women
Australia	71	74	Mexico	63	68
Austria	69	74	Netherlands	70	73
Canada	70	74	New Zealand	69	72
China	63	65	Norway	70	74
Cuba	67	70	Russian Federation	53	64
Denmark	69	71	Spain	70	75
France	69	75	Sweden	72	75
Germany	70	74	Switzerland	71	75
Italy	71	75	United Kingdom	69	72
Japan	72	78	United States	67	71

Source: World Health Organization (2009) Statistical Information System. Core Health Indicators, Accessed January 2, 2012 from www.who.int/whosis/database/core/core_select.cfm

Table 2–3: Infant Mortality Rate in the United States and Selected Countries, 2009 Estimates

Country	IMR	Country	IMR
Japan	2.79	Austria	4.42
Sweden	2.75	United Kingdom	4.85
Saudi Arabia	11.57	China	20.25
Canada	5.04	Angola	180.21
Cuba	5.82	United States	6.69 (2006)*
Germany	3.99	U.S. black	13.29 (2006)*
Russian Federation	10.56	U.S. white	5.56 (2006)*

*Sources: Central Intelligence Agency (CIA). World Factbook. 2009 estimates. Accessed January 2, 2012 from https://www.cia.gov /library/publications/the-world-factbook/rankorder/2091rank.tml; *National Vital Statistics Report, Deaths: Final Data for 2006, 57(14), April 17, 2009, http://www.cdc.gov/nchs/data/nvsr/nvsr57/nvsr57_14pdf.*

mortality, the United States ranks low relative to other industrialized nations. As seen in Table 2–1, the life expectancy in the United States in 2006 was 75 years for men and 80 years for women (WHO, 2009). All other countries listed in Table 2–1, except for China, Cuba (women only), Mexico, and the Russian Federation, have higher life expectancies. The same is true for healthy life expectancy, shown in Table 2–2. As with life expectancy and healthy life expectancy, the U.S. infant mortality rate compares unfavorably with all other industrialized nations, higher than that of Sweden, Germany, Japan, Canada, Austria, and the United Kingdom (see Table 2–3).

The World Health Organization (WHO) published a comparison and rankings of 191 nations' health care systems in 2000 (WHO, 2000). The United States ranked 37th among nations. France has the highest rated health care system, the British system is 18th, and the Canadian system is 30th. Surprisingly, Morocco is ranked above Canada and the United States at 29th. Selected rankings are presented in Table 2–4. But why does the United States rank below Morocco, which is ranked at 110th in disability-adjusted life expectancy? The WHO used a formula comprised of many components. WHO ranked countries on the following attributes:

1. *Health*—Disability-adjusted life expectancy (DALE) and the distribution of life expectancy at birth throughout the population. WHO calculated measures such as the number of people who survived at age 1, age 2, and so on, over the entire population, how many people had each of a set of previously identified disabilities at age 1, age 2, and so on. These sets were weighted and disability was calculated by summing each of these measures with the weight. Survival at each age was then reduced by this disability figure, producing a range for the DALE and DALE distribution. According to WHO, the wider the distribution on this measure, the lower a country ranked. So if the lowest DALE and the highest DALE calculated were close together (Japan, ranked number one, was 6 years) then they were ranked higher than a country with a wider difference (the United States was 18 years).

Table 2–4: World Health Organization Rankings Data, 2000

Nation	Attainment of Goals						Health Expenditures per Capita	Performance	
	Health		Responsiveness		Fairness in Financial Contribution	Overall Goal Attainment		Level of Health	Overall Health System
	Level	Distribution	Level	Distribution					
United States	24	32	1	3–38	54–55	15	1	72	37
France	3	12	16–17	3–38	26–29	6	4	4	1
Germany	22	20	5	3–38	6–7	14	3	41	25
Cuba	33	41	115–117	98–100	23–25	40	118	36	39
Canada	12	18	7–8	3–38	17–19	7	10	35	30
Chile	32	1	45	103	168	33	44	23	33
Colombia	74	44	82	93–94	1	41	49	51	22
Japan	1	3	6	3–38	8–11	1	13	9	10
Morocco	110	111	151–153	67–68	125–127	94	99	17	29
Spain	5	11	34	3–38	26–29	19	24	6	7
United Kingdom	14	2	26–27	3–38	8–11	9	26	24	18

Source: World Health Organization (WHO). (2000). World health report 2000—Health systems: Improving performance. Geneva, Switzerland: Author.

2. *Responsiveness*—The level of responsiveness was based on "respect for the person, confidentiality, autonomy, prompt attention, proper amenities, access to social support networks, and choice of provider." Members of the WHO team surveyed almost 1,800 key informants from 35 countries and conducted an Internet survey of over 1,000 others. The distribution was also determined by key informant interviews. Most European countries, the United States, and Canada were ranked the same in distribution of responsiveness from 3–38, meaning the WHO could not distinguish between them.

3. *Fairness in Financial Contribution*—"The way health care is financed is perfectly fair if the ratio of total health contribution to total non-food spending is identical for all households, independently of their income, their health status or their use of the health system" (WHO, 2000). The description focuses on prepayment of health care rather than out-of-pocket payment, and government financing of a "progressive" system where the wealthier pay more than the nonwealthy.

4. *Overall Goal Attainment*—A measure that takes into consideration all three criteria.

5. *Health Care Expenditure per Capita*—International dollar estimate of average amount spent per person in a nation on health care.

6. *Performance on Level of Health*—A subjective ranking of a nation's "achievement relative to their resources."

7. *Performance on Health System*—Five components are weighted: 25 percent for level of health, 25 percent for distribution of health, 12.5 percent for level of responsiveness, 12.5 percent for distribution of responsiveness, and 25 percent for fairness of financial contribution (WHO, 2000).

However, it is important to point out that rankings are affected by the factors used in the comparisons. Previous studies sited have been critized in leading academic journals for gross distortions from severe methodological flaws, including huge measurement errors that produce results with no statistical significance, data missing from dozens of countries, biased assumptions, and extreme subjectivity. For example, comparisons with countries for which data are available suggest that low birth weight newborns have better chances of survival in the United States than elsewhere. So, although the United States has a higher infant mortality rate, some of this mortality comes from attempts to increase survival of very high-risk births. In addition, blunt instruments like overall life expectancy do not take social factors, like violent crime and obesity, into account.

Another approach is to examine survival rates after a serious diagnosis has been made: for example, how long does the average patient live after being diagnosed with a stroke, heart attack, or breast cancer? This approach has several qualities in its favor: it is quantitative; it can control for population disparities between countries by focusing on a particular disease; and, it focuses on the actual purpose of delivering health care—treating disease. These studies have found that, in all cancers studied, 91.9 percent of Americans survived for 5 years after diagnosis, compared to 57.1 percent for Europeans. These studies further reveal that the United States has better access to treatment for the most prevalent chronic diseases; wider access to preventive care and cancer screening; broader availability of the newest life-changing health care technology; wider access to the most accurate diagnostic technology; quicker access to innovative, life-saving cures and safer, less invasive treatments; more rapid access to highly trained specialists; and ultimately, far better access to the world's leading doctors and medical scientists who themselves are the source of the world's leading innovations by any metric examined (Atlas, 2010).

Americans have better survival rates than Europeans for most common as well as rare cancers. Among more common cancers, the breast cancer mortality rate is 52 percent higher in Germany than in the United States, and 88 percent higher in the United Kingdom. Prostate cancer mortality is strikingly higher in the United Kingdom and in Norway. Age-standardized death rates from prostate cancer from 1980–2005 have been reduced far faster in the United States than in the 15 other developed nations studied, attesting to superior outcomes in what is the most common cancer among men. The mortality rate for colorectal cancer among British men and women is about 40 percent higher. Americans, whether men or women, enjoy superior overall survival from cancer than western Europeans (Atlas, 2010).

Lower-income Americans are in better health than comparable Canadians. It is often claimed that government-financed health care systems, such as Canada's, eliminate income-related barriers to health. The "health–income gradient" (i.e., the concept that higher income achieves better health, and lower income means worse health) for adults 16 to 64 years old reveals a more severe disparity in Canada than in the United States. Specifically, twice as many American seniors with below-median incomes self-report "excellent" health compared to Canadian seniors (11.7% vs. 5.8%). Conversely, white Canadian young adults with below-median incomes are 20 percent more likely than lower-income Americans to describe their health as "fair or poor."

Americans spend much less time waiting than patients in Canada and the United Kingdom—to see a specialist, to have life-changing elective surgery like hip replacements or cataract removal, or to obtain radiation treatment for cancer. In total, 827,429 people were found to be waiting for some type of procedure in Canada. In England, nearly 1.8 million people were waiting for a hospital admission or outpatient treatment (Atlas, 2010).

Finally, by any variety of measures, Americans are responsible for the vast majority of all health care innovations from which the entire world benefits. The top five U.S. hospitals conduct more clinical trials than all the hospitals in any other single developed country. Since the mid-1970s, the Nobel Prize in medicine or physiology has gone to American residents more often than recipients from all other countries combined. From 1969 to 2008, Americans (2009 population, 307 million) won or shared the Nobel Prize in Medicine and Physiology 57 times compared with 40 times by medical scientists from the European Union, Switzerland, Japan, Canada, and Australia combined (2009 combined population, 681 million). Indeed, of the past 34 years, there were only 5 years in which a scientist living in America did not either win or share in the prize (Atlas, 2010).

So, do these statistics mean that the United States has poorer care than other countries? Health status measures are used to justify particular social and political systems such as capitalism, socialism, or communism. For example, proponents of capitalistic, free-market systems would often point to the dismal health status statistics in the former Soviet Union to argue that the United States' largely free-market system was better than "socialized" medicine (see Table 2–4). On the other hand, Michael Moore, in his movie *Sicko*, used the example of Cuba to argue that this communist system's provision of health care is much better than that of the United States. In Tables 2–1 to 2–4, Cuba is very similar to the United States and a great deal better than all other developing countries. Similarly, Canada, the United Kingdom, and France, although democratically governed, all have "socialized" medicine or universal health care. But should we use health status measures to validate or criticize political systems? And do these statistics truly reflect the relationship between the health care system and the population's health? We discuss this issue in the next Your Opinion Matters section.

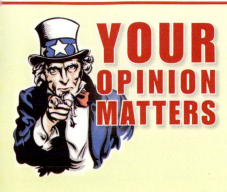

YOUR OPINION MATTERS

Does the United States Have a Poorer Quality of Care Than Other Industrialized Nations? Should We Use Health Status Measures to Validate or Criticize Political Systems? Do These Statistics Truly Reflect the Relationship Between the Health Care System and the Population's Health?

Yes

As seen in the tables presented earlier in the chapter, Americans do not live as long or as healthy lives as people in other industrialized nations. A 2007 study by the Commonwealth Fund found that the United States ranks the lowest out of 14 countries compared international rates of "amenable mortality"—that is, deaths from certain causes before age 75 that are potentially preventable with timely and effective health care (Nolte & McKee, 2008). In addition, the United States also ranks low on patient perceptions of care compared to other countries. In another Commonwealth Fund study of developed nations comparative systems, the United States ranked sixth out of six nations (Australia, Canada, Germany, New Zealand, and the United Kingdom were compared). The United States ranked last on patient safety, patient-centeredness, efficiency, and equity (Davis et al., 2007). For example, 13 percent of U.S. respondents believed that they had been given the wrong medication or wrong dose of a medication in the past 2 years compared to 9–10 percent of respondents in other countries (patient safety) (Davis et al., 2007). Our mortality rates, especially for infant mortality, are much higher than in other countries. Our system is also the least equitable by any standard. Because we do not have a system with universal coverage, many poorer people cannot access health care. Over 40 percent of people surveyed in the Commonwealth Fund study who had below average incomes said that they did not go to a doctor during the past year because of the cost, compared to 17 percent with incomes above average (Davis et al., 2007). This 27 percentage point difference was by far the largest among the six nations. Poorer people are usually sicker, and yet they have more trouble accessing care in the United States than in other countries. High-quality systems are equitable as well as efficient and effective. The United States system only ranks highly on one aspect and therefore provides poor quality overall.

No

Mark Twain once said, "There are lies, damn lies, and statistics." There are problems with many of the statistics that various studies use to compare the United States to other countries. First, the United States has a shorter life expectancy because of more deaths from car accidents and homicides that disproportionately affect the young. The infant mortality rate is also measured differently in the United States than in other countries. In the United States, we deliver more high-risk and premature babies than in other countries, and all births where the babies draw a breath are counted as live births. Some countries do not count babies who are born below a certain birth weight or gestational period (MacDorman & Mathews, 2009). And although, according to the WHO, the United States ranks 37th compared to other countries, our system was ranked first in responsiveness. Most people receiving care would rate highly responsive care as high-quality care. Even the study conducted by the Commonwealth Fund found that the United States ranked first in effectiveness measures. People in the United States are receiving more preventive care and chronic disease treatment than in other countries. Finally, the United States has better survival rates for cancer than most other countries and lower cancer mortality rates. If a person has cancer in the United States, he or she is more likely to survive it than those with cancers living in other countries. No one should be denied care based on income, but quality care should not be measured by equity, but by responsiveness and effectiveness. On those rankings, the United States has the best quality care in the world.

You decide:

1. What are the components of US health care that are best in the world?

2. What services provided by the US health care system are considered not the best among first world countries?

3. Will all US citizens be covered with health insurance after additional requirements of the Patient Protection and Affordable Care Act are implemented in 2014?

4. In what are areas of the US health care system have there been attempts to improve the quality of care delivered?

▪ Causes of Death and Actual (Underlying) Causes of Death

Major causes of death have changed over time. In the late 1800s and early 1900s, infectious diseases caused most deaths. Now, the major killers are chronic diseases, which are caused by way-of-life factors and are thus often preventable. The top causes of death in the United States are heart disease, cancer, and stroke. Although these diseases are the reported causes of death, the major underlying causes of death were tobacco, obesity (diet/inactivity), and alcohol. It is estimated that 435,000 deaths in the year 2000 resulted from tobacco use and 300,000 resulted from obesity (Mokdad et al., 2004). These numbers have not changed much over time. There has been a 30 percent drop in death rates from heart disease and stroke over the past 60 years. Although it is true that health care technology has improved and we have made many advances in treating heart disease, the decline in heart disease mortality has also been affected by changes in diet, a decrease in smoking rates, and better control of hypertension.

▪ Smoking and Health Status

As mentioned above, smoking is the number one risk factor for premature death. The heart attack rate is two to five times greater for smokers than nonsmokers, depending on age (Parish et al., 1995). Smoking also has a dose-response effect, meaning the higher the dose (or the more you smoke), the more likely the outcome (heart attack rate). Smoking has a great impact on health care costs. Smokers age 50 and older are two times more likely than former smokers to die within the next 15 years (Surgeon General, 1990).

It is indisputable that smoking has serious consequences for a person's health. Many believe that smoking should be banned altogether in the same manner that illegal drugs are prohibited. This position makes sense for improving health status; however, it is also a double-edged sword. If everyone quit smoking, our Social Security payments would increase because people would live longer. Smokers pay into Social Security once they begin working, until retirement at age 62–65. Smokers pay into the system and die early without receiving its full benefits. Therefore, if everyone quit smoking, our taxes would increase. If more people start living longer, most likely they will develop other chronic conditions and limitations and will require more health care treatment, leading to higher health care costs and a larger burden on the Medicare program. Smokers also help to pay for many governmental programs through taxes paid on cigarettes (also called a sin tax). Were smoking to be eliminated, the government would have to end many of its programs or find another tax base. Therefore, there are many considerations to changing a law that many agree would improve health status.

▪ Leading Causes of Death by Age

Overall, the leading causes of death are heart disease, cancer, and stroke. However, leading causes of death vary by age. Infant deaths are mostly caused by congenital anomalies, sudden infant death syndrome (SIDS), and short gestation. Young children are more likely to die because of injuries, cancer, and congenital anomalies. Teens and adults up to age 35 suffer mostly violent deaths from unintentional injury, homicide, and suicide. Adults ages 35–54 usually die from unintentional injuries, cancer, or heart disease. Finally, adults 55 and over usually die from chronic disease–related conditions: heart disease, cancer, and stroke (CDC, 2009). The leading causes of death by age group are listed in Table 2–5.

Table 2–5: Leading Causes of Death by Age	
Age	**Leading Cause of Death**
<1	Congenital anomalies, short gestation, SIDS (sudden infant death syndrome), maternal pregnancy complication
1–14	Injuries, cancer, congenital anomalies, homicide
15–34	Injury, homicide, suicide, cancer, heart disease, HIV, congenital anomalies, stroke
35–44	Unintentional injury, cancer, heart disease, suicide
45–54	Cancer, heart disease, unintentional injury, liver disease
55+	Heart disease, cancer, stroke

Source: *Centers for Disease Control and Prevention (2009). Ten Leading causes of death and injury 2006; August 20; Retrieved February 5, 2010 from http://www.cdc.gov/injury/wisqars/LeadingCauses.html*

Other Factors Influencing Health Status

Age

In general, as adults grow older, their health status deteriorates, and they need more health care services. After the age of 65, chronic conditions such as arthritis, hypertension, hearing impairment, heart disease, orthopedic problems, cataracts, and diabetes increase. This rise results in an increase in health care expenditures for these conditions. Three-fourths of people age 65 or older do not have any significant disabilities and 5 percent are nursing home residents. As people increase in age (after age 75), limitation of activity increases.

Gender

Other than mortality measures, women on most other measures of health status are less "healthy" than males, but women live longer than men. Many believe that this difference is not due to true biological differences favoring men. Rather, it is an artifact (i.e., it is not real). These differences are explained by the care-seeking behavior of women who go to physicians more often than men so that they are more likely to be diagnosed with an illness. In addition, many believe that society "allows" women more than men to adopt the sick role (discussed in Chapter 1).

Poverty and Health Status

As mentioned in the discussion of infant mortality, poor people are sicker than non-poor people throughout the world. Poorer nations (developing countries) have substantially higher mortality and morbidity rates than wealthier nations (developed countries). Poverty can adversely affect health by several mechanisms: inadequate physical/social environment, inadequate information and knowledge, a risk-promoting lifestyle or unhealthy attitudes and behaviors, and through diminished access to health care. The result of the combination of these factors is decreased survival rates and an increase in the incidence of diseases.

Mortality data by income show that poor people tend to die at a greater rate than non-poor. For example, lower-income people have a higher rate of serious chronic health conditions. This higher rate may exist because low-income people tend to have jobs that are more dangerous. Low-income people are twice as likely to have heart disease, arthritis, and hypertension when compared to "all income" groups. Low-income people also experience a twofold difference in limitation of activity. Finally, across all racial groups, poor people are significantly more likely to perceive their health as poor or fair than is the case for the non-poor (Marmot, 2002).

■ Health Status and Race and Health Disparities

Vignette

Elizabeth is a 35-year-old Caucasian woman. She works for the Veterans Administration and has Blue Cross Blue Shield insurance through the Federal Employee Health Benefits Plan. She sees a gynecologist, Dr. Smith, yearly for an exam that includes a preventive Pap smear. She has a family history of breast cancer and recently noticed a lump in her breast. Her yearly visit was 3 weeks away, so she waited to report it during that visit. When she sees Dr. Smith, he examines her breasts, and he decided to send Elizabeth for a mammogram. After the mammogram, Elizabeth is then sent for a biopsy. The lump is ruled benign.

Joyce is a 35-year-old African American woman. She works for the Social Security Administration and has Blue Cross Blue Shield insurance through the Federal Employees Health Benefit Plan as well. She sees Dr. Smith every year for an exam and preventive Pap smear. During the last month, Joyce noticed what she thought might be a lump in her breast. However, her appointment was only a few weeks away, so she decided to report the lump during her visit. Joyce has no known family history of breast cancer. Dr. Smith examines her breasts and believes that Joyce has fibrocystic tissue in her breasts. He recommends that Joyce reduce her caffeine and salt intake. On leaving the doctor's office, Joyce schedules her exam for the next year.

1. Does this situation represent a health disparity?

2. Should Joyce have been sent for a mammogram too? Why or why not?

3. Do you think that the race of the patient should play a part in whether the physician refers for a follow up mammogram in this case?

4. Do you think that patients are treated differently by clinicians based on their race, national origin, insurance status, or whether they are obese?

Blacks have higher rates of heart disease and stroke than do whites. Some postulate that there is likely a biological explanation given the high prevalence of hypertension among blacks. This increase may be attributable to true physical/biological differences (elasticity of arteries) between the races, and to a lesser extent, to differences in health behavior (Din-Dzietham et al 2004).

Hispanics and blacks are more likely to report fair or poor health. Black males are more susceptible to firearm-related deaths and HIV infection. Whites have a substantially lower incidence of cancer than blacks in general, and a majority of this difference is due to poverty-related behavior. Five-year survival rates for non-whites are much lower as well for most conditions than for whites. Overall, most of the morbidity and mortality difference between the races is due to socioeconomic status, less access to care, and behavioral factors—not race per se (Marmot, 2002).

However, as a nation we are very concerned about disparities in the treatment of disease. The Institute of Medicine (IOM), a nonprofit part of the Academies of Science, released a definitive report on disparities in America in 2002. The report, "Unequal Treatment: Confronting Racial and Ethnic Disparities in Health Care," showed that minorities receive fewer treatments and procedures than whites for a multitude of conditions. The IOM model "views health care disparities as resulting from characteristics of the health care system, the society's legal and regulatory climate, discrimination, bias, stereotyping and uncertainty. Not all dissimilarities in care are necessarily a disparity."

For example, among patients who were appropriate candidates for coronary angiogram, 82.4 percent of whites received the procedure compared to only 58.7 percent of African Americans (LaVeist et al., 2002). Similarly, only 62.9 percent of African American women over age 65 in Medicare-managed care plans received mammograms compared to 70.9 percent of white women (Schneider, Zaslavsky, & Epstein, 2002). These differences in treatment may be the result of patient or provider preferences, but they could indicate disparities in treatment as well. At this time, it is very difficult to determine the cause of disparities and, therefore, how to improve them.

▪ Mental Illness

Up to this point, this chapter has focused mostly on physical measures of health status. However, mental illness is a significant problem in the United States. It is estimated that mental disorders and illnesses have the second highest disease burden of any chronic disease, mental or physical (NIMH, 2009). The National Institute of Mental Health estimates that one in four adults suffer from any mental disorder, and about 6 percent suffer from a major mental illness (NIMH, 2009). It is estimated that mental disorders lead to approximately $193.2 billion in lost productivity (Kessler et al., 2008).

Chronic mental illness can have a serious impact on health status because it may cause increased utilization of all types of health care services. People who are mentally ill use more health care services, not only mental health services. In 1996, the last year for which estimates are available, the direct cost alone of treating mental disorders, including substance abuse, Alzheimer's, and dementia, was greater than $99 billion (U.S. DHHS, 1999). Mental health, mental illness, and the mental health care system are discussed in more detail in Chapter 8.

▪ Summary

In this chapter, we discussed the definition of health, how health status is measured, how health status measures are used to influence health care systems and compare different countries, challenges to measuring health status, other factors that influence health status, the existence of disparities in health care, and mental illness in the United States. Measuring health status is complicated, but it is vital to organizing our health care system and improving the health of our nation. We must know the health care needs of the nation's subpopulations to provide the appropriate treatment options and be able to plan for the health needs of future generations.

▪ Review Questions

1. How is health defined? What aspects are incorporated into the World Health Organization definition?

2. What is health status? What are some of the ways to measure health status?

3. What is a mortality rate? How is it measured? How do mortality rates differ by subgroups?

4. What is the infant mortality rate, and how it is used?

5. Explain why the U.S. infant mortality rate may be so different from other countries'. Why does the United States have such large racial differences in infant mortality?

6. What are morbidity rates, and how are they measured?

7. How do we measure disability? Why is it necessary to measure disability as well as mortality and morbidity?

8. What are the nontraditional measures of health?

9. What are some challenges to using quality-adjusted life years?

10. What are some of the reasons for measuring health status of groups and populations?

11. Explain how the WHO compares health care systems across countries. What are the advantages to using these measures? What are the disadvantages?

12. What are the top causes of death by age group? How do these change across age groups?

13. What role does smoking have on health status? What are the implications of outlawing smoking?

14. Explain the influence of age, sex, race, and poverty on health status.

15. What are health disparities? Describe the difference between differences and disparities.

▪ Additional Resources

Organization of Economic Co-operation and Development http://www.oecd.org

Commonwealth Fund http://www.cmwf.org

Centers for Disease Control and Prevention http://www.cdc.gov

Institute of Medicine http://www.iom.edu

World Health Organization http://www.who.org

References

Atlas, L. (2010). The ignored facts of American health care. *Defining Ideas; A Hoover Institute Journal*, December 13.

Centers for Disease Control and Prevention (CDC). (2009). Ten leading causes of death and injury, 2006. August 20. Retrieved February 5, 2010, from http://www.cdc.gov/injury/wisqars/LeadingCauses.html.

Centers for Disease Control and Prevention (CDC). (2010). *Deaths: Final data for 2007, National Vital Statistics Reports, 58*(19); May 2010.

Central Intelligence Agency (CIA). The World Factbook. 2009 estimates. Retrieved January 2, 2012, from https://www.cia.gov/library/publications/the-world-factbook/rankorder/2091rank.tml.

Davis, K., Schoen, C., Schoenbaum, S. C., Doty, M. M., Holmgren, A. L., Kriss, J. L., et al. (2007). *Mirror on the wall: An international update on the comparative performance of American health care*. The Commonwealth Fund, May 15, 2007, vol. 59.

Din-Dzietham, R., Couper, D., Evans, G., Arnett, D., Jones, D. (2004 April). Arterial stiffness is greater in AfricanAmericans than in whites: Evidence from the Forsyth County, North Carolina, ARIC cohort. *American Journal of Hypertension*, 17(4), 304–313.

Draper, D., Kahn, K. L., Reinisch, E. J., Sherwood, M. J., Carney, M. F., et al. (1990). Studying the effects of the DRG-based prospective payment system on quality of care: Design, sampling, and fieldwork. *Journal of the American Medical Association, 264*(15), 1956–1961.

Kahn, K. L., Keeler, E. B., Sherwood, M. J., Rogers, W. H., Draper, D., et al. (1990a). Comparing outcomes of care before and after implementation of the DRG-based prospective payment system. *Journal of the American Medical Association, 264*(15), 1984–1988.

Kahn, K. L., Rogers, W. H., Rubenstein, L. V., Sherwood, M. J., Reinisch, E. J., et al. (1990b). Measuring quality of care with explicit process criteria before and after implementation of the DRG-based prospective payment system. *Journal of the American Medical Association, 264*(15), 1969–1973.

Kessler, R. C., Heeringa, S., Lakoma, M. D., Petukhova, M., Rupp, A. E., et al. (2008). Individual and societal effects of mental disorders on earnings in the United States: Results from the national comorbidity survey replication. *American Journal of Psychiatry, 165*(6), 703–711.

LaVeist, T. A., Morgan, A., Arthur, M., Planthol, S., & Rubinstein, M. (2002). Physician referral patterns and race difference in receipt of coronary angiography. *Health Services Research*, 37(4), 949–962.

MacDorman, M. F., & Mathews, T. J. (2009). *Behind international rankings of infant mortality: How the United States compares with Europe*. NCHS Data Brief No. 23. November. Hyattsville, MD: Centers for Disease Control and Prevention.

Maciejewski, M., Call, K. T., Dowd, B., & Feldman., R. (2001). Comparing mortality rates and days of survival for HMO enrollees fee-for-service beneficiaries. *Health Services Research, 35*(6), 1245–1265.

Marmot, M. (2002). The influence of income on health: Views of an epidemiologist. *Health Affairs, 21*(2), 31–46.

Miilunpalo, S., Vuori, I., Oja, P., Pasanen, M., & Urponen, H. (1997). Self-rated health status as a health measure: The predictive value of self-reported health status on the use of physician services and on mortality in the working-age population. *Journal of Clinical Epidemiology, 50*(5), 517–528.

Mokdad, A. H., Marks, J. S., Stroup, D. F., & Gerberding, J. L. (2004). Actual causes of death in the United States, 2000. *Journal of the American Medical Association, 291*(10), 1238–1245.

Mukamel, D. B., Zwanziger, J., & Tomaszewski, K. J. (2001). HMO penetration, competition, and risk-adjusted hospital mortality. *Health Services Research, 36*(6, Part 1), 1019–1035.

National Institute of Mental Health (NIMH). (2009, August 6). Statistics. Retrieved February 4, 2010, from http://www.nimh.nih.gov/health/topics/statistics/index.shtml.

National Vital Statistics Report, Deaths: Final data for 2006, 57(14), April 17, 2009, http://www.cdc.gov/nchs/data/nvsr/nvsr57/nvsr57_14.pdf.

Nolte, E., & McKee, C. M. (2008). Measuring the health of nations: Updating an earlier analysis. *Health Affairs, 27*(1), 58–71.

Parish, S., Collins, R., Peto, R., Youngman, L., Barton, J., Jayne, K., et al. (1995). Cigarette smoking, tar yields, and non-fatal myocardial infarction: 14 000 cases and 32 000 controls in the United Kingdom. *British Medical Journal, 311*(7003), 471–477.

Schneider, E. C., Zaslavsky, A. M., & Epstein, A. M. (2002). Racial disparities in the quality of care for enrollees in medicare managed care. *Journal of the American Medical Association, 287*(10), 1288–1294.

Surgeon General. (1990). *The health benefits of smoking cessation: A report of the surgeon general.* Rockville, MD: Centers for Disease Control, Center for Chronic Disease Prevention and Health Promotion, Office on Smoking and Health.

U.S. Department of Health and Human Services (U.S. DHHS). (1999). *Mental health: A report of the surgeon general—executive summary.* Rockville, MD: U.S. Department of Health and Human Services, Substance Abuse and Mental Health Services Administration, Center for Mental Health Services, National Institutes of Health, National Institute of Mental Health.

World Health Organization (WHO). (1946). Preamble to the Constitution of the World Health Organization as adopted by the International Health Conference, New York, June 19–July 22, 1946; signed on July 22, 1946 by the representatives of 61 states (Official Records of the World Health Organization, no. 2, p. 100) and entered into force on April 7, 1948. Page 2.

World Health Organization (WHO). (2000). *World health report 2000—Health systems: Improving performance.* Geneva, Switzerland: Author.

World Health Organization (WHO). (2009). Statistical information system. Core health indicators, Retrieved January 2, 2012, from http://www.who.int/whosis/database/core/core_select.cfm.

Health Services in Perspective

Key Terms

defensive medicine

diminishing marginal returns

disability rates

"flat-of-the-curve" medicine

inertia

leading causes of death

mechanistic approach to the treatment of disease

medical care

preventive public health

space shot mentality

"way-of-life factors"

zero sum game

Learning Objectives

- Discuss whether the United States receives adequate "value" for the amount of health spending.

- Describe trends in life expectancy, mortality, disability, and chronic diseases over time.

- Discuss the concept of diminishing marginal returns as it relates to health care.

- Describe the successes of the health care system.

- Discuss the strategies that Americans use to cope with disease.

▪ Introduction

The last chapter discussed measures of health status and their uses. In this chapter, we discuss trends in health status in the United States and how the health care system has evolved to respond to those trends. We also discuss whether the United States receives commensurate "value" for the amount that it spends on health care.

▪ Impact of Modern Medicine on Health

Is modern medicine effective in improving health? Compared to its accomplishments in the early twentieth century, modern medicine may have relatively little impact on health today. In 2008, the United States spent $2.3 trillion on health care—$7,861 per capita, or 16.2 percent of the gross domestic product (GDP) (Hartman et al. & the National Health Expenditure Accounts Team, 2010). Health care costs have increased faster than general inflation almost every year (see Figure 3–1). We spend about 2½ times more on health care per capita than other developed countries (participants in

Medical care services, medical care, and all items
Annual average percent change in consumer price index

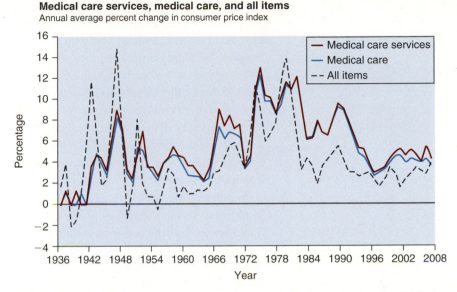

Figure 3–1 Medical service, medical care inflation compared to general inflation.
Source: U.S. Bureau of Labor Statistics.

the Organization for Economic Co-operation and Development). In 1940, 4 percent ($4 billion) of our GNP/GDP was spent on health care. By 1987, that percentage nearly tripled to 11 percent ($500 billion), and by 2008 the 1940 percentage more than quadrupled, to 16.2 percent ($2.3 trillion) of our GDP (CMS, 2010). Are we spending too much? Are we receiving value from our health care system that parallels these geometric increases in expenditures? What type of value do we receive for our health spending?

Many health care professionals and politicians have decried the amount that the United States spends on health care, especially relative to other countries (Boden-heimer, 2005; Davis et al., 2007; Davis, Schoen, & Stremikis, 2010; Marmot, 2002; WHO, 2000). In addition, forecasters are troubled because we cannot sustain these increases without draconian shifts in spending away from other essential budget priorities. However, the amount that we spend as a nation may not be the best predictor of value in health care. Recent studies have estimated substantial life expectancy gains and decreases in mortality that outweigh the costs. About 50 percent of the life expectancy gains from 1960–2000 (almost 7 years for newborns) were attributable to **medical care**. Cutler and colleagues (2006) further estimated that we spent, on average, $19,900 per year of life gained from birth. From a cost-effectiveness standpoint, $20,000 per year of life gained is well worth the cost. Yet, the cost of a year of life gained has increased over time and increases with age. The cost for a year of life gained from 1960 to 1970 was $75,100 for people over age 65. This figure increased to $145,000 from 1990 to 2000 (Cutler, Rosen, & Vijan, 2006).

Further, health care expenditures are not necessarily greater for those who live longer, at least past the age of 70, unless that person is institutionalized (living in a nursing home) at age 70. Those who are healthier generally live longer than those who are sicker, but by the end of their lives, their cumulative health expenditures are about the same. Those who are in good health at age 70 live approximately 14.3 years longer and have cumulative health expenditures of approximately $136,000 (in 1998 dollars). Those who are sicker have a shorter life expectancy and spend cumulatively about $145,000 (in 1998 dollars). These findings contradict many previously held assumptions that the longer we live, the more we will spend on health care (Lubitz et al., 2003).

Yet not all studies reach the same conclusion. Advances were made in the treatment of acute myocardial infarction (AMI), or heart attacks, in the 1980s and 1990s. Significant gains in survival rates were achieved in the 1980s and early 1990s, but survival rates have remained much the same since 1996 (Skinner, Staiger, & Fisher, 2006). This study also found that higher spending was actually associated with lower survival rates. Cost-effectiveness of treatments may have also changed over time. Skinner and his colleagues estimated that we now spend $300,000 per year of life gained for AMI patients.

In general, the prevailing message has been that we are not receiving adequate "returns" on our investment in health care. At the same time, demand for health care is increasing. So, why is there a sustained increase in demand for health care services when those funds could be spent elsewhere and produce better returns? There are several reasons for this increase in demand: (1) Patients are not rational consumers. They do not always know the "value" of health care services that they demand. However, patients will utilize them anyway for *any* perceived benefit. (2) Patients do not usually pay for care at the time they receive it. When insurance is paying for care, patients are less likely to question if they are receiving enough "value" for the service, (i.e., if it is worth purchasing). (3) Health care is a business, and providers are willing to offer services that may be of marginal value in the aggregate but may benefit an individual patient. Hospitals, doctors, and other providers have to sell services to make money and keep people employed. (This is not to say that most providers do not choose careers in the health professions out of their compassion for others, but all providers must also earn a living).

Why should we be concerned that some treatments are not cost-effective or that we are not realizing a reasonable "return on investment" in health care? The answer is, because we not only incur direct expenses for care, but we also incur opportunity costs. An opportunity cost is the value of an alternative decision that was forgone once a choice has been made. For example, when we go to the doctor, we incur many opportunity costs such as our time spent elsewhere. We could be working and earning money, and those lost wages become an opportunity cost. Another opportunity cost would be our copayment and any parking fees we might incur. The cost of visiting the doctor is equivalent to money that could be spent buying something else. For small health care needs, we may behave in a more rational manner regarding opportunity costs. We may be able to understand that a $20 copayment at the doctor's office does result in foregoing a trip to the movies or dinner at a restaurant. If the condition is not serious, then we may choose the movies or dinner over the doctor visit. However, for more serious health care issues, where there may be fewer alternatives and larger payments, we may not be able to weigh the opportunity costs. For example, if you are not alive, there is little or no opportunity to spend your time or money elsewhere. We may not be able to weigh having heart surgery versus buying a car or house, largely because many of these services and illnesses cannot be anticipated as well as the human emotion surrounding the illness. Also, we do not pay the full cost of any of these goods or services, especially those involving life-threatening conditions, at the time of purchase, so we are less sensitive to the overall price.

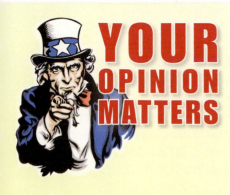

Are We Getting Enough "Value" Out of the Health Care Dollars That We Spend?

Yes

Despite what many critics say and despite its expense, health care in the United States is of great value. We are getting the "bang for our buck." Researchers have discovered many life-saving, life-extending, and quality-of-life-enhancing treatments and procedures. Many of these interventions were very expensive at first but became cost-effective over time as their awareness and use expanded. Their utilization became more frequent, and generic drugs were produced and substituted for the more expensive brand names. Treatment for heart attacks today is vastly different that it was in the 1980s, predominantly as a result of better technology. In the mid-1980s, only about 10 percent of heart attack patients were treated with intensive methods, even though bypass surgery was first developed in the 1960s (Cutler & McClellan, 2001). Use of several intensive procedures increased throughout the 1980s and 1990s, including bypass surgery, cardiac catheterization, and angioplasty. Angioplasty with stents was first used in 1995 and has grown in use more dramatically than any other procedure. More than half of heart attack patients now undergo at least one intensive procedure, and many are prescribed medications to help manage their conditions as well. On the whole, these developments have resulted in a $60,000 benefit per patient, or about $7 gained for every $1 spent. Even more impressive are the gains from better treatment of low birth weight infants, largely the result of better perinatal technology. In 1990, the cost of treating premature infants was $40,000 more than in 1950 (comparing 1950–1990 in present value). However, life expectancy increased by over 12 years, and it is estimated that gains are about $6 for every dollar invested. Research has uncovered highly successful disease management strategies for asthma, congestive heart failure, and diabetes that have added value to the health care system.

Although the amount spent on health care as "real" income has increased over time, so has the amount spent on other budget items. We are spending more on goods and services, as reflected in our growing GDP. Health care spending per capita increased about 70 percent from 1960 to 2000 but only accounted for about one-quarter of the increase in per capita income. The rest of the per capita income increase went to non–health care spending. We can afford to spend more on health care because we are making more money in real terms (Chernew, Hirth, & Cutler, 2009). In fact, with only one-quarter of our increased income allotted to health care, we could potentially afford to spend even more.

(Continued)

No

We are not receiving enough value for our health care spending. We spend more than any other country per capita on health care yet have higher infant mortality, lower life expectancy, and more disability than many countries that spend less and manage to insure their entire populations. Canada spent 43 percent less per capita on health care in 2000 than the United States after controlling for purchasing parity (Reinhardt, Hussey, & Anderson, 2004). Much of the amount that we spend is considered administrative overhead, which includes regulation, fraud, abuse and waste. Researchers have estimated that 25 percent of the cost of health care is attributed to regulation and 31 percent to administration alone (Conover, 2004; Woolhandler, Campbell, & Himmelstein, 2003). To what extent these overlap (administrative costs imposed by regulations) is unknown; however, whether the figure is 25 or 31 percent or some combination of both estimates, a significant percentage of the health care dollar does not provide any direct benefit to patients. Also, many patients in different parts of the country receive different levels of treatment for the same problem, yet patients in high-cost and high-use areas do not report better satisfaction with or quality of their care. Most of the spending is attributed to unnecessary procedures or tests or longer hospitals stays, which may place the patient at risk of hospital acquired infections or complications. Technology is expensive and there is no rational system in place for determining when expensive procedures should be used and when a lower-cost approach is better. Instead we tend to provide more technology to everyone regardless of the cost-effectiveness of the treatment or diagnostic procedures. For example, most spinal-fusion surgery is not cost-effective. These procedures are very expensive and may not result in improved outcomes for patients. Pain rehabilitation is much more cost-effective, yet spinal fusion surgery increased 77 percent between 1996 and 2001 (Deyo, Nachemson, & Mirza, 2004). More spending on health is justified as long as we can improve our mortality, life expectancy, or quality of life. However, far too many treatments and procedures do not produce enough "Bang for Our Buck" and therefore, the public dollar should not continue to be used for those interventions.

You decide:

1. How is value measured?

2. What should be the focus of measuring value as health care's share of GDP grows

3. What are the assets of the US health care system

4. What are the major problems with the US health care system

▪ Diminishing Marginal Returns

Health care, like most other goods and services, has **diminishing marginal returns**. For each additional dollar spent, we obtain less of a gain in output, whether it is measured by increased life expectancy, lower mortality, or better quality of life (See Figure 3–2). Part of the reason for this diminishing marginal return is that there is a distinction between health care and medical care. Modern medicine is not synonymous with health care. Health care includes factors that affect lifestyle, genetics and socioeconomic factors (Fuchs, 2004). Medical care in general has less impact on overall health, with many differences in outcomes attributable to other factors such as genetics and lifestyle.

Yet, each year we spend more on health care but the returns decrease over time. As stated earlier, an estimated 25 percent of health care spending is the result of regulation, which arguably produces little or no marginal benefit and may, in fact, harm people (Conover, 2004). Waste, fraud, and defensive medicine direct the health care dollar away from payment for services that bring real returns. Yet it is very difficult to precisely estimate the costs of fraud, waste, and defensive medicine. **Defensive medicine** occurs when providers order additional or "unnecessary" tests to protect themselves in case of a lawsuit. Defensive medicine increases costs, but does not really help the practitioner treat the patient and may even harm the patient. These expenses add to the cost of health care without producing positive returns (improved health status).

When observing level of disability as an outcome for treatments to reduce disability, there is also no indication that returns are positive. In fact, disability and activity limitations, as well as the number of people with chronic conditions have been increasing over time (see Table 3–1, Figure 3–3).

Diminishing marginal returns have always existed in health care and can be observed historically by examining the performance of public health measures against those of some acute care treatments. The first advances in increasing life expectancy came from public health efforts such as sanitizing the water supply and creating adequate sewage systems. For very little money, relatively, these inputs led to

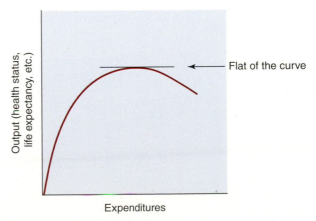

Figure 3–2 Diminishing marginal returns.
© Cengage Learning 2013

Table 3–1: Chronic Disease: Current and Projected Burden, United States, 2003–2023

Chronic Disease	Increase in Prevalence (2003–2023)[a]	Current Cost (2003)	Future Cost (2023)
Overall chronic illness[b]	42%	$1.3 trillion	$4.2 trillion
Cancers[c]	62	$319 billion	$1,106 billion
Diabetes	53	$132 billion	$430 billion
Hypertension	39	$312 billion	$927 billion
Pulmonary conditions	31	$139 billion	$384 billion
Heart disease	41	$169 billion	$927 billion
Mental disorders	54	$217 billion	$704 billion
Stroke	29	$36 billion	$98 billion

Source: R. DeVol and A. Bedroussian, An Unhealthy America: The Economic Burden of Chronic Disease *(Santa Monica, Calif.: Milken Institute, October 2007).*

Note: Cost figures include medical costs plus reduced on-the-job productivity.

[a]Population is expected to grow 19 percent from 2003 to 2023.

[b]These figures do not include all chronic conditions but are based on data for the seven most common chronic diseases: cancers, diabetes, hypertension, stroke, heart disease, pulmonary conditions, and mental disorders.

[c]Includes breast, colon, lung, prostate, and other cancers.

tremendous gains in health status. However, once the major efforts at improving sanitation occurred, further efforts brought less benefit. Similarly, reducing air pollution in the early 1900s had a much larger impact on improving health status than reductions of air pollution in the 1970s and 1980s because the air was already much cleaner than it had been.

What is the cause of the diminishing marginal returns? Some suggest that spending large amounts on cures after the presence of illness, rather than spending scarce dollars on less-expensive preventive measures and education, produces the diminishing

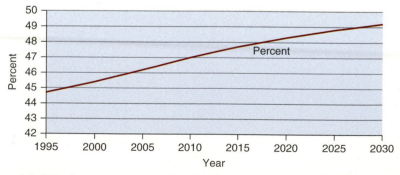

Figure 3–3 Projected percent of population with chronic condition, 1995–2030.
© *Cengage Learning 2013*

returns. We spend about 90 percent of our health care dollars on acute and chronic care treatment, 10 percent on prevention and education, and only 3 percent on public health measures (Beitsch et al., 2006). We (as individuals) control a vast majority of our risky behaviors that have real impact on health status such as diet, exercise, smoking, and drinking. Our top three causes of death (heart disease, cancer, and stroke) are largely related to lifestyle factors, yet we do not focus the efforts of our health care system on health promotion and disease prevention programs, many of which target lifestyle factors. For some treatments, we have made huge gains in the past, but relatively few new treatments or technologies have made substantial additional advances in effectiveness. As Skinner and colleagues noted above, we are not obtaining as much value out of treatments for heart attacks as we did 20 years ago. We practice what Enthoven coined, in the 1970s, as **"flat-of-the-curve" medicine**. He posited that we have reached the point in many health care treatments where we do not experience any additional increase in health status for additional spending. However, we continue to supply and demand these services despite having no gains in health status.

Increased Input Despite Decreased Output

As a nation, we have experienced an increasing demand for health services coupled with increasingly higher expectations of the results. Yet, the evidence suggests that we are receiving less marginal value for our health care dollars over time. This pattern is not unique to the United States but is observed in all developed countries. Why does this seemingly irrational spending continue to occur? Ironically, one of the "outcomes" of successful outcomes is the further need for care. For example, patients who receive transplants must use anti-rejection drugs for long periods following the transplant, and the number of successful transplants is increasing (see Figure 3–4). Also, some successful outcomes are not well measured. For example, an HIV-positive patient today lives longer than in the past, which results in incurring additional care costs during the prolonged life (see Figure 3–5). The value of those costs is high from a cost-effectiveness

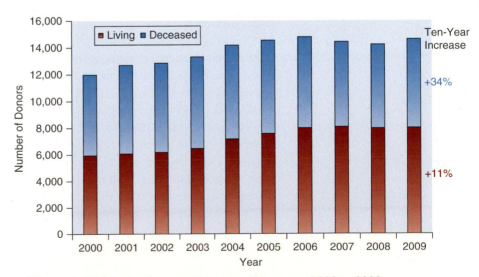

Figure 3–4 Living and deceased donors: All organs, 2000 to 2009.
Source: OPTN/SRTR Annual Report, Table 1.1.

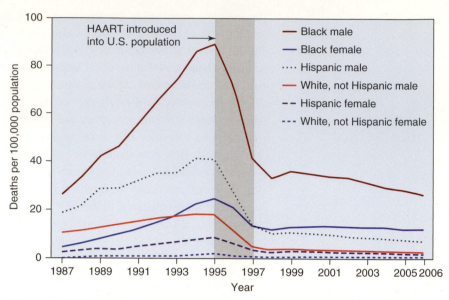

Figure 3–5 HIV death rates and introduction of highly active antiretroviral therapy (HAART).

Source: From Health, United States, 2009. In Brief—Medical Technology. *(2009). Hyattsville, MD: U.S. Department of Health and Human Services, Centers for Disease Control and Prevention, National Center for Health Statistics.*

standpoint, however, because HIV positive patients tend to be younger and have additional productive years.

However, in balance we are still receiving decreased returns for our increasing investments in health services as measured by mortality and morbidity trends compared to the results of early public health interventions. The major causes of death from the sixteenth to the early twentieth centuries were infectious diseases such as pneumonia, tuberculosis, diarrhea and enteritis, cholera, and diphtheria. However, trends over time demonstrate that mortality from these diseases was in rapid decline before medical interventions such as antibiotics and vaccinations were available. In England and Wales, the death rates for children under age 15 from scarlet fever, diphtheria, whooping cough, and measles declined from over 6,000 deaths per million children in 1860 to just over 1,000 deaths by the 1930s. Antibiotics and compulsory immunization for diphtheria were not introduced until the 1940s. In fact, 90 percent of the decline in mortality between 1860 and 1965 can be attributed to factors other than medical treatment (Porter, 1972). Similarly, death rates for tuberculosis (also called consumption) in New York declined from over 700 deaths per 10,000 people in the early 1800s to 180 per 10,000 by 1910, when the first sanatorium for tuberculosis treatment was opened (Porter, 1972). Factors such as improved *nutrition, clean water, and appropriate sewage disposal as well as declining birth rates were responsible for the decline in mortality* and improvement in health status currently enjoyed in the twenty-first century (McKeown, 1978). Although our mortality rates have continued to decline during the twenty-first century, the rate of decline has decreased, with the majority of the early overall gains the result of a drop in mortality from infectious disease, especially among infants.

■ Why the Mixed Results of Modern Medicine?

The experts disagree about the impact of modern medicine on improved health status in part because medicine's effectiveness is dependent on the way that it is measured. In chapter 2, we discussed the many ways of measuring health status. These proxy indicators included overall morbidity rates, mortality rates, life expectancy, infant mortality, and others. Yet there are still other ways that the success or failure of the United States health care system can be assessed. In addition to overall rates, we can observe changes over time in mortality and morbidity rates, changes in life expectancy, disability, and chronic conditions. Because the collective investment in health care is large, we would expect death rates, morbidity, and life expectancy to have improved over time.

■ Trends in Current Health Status

Many positive trends can be seen in our current health status as measured by life expectancy and infant mortality. As Table 3–2 illustrates, this nation has enjoyed increases in life expectancy at 65 years of age for both genders from 1970 through 2007.

Disability rates have also declined for the population over age 65. However, numbers of people with chronic conditions are increasing for all adults over age 45, and disability rates are increasing for the age group 50–64 years old. Rates of neck and back problems among 50–64 year olds increased over 30 percent between 1997 and 1999, and again between 2005 and 2007 (Martin et al., 2010). Rates of diseases such as diabetes, hypertension, and neurological conditions have increased as well. Americans also need more assistance with activities of daily living and instrumental activities of daily living at younger ages (Martin et al., 2010). These trends indicate that the burden of disease is growing as well as the prevalence, with more individuals requiring assistance in the form of canes, walkers, wheelchairs, or other medical equipment. Rates of overweight and obesity are increasing as well, contributing to increases in chronic conditions (see Figure 3–6). We are living longer, but we are producing more, not fewer, disabled or chronically ill individuals who are living longer and consuming even more health resources—we are not curing disease.

■ Other Outcome Measures

As discussed in Chapter 2, life expectancy is an important and frequently used outcome measure. Although we are living longer, our life expectancy is not increasing at anywhere near the same rate as our expenditures on health care. Health care expenditures have more than tripled since 1990 (CMS, 2010) but have only added 2.7 additional years to our life expectancy (Bell & Miller, 2002). The percentage change in outcome (life expectancy, 3.5%) does not match the percentage change in input (dollars we invest, 70.5% total, or 3.9% of our GDP). However, this outcome measure is purely quantitative and is *not sensitive* to improvements in the quality of life. Many treatments improve our daily quality of life without contributing to gains in life expectancy, such as treatments for allergy relief, heartburn/acid reflux, and erectile dysfunction.

In sum, **preventive public health** measures have been the most cost-effective health care interventions to date. The returns on investment for immunizations, prenatal care, smoking cessation, and cholesterol control are relatively high. Some health screening programs and many disease management programs have been proven to be

Table 3–2: Life Expectancy at Birth, and at 65 Years of Age, by Race and Sex: United States, Selected Years 1970–2007
[Data are based on death certificates]

Specified Age and Year	All Races			White			Black or African American[1]		
	Both Sexes	Male	Female	Both Sexes	Male	Female	Both Sexes	Male	Female
At Birth				**Remaining Life Expectancy in Years**					
1970	70.8	67.1	74.7	71.7	68.0	75.6	64.1	60.0	68.3
1980	73.7	70.0	77.4	74.4	70.7	78.1	68.1	63.8	72.5
1990	75.4	71.8	78.8	76.1	72.7	79.4	69.1	64.5	73.6
1995	75.8	72.5	78.9	76.5	73.4	79.6	69.6	65.2	73.9
1999	76.7	73.9	79.4	77.3	74.6	79.9	71.4	67.8	74.7
2000	76.8	74.1	79.3	77.3	74.7	79.9	71.8	68.2	75.1
2001	76.9	74.2	79.4	77.4	74.8	79.9	72.0	68.4	75.2
2002	76.9	74.3	79.5	77.4	74.9	79.9	72.1	68.6	75.4
2003	77.1	74.5	79.6	77.6	75.0	80.0	72.3	68.8	75.6
2004	77.5	74.9	79.9	77.9	75.4	80.4	72.8	69.3	76.0
2005	77.4	74.9	79.9	77.9	75.4	80.4	72.8	69.3	76.1
2006	77.7	75.1	80.2	78.2	75.7	80.6	73.2	69.7	76.5
2007	77.9	75.4	80.4	78.4	75.9	80.8	73.6	70.0	76.8
At 65 years									
1970	15.2	13.1	17.0	15.2	13.1	17.1	14.2	12.5	15.7
1980	16.4	14.1	18.3	16.5	14.2	18.4	15.1	13.0	16.8
1990	17.2	15.1	18.9	17.3	15.2	19.1	15.4	13.2	17.2
1995	17.4	15.6	18.9	17.6	15.7	19.1	15.6	13.6	17.1
1999	17.7	16.1	19.1	17.8	16.1	19.2	16.0	14.3	17.3
2000	17.6	16.0	19.0	17.7	16.1	19.1	16.1	14.1	17.5
2001	17.7	16.2	19.0	17.8	16.3	19.1	16.2	14.2	17.6
2002	17.8	16.2	19.1	17.9	16.3	19.2	16.3	14.4	17.7
2003	17.9	16.4	19.2	18.0	16.5	19.3	16.4	14.5	17.9
2004	18.2	16.7	19.5	18.3	16.8	19.5	16.7	14.8	18.2
2005	18.2	16.8	19.5	18.3	16.9	19.5	16.8	14.9	18.2
2006	18.5	17.0	19.7	18.6	17.1	19.8	17.1	15.1	18.6
2007	18.6	17.2	19.9	18.7	17.3	19.9	17.2	15.2	18.7

---Data not available.

[1]Data shown for 1900–1960 are for the nonwhite population.

Notes: Populations for computing life expectancy for 1991–1999 are 1990-based postcensal estimates of U.S. resident population. See Appendix I, Population Census and Population Estimates. In 1997, life table methodology was revised to construct complete life tables by single years of age that extend to age 100 (Anderson RN. Method for constructing complete annual U.S. life tables, NCHS, Vital Health Stat 2(129), 1999). Previously, abridged life tables were constructed for 5-year age groups ending with 85 years and over. Life table values for 2000 and later years were computed using a slight modification of the new life table method due to a change in the age detail of populations received from the U.S. Census Bureau. Values for data years 2000–2007 are based on a newly revised methodology that uses vital statistics death rates for ages under 66 and modeled probabilities of death for ages 66 to 100 based on blended vital statistics and Medicare probabilities of dying and may differ from figures previously published. The revised methodology is similar to that developed for the 1999–2001 decennial life tables. Starting with 2003 data, some states allowed the reporting of more than one race on the death certificate. The multiple-race data for these states were bridged to the single-race categories of the 1977 Office of Management and Budget Standards for comparability with other states. See Appendix II, Race. Some data have been revised and differ from previous editions of *Health, United States*. Data for additional years are available. See Appendix III.

Source: CDC/NCHS, National Vital Statistics System; Grove RD, Hetzel AM. Vital statistics rates in the United States, 1940–1960. Washington, DC: U.S. Government Printing Office, 1968; Arias E, Rostron BL, Tejada-Vera B. United States life tables, 2005. National vital statistics reports; vol 58 no 10. Hyattsville, MD: NCHS, 2010. Xu J, Kochanek KD, Murphy SL, Tejada-Vera B. Deaths: Final Data for 2007. National vital statistics reports; vol 58 no 19. Hyattsville, MD: NCHS, 2010.

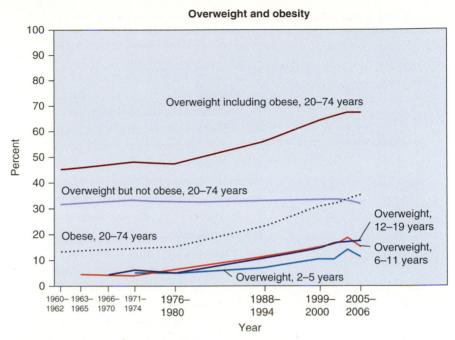

Figure 3–6 Percent of population overweight and obese by age groups, 1960–2006.
Source: National Center for Health Statistics. Chartbook on Trends in the Health of Americans. Health, United States, 2006. Hyattsville, MD: Public Health Service. 2006.

cost-effective. Disease management for asthma, diabetes, and congestive heart failure often results in better outcomes and lower overall costs for patients who are enrolled in those programs.

The health care system has also made great technological strides in a number of areas such as decreasing infant mortality as a result of increased survival of low-birth-weight and premature infants, improving quality of life for women through improved birth control methods, fighting infectious diseases through use of antibiotics, increasing survival rates for some cancers (skin cancer, leukemia, colorectal cancer, breast cancer, testicular cancer), saving lives through improved expertise in trauma care, and extending life through treatments such as angioplasty for heart disease or organ transplants. However, as successful as many of these treatments have been, some experts have questioned the cost-effectiveness of their broad application (Nagle and Smith, 2004).

▪ Why Are Chronic Diseases Increasing?

The human species is not genetically suited to living in a high-technology-driven society. For 99 percent of the duration of man on Earth, they have been hunter-gatherers. In addition, the advent of agriculture brought dramatic changes in diet, population density, and patterns of daily life. Nutrition levels dropped and infection rates increased in early agricultural development because we were inferior farmers living closer together. In fact, most infectious diseases were not prevalent until after the agricultural revolution. McKeown (1978) attributed most of the improvements in deaths from infectious disease to better sanitation, improved nutrition, and declining birth rates.

▪ Leading Causes of Death

Today, the **leading causes of death** are heart disease, cancer, and stroke. These chronic diseases are the main killers of the last half of the twentieth century into the twenty-first century. These diseases result from mal-adaptation to our environment and to an increasingly sedentary lifestyle. Humans are not genetically programmed to endure the stresses and consequent illness of life in an industrialized, high-tech society. These diseases are primarily behavior related.

Previously, many of our most prevalent diseases and causes of death were due to acute illnesses with rapid onset, severe symptoms, and a short course. Most of our burden of disease and causes of death now are related to chronic illnesses with long durations and few changes or slow progressions. These chronic diseases are not a natural part of aging, but occur because of the way we live. For example, an increase in blood pressure and an increase in cholesterol level are not normal age-related factors; rather they are lifestyle or behavioral factors. By having examined modern day hunter-gatherers such as some African tribesmen from studies from the 1940s and 1950s, we observed that the blood pressures and cholesterol levels of these populations *did not increase* with age.

Figure 3–7 presents the top 10 leading causes of death by race for the United States for the twentieth century. The leading causes of death have not changed in the twenty-first century. In 1900, the crude death rate was approximately 17 per 1,000. In 2010, the crude death rate in the United States was estimated to be 8.38 per 1000 (Central Intelligence Agency (CIA), 2010). Most of our decline in age-adjusted mortality came from 1936–1954 due to decreased mortality in children and younger adults (Bell & Miller, 2002). Table 3–3 shows the leading causes of death in the twenty-first century.

Trends in **"way-of-life" factors** over the past 20 years show a decrease in the number of motor-vehicle deaths, especially those related to alcohol (see Table 3–4).

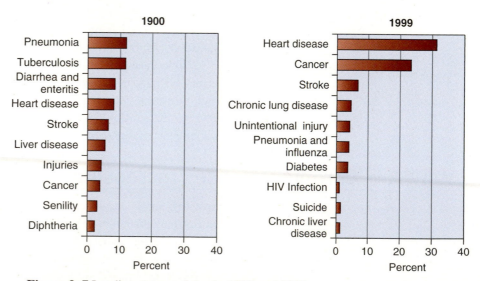

Figure 3–7 Leading causes of death, 1900 and 1999.

Source: Centers for Disease Control and Prevention (CDC). (1999). Control of infectious diseases 1900–1999. Morbidity and Mortality Weekly Report, 48, *621–629.*

Table 3–3: Deaths and Percentage of Total Deaths for the 10 Leading Causes of Death by Sex, United States, 2006

[The asterisk (*) preceding cause-of-death codes indicates they are not part of the *International Classification of Diseases, Tenth Revision* (ICD–10), Second Edition; see "Technical Notes"]

Cause of Death (based on ICD–10, 2004)		Males			Females		
		Rank[1,2]	Deaths	Percent of Total Deaths	Rank[1,2]	Deaths	Percent of Total Deaths
All causes		. . .	1,201,942	100.0	...	1,224,322	100.0
Diseases of heart	(I00–I09, I11, I13, I20–I51)[3]	1	315,706	26.3	1	315,930	25.8
Malignant neoplasms	(C00–C97)	2	290,069	24.1	2	269,819	22.0
Accidents (unintentional injuries)	(V01–X59, Y85–Y86)	3	78,941	6.6	6	42,658	3.5
Chronic lower respiratory diseases	(J40–J47)	4	59,260	4.9	4	65,323	5.3
Cerebrovascular diseases	(I60–I69)[3]	5	54,524	4.5	3	82,595	6.7
Diabetes mellitus	(E10–E14)	6	36,006	3.0	7	36,443	3.0
Intentional self-harm (suicide)	(*U03, X60–X84, Y87.0)	7	26,308	2.2	16	6,992	0.6
Influenza and pneumonia	(J10–J18)	8	25,650	2.1	8	30,676	2.5
Nephritis, nephrotic syndrome and nephrosis	(N00–N07, N17–N19, N25–N27)[3]	9	22,094	1.8	9	23,250	1.9
Alzheimer's disease	(G30)	10	21,151	1.8	5	51,281	4.2
Septicemia	(A40–A41)	12	15,522	1.3	10	18,712	1.5

...Category not applicable.

[1]Rank based on number of deaths.

[2]Ranks above 10 are provided for informational purposes when a cause is among the top 10 for one of the groups being compared.

[3]Cause-of-death coding changes in 2006 may affect comparability of data between 2006 and previous years; see "Technical Notes."

Source: *Center for Disease Control and Prevention: http://www.cdc.gov/nchs/hus/contents2010.*

Table 3–4: Age-Adjusted Death Rates for Selected Causes of Death by Sex, Race, and Hispanic Origin: United States, Selected Years 1950–2007
[Data are based on death certificates]

Sex, Race, Hispanic Origin, and Cause of Death[1]	1950[2,3]	1960[2,3]	1970[3]	1980[3]	1990	2000[4]	2005[4]	2006[4]	2007[4]
All persons	Age-adjusted death rate per 100,000 population[5]								
All causes	1,446.0	1,339.2	1,222.6	1,039.1	938.7	869.0	798.8	776.5	760.2
Diseases of heart	588.8	559.0	492.7	412.1	321.8	257.6	211.1	200.2	190.9
Ischemic heart disease	---	---	---	345.2	249.6	186.8	144.4	134.9	126.0
Cerebrovascular diseases	180.7	177.9	147.7	96.2	65.3	60.9	46.6	43.6	42.2
Malignant neoplasms	193.9	193.9	198.6	207.9	216.0	199.6	183.8	180.7	178.4
Trachea, bronchus, and lung	15.0	24.1	37.1	49.9	59.3	56.1	52.6	51.5	50.6
Colon, rectum, and anus	---	30.3	28.9	27.4	24.5	20.8	17.5	17.2	16.9
Chronic lower respiratory diseases	---	---	---	28.3	37.2	44.2	43.2	40.5	40.8
Influenza and pneumonia	48.1	53.7	41.7	31.4	36.8	23.7	20.3	17.8	16.2
Chronic liver disease and cirrhosis	11.3	13.3	17.8	15.1	11.1	9.5	9.0	8.8	9.1
Diabetes mellitus	23.1	22.5	24.3	18.1	20.7	25.0	24.6	23.3	22.5
Human immunodeficiency virus (HIV) disease	---	---	---	---	10.2	5.2	4.2	4.0	3.7
Unintentional injuries	78.0	62.3	60.1	46.4	36.3	34.9	39.1	39.8	40.0
Motor vehicle-related injuries	24.6	23.1	27.6	22.3	18.5	15.4	15.2	15.0	14.4
Poisoning	2.5	1.7	2.8	1.9	2.3	4.5	7.9	9.1	9.8
Suicide[6]	13.2	12.5	13.1	12.2	12.5	10.4	10.9	10.9	11.3
Homicide[6]	5.1	5.0	8.8	10.4	9.4	5.9	6.1	6.2	6.1

Source: Center for Disease Control and Prevention: http://www.cdc.gov/nchs/hus/contents2010.htm#table024

However, we also have experienced an increase in the prevalence of overweight and obese adults and children. It seems that gains that result from improvements in one behavioral risk factor are mitigated by changes in other behavioral factors.

Modern Medicine's Strategy Against the Diseases of Civilization (Largely a High-Tech Approach)

Vignette

Charlie is a 40-year-old Caucasian man. He was an athlete in high school and exercised regularly when he was in college, but since then has not eaten well or exercised on a regular basis. Every once in a while, Charlie will get motivated to lose weight and will start eating better and exercising. Once he attains his goal, he usually goes back to his old habits. He knows he has a history of diabetes and heart disease in his family but would rather eat what he wants and enjoy life while he is young. Charlie goes for a yearly check-up with his doctor and has blood work done. The doctor tells him that his HbA1C, cholesterol, and triglycerides are all too high and that he needs to lose weight. A year passes, and Charlie's results are the same. The doctor prescribes metformin for Charlie's Type II diabetes and a statin for his cholesterol and triglycerides. The doctor also refers Charlie to a dietitian. Charlie schedules a follow-up appointment for three months. At the next appointment, Charlie's values are a little better, but he admits that he is not following what the dietitian is asking him to do. The metformin is causing him to lose weight, even without watching what he eats too closely. The doctor encourages him to keep working with the dietitian anyway. She tells him that if he doesn't change his lifestyle, his health could worsen and lead to requiring insulin for his diabetes or putting him at risk for a heart attack. Charlie knows that pharmaceutical companies are always coming out with new and better drugs. He believes that by the time he needs to be concerned, there will probably be other treatments available to him.

1. What strategy or strategies of coping with illness are illustrated in this story?

2. Should we hold Charlie accountable for his personal decisions that are contributing to his obesity and high cholesterol by asking him to pay more health insurance to cover his prescriptions?

3. Which scenario would cost society less? Charlie suffering complications from his diabetes and obesity, losing his job and health insurance, and require inpatient hospital care. Or, Charlie eating a healthy diet, exercising, losing weight, and following all the recommendations of his dietitan.

4. Who **utlimately** decides which of the above scenarios described in Question 3 occurs?

Modern medicine approaches the treatment of diseases using sophisticated technology, investing large amounts of money, and focusing on curative treatments. There are five main reasons for our reliance on the high-tech approach.

Technical Response

We rely on a **mechanistic approach to the treatment of disease** because it is consistent with the historical evolution of medical science. This treatment approach is based on the assumption that humans operate as "machines." We can disassemble machines and repair them, so medicine should be able to apply this capability to human beings. We view many parts and organ systems as parts of a machine and use invasive techniques such as replacing valves or lenses, transplants, by-pass grafts, and other techniques to treat conditions.

Space Shot Mentality

In some human endeavors, investments of large amounts of money have been successful. President Kennedy set a goal of having a man on the moon by the end of the 1960s, and with the backing of Congress and the American people, put enormous sums into funding NASA. Why should this **space shot mentality** not work for cancer, HIV/AIDS, or other health problems?

It should be noted that much of the capability to launch a man on the moon was already present when President Kennedy set the goal in the early 1960s. We are still discovering the causes and mechanisms of some diseases. Nevertheless, we tend to believe that technology can achieve anything. Even our emphasis on and funding of medical education is concentrated on acute care settings rather than in prevention, disease management, or long-term care. In addition, our medical research focus is often on finding medicinal or surgical cures for idiosyncratic or rare diseases rather than on the effects of changing behaviors on mortality and morbidity. Of the $2.3 trillion in health care spending in 2008, less than 10 percent was spent on preventive measures.

Cure More Palatable Than Prevention

The high-tech response is not just a result of the mechanistic, technical response to problems. Many people continue to engage in unhealthy behaviors with the hope that they will not develop problems or if they do, a treatment (cure) will be available. Most people want to enjoy what they can in the short term, hoping that any damage will be repaired in the long term. Ironically, individuals who are likely to suffer from chronic diseases such as diabetes, hypertension, or heart disease are our decision makers and leaders.

"Many people mistakenly believe that health care is synonymous with medical care. Health is, to a large degree, a matter of personal responsibility that must be exercised within limits of genetic endowment. Educational achievement, income, and environment are also important factors. As a general rule, however, medical care has relatively little impact on health."

William R. Barclay, MD (1976)
Editor, Journal of the American Medical Association

▪ Inertia

Inertia is a law of physics that states that a body in motion, left to itself, will keep moving (similarly, a body at rest will stay at rest if it is left to itself). The nation's health care system is a complex and multifaceted entity that cannot accommodate draconian changes. Alterations occur slowly and incrementally and can take many years to implement. The health care industry is a huge employer; accounting for 10 percent of jobs and 16 percent of production in the United States (Bureau of Labor Statistics & U.S. Department of Labor, 2010a, 2010b). Our current system, both in its education of professionals and its modes of delivery, are geared toward curing rather than preventing. It will be difficult to change the way we think and behave let alone change the direction of medical thinking.

▪ Zero Sum Game

The biomedical research industry is interested in self-preservation, which includes its continued quest for cures, as opposed to emphasizing prevention. No individual or industry is going to agree to put themselves out of work because societal money could be better spent elsewhere. After all, there is no guarantee that money that is not spent on researching cures, symptomatic treatments, or treatments to manage chronic conditions would be spent on prevention and not on education or defense. Money is a scarce resource, and there is a finite amount that can be spent—a **zero sum game**. We must decide how much to spend on health care, research, defense, and education, from a societal perspective. At the same time, we often make health care decisions as individuals and then criticize those decisions from a societal perspective. For example, many people would choose life-sustaining health care treatment for their parents or grandparents (not curative treatment, just sustaining) while at the same time decrying the amount spent on the elderly in their last days of life. This dichotomy will make shifting scarce resources from acute care to preventive care very difficult.

The high-tech approach has its consequences, including rapidly rising expenditures, a concentration of resources in acute hospitals, a concentration of resources on "interesting" medical conditions at the expense of the elderly, disabled, and mentally ill, and a medical education system that emphasizes specialty training and cures rather than primary care and prevention.

▪ How Do We Deal with Disease?

Often how we deal with diseases as individuals and patients is at odds with modern medicine's approaches to disease treatment. Human beings use five modes of mediation between them and their vulnerability to disease. These modes are divided into two main categories: nontechnical and technical. The nontechnical category includes interventions such as magic, religion, or an appeal to supernatural power(s) for a cure; compassion or helping others in their time of need; and stigmatizing certain diseases (most commonly deformity and serious mental illness). These first three modes of mediation assist in coping with disease but have not altered its natural course in any consistent way.

The technical category includes modern scientific medicine. Only by this mode do we see disease altered in a predictable way. However, even in the twenty-first century relatively few health care treatments have been subjected to rigorous evaluation. Randomized clinical trials, which are the gold standard for evaluating the efficacy of a treatment, have only been conducted on a minority of modern health care treatments, mostly related to pharmaceuticals. The rest of modern medicine falls into a large gray area where doctors practice from training, experience, and clinical intuition.

However, we frequently use modern scientific medicine whether or not it is effective as a means of coping with disease. After all, doing something may be better than doing nothing, regardless of the odds of success. Many providers, patients, and their families often subscribe to this philosophy. For example, we aggressively treat liver cancer even though it has an exceedingly low cure rate. For some, a one-in-one-hundred chance is better than no chance at all. Patients may reason, "What do I have to lose?" They are informed they are going to die anyway, and they often do not have to pay for "heroic" high-tech interventions because third-party payers most likely pay the bill. This behavior is made possible by substantial variation in the practice of medicine and in various incentives in the health care system, including third-party reimbursement. Clinical trials can possibly reduce this variation by proving or disproving the efficacy of any given treatment method. However, we still have many treatments whose efficacy is often questionable that are still being used (e.g., back surgery, arthroscopic knee surgery).

In response to the increased costs associated with health care, the United States health care system has employed the following strategies: (1) shifting from fee-for-service and indemnity coverage to managed care; and (2) standard protocols and formularies of treatment. These strategies conflict with the use of ineffective health care treatments to help individuals cope with disease. In fact, these strategies were designed to limit the amount of ineffective health care treatments that are used as coping mechanisms.

■ Summary

We started the chapter by examining whether modern medicine has relatively little impact on health today. We examined the questions of whether we are spending too much on health care and whether we are receiving value from our expenditures in improved health and longer life expectancy. What type of value do we receive for our health spending? The United States spends an enormous amount of money on health care services; however it is unclear whether we receive appropriate value for our investment. In addition, experts are troubled because we cannot sustain these increases without draconian shifts in spending away from other essential budget priorities. Further, health care expenditures are not necessarily greater for those who live longer or are healthier. Overall, we are not getting adequate returns on our investment in health care, although demand for health care is increasing.

There are several reasons for this increase in demand, including these: (1) Patients are not rational consumers; (2) patients do typically bear the full cost of the care at the time they receive it; and, (3) health care is a profit-driven business, and providers are willing to offer services that may provide minimal value overall even though they benefit an individual patient.

Health care services, like many other goods and services, have diminishing marginal returns. For each additional dollar spent, we obtain less of a gain in output, whether it is measured by increased life expectancy, lower mortality, or better quality of life. In other words, each year we spend more on health care, but the returns decrease over time. This may be due to waste, fraud, and defensive medicine that direct money away from payment for services that bring real returns.

Despite these challenges, there are many positive trends in our health status as measured by life expectancy and infant mortality. We have experienced increases in life expectancy at 65 years of age for both genders from 1970 through 2007, and disability rates have also declined for the population over age 65. However, while we are living longer, we are also experiencing more, not fewer, chronically ill individuals who are living longer and consuming even more health resources.

Today, the leading causes of death are heart disease, cancer, and stroke. These chronic diseases are the main killers of the last half of the twentieth century into the twenty-first century and result from the mal-adaptation to our environment and to an increasingly sedentary lifestyle.

Many of the issues that we face regarding health status are a reflection of modern medicine. The modern health care industry focuses on using sophisticated technology to cure diseases, investing large amounts of money to treat conditions that are a result of lifestyle choices, and emphasizing curative rather than preventive treatments.

▪ Review Questions

1. Has modern medicine been effective in the late twentieth century and early twenty-first century? Explain.

2. Explain why we see increasing demand for health care despite some inadequate returns on investment.

3. Define *opportunity cost*, and give an example of your own of an opportunity cost in health care.

4. Discuss the concept of diminishing marginal returns in health care and why this is a concern for the U.S. health care system.

5. Explain the decline in infectious diseases in the 1800s and what factors contributed to this decline.

6. Discuss the trends in our current health status related to mortality, chronic diseases, disability, and so forth.

7. Explain why chronic diseases have increased over time.

8. Describe modern medicine's strategy against diseases.

9. Describe how we use modern medicine to cope with disease.

▪ Additional Resources

Bureau of Labor Statistics http://www.bls.gov

National Center for Health Statistics http://www.cdc.gov/nchs

World Health Organization http://www.who.org.

▪ References

Beitsch, L. M., Brooks, R. G., Menachemi, N., & Libbey, P. M. (2006). Public health at center stage: New roles, old props. *Health Affairs, 25*(4), 911–922.

Bell, F. C., & Miller, M. L. (2002). *Life tables for the United States Social Security area 1900–2100*. Actuarial Study No. 116. Retrieved January 02, 2012, from http://www.socialsecurity.gov/OACT/NOTES/as120/TOCX.html.

Bodenheimer, T. (2005). High and rising health care costs. Part 1: Seeking an explanation. *Annals of Internal Medicine, 142*(10), 847–854.

Bureau of Labor Statistics & U.S. Department of Labor. (2010a). *Career guide to industries, 2010–11 edition*. Health Care. Retrieved July 20, 2010, from http://www.bls.gov/oco/cg/cgs035.htm.

Bureau of Labor Statistics & U.S. Department of Labor. (2010b). Employment, hours, and earning from the current employment statistics survey. Retrieved July 20, 2010, from http://www.bls.gov/news.release/empsit.toc.htm.

Centers for Disease Control and Prevention (CDC). (1999). Control of infectious diseases 1900–1999. *Morbidity and Mortality Weekly Report, 48*, 621–629.

Centers for Medicare and Medicaid Services (CMS). (2010). National health expenditures, 2008, historical. Retrieved February 3, 2010, from https://www.cms.gov/NationalHealthExpendData/02_NationalHealthAccountsHistorical.asp

Central Intelligence Agency (CIA). (2010). The World Factbook—Country comparison: Death rate. Retrieved July 2, 2010, from https://www.cia.gov/library/publications/the-world-factbook/rankorder/2066rank.html

Chernew, M. E., Hirth, R. A., & Cutler, D. M. (2009). Increased spending on health care: Long-term implications for the nation. *Health Affairs, 28*(5), 1253–1255.

Conover, C. J. (2004). *Health care regulation: A $169 billion hidden tax*. The Cato Institute. Retrieved January 2, 2012, from http://www.cato.org/pub_display.php?pub_id=2466.

Cutler, D. M., & McClellan, M. (2001). Is technological change in medicine worth it? *Health Affairs, 20*(5), 11–29.

Cutler, D. M., Rosen, A. B., & Vijan, S. (2006). The value of medical spending in the United States, 1960–2000. *New England Journal of Medicine, 355*(9), 920–927.

Davis, K., Schoen, C., Schoenbaum, S. C., Doty, M. M., Holmgren, et al. (2007). *Mirror on the wall: An international update on the comparative performance of American health care*. New York, NY: The Commonwealth Fund.

Davis, K., Schoen, C., & Stremikis, K. (2010). *How the performance of the U.S. health care system compares internationally: 2010 update.* New York, NY: The Commonwealth Fund.

Deyo, R. A., Nachemson, A., & Mirza, S. K. (2004). Spinal-fusion surgery—The case for restraint. *New England Journal of Medicine, 350*(7), 722–726.

Fuchs, V. R. (2004). Perspective: More variation in use of care, more flat-of-the-curve medicine. *Health Affairs*, published ahead of print October 7, 2004, doi:10.1377/hlthaff.var.104. Retrieved January 2, 2012 from http://content .healthaffairs.org/content/early/2004/10/07/hlthaff.var.104.citation.

Hartman, M., Martin, A., Nuccio, O., Catlin, A., & the National Health Expenditure Accounts Team. (2010). Health spending growth at a historic low in 2008. *Health Affairs, 29*(1), 147–155.

Lubitz, J., Cai, L., Kramarow, E., & Lentzner, H. (2003). Health, life expectancy, and health care spending among the elderly. *New England Journal of Medicine, 349*(11), 1048–1055.

Marmot, M. (2002). The influence of income on health: Views of an epidemiologist. *Health Affairs, 21*(2), 31–46.

Martin, L. G., Freedman, V. A., Schoeni, R. F., & Andreski, P. M. (2010). Recent trends in disability and related chronic conditions among people ages fifty to sixty-four. *Health Affairs, 29*(4), 725–731.

McKeown, T. (1978). Determinants of health. *Human Nature* (1), 57–62.

Nagle, P., & Smith, A. (2004). Review of recent U.S. cost estimates of revascularization. *American Journal of Managed Care, 10*, S370–S376).

Porter, R. R. (1972). *The contribution of the biological and medical sciences to human welfare.* Paper presented at the Presidential Addresses of the British Association for the Advancement of Sciences, Swansea Meeting. London: Author.

Reinhardt, U. E., Hussey, P. S., & Anderson, G. F. (2004). U.S. health care spending in an international context. *Health Affairs, 23*(3), 10–25.

Skinner, J. S., Staiger, D. O., & Fisher, E. S. (2006). Is technological change in medicine always worth it? The case of acute myocardial infarction. *Health Affairs, 25*(2), w34–47.

U.S. Department of Health and Human Services (U.S. DHHS). (2009). *Health, United States, 2009. In Brief—Medical Technology.* Hyattsville, MD: U.S. Department of Health and Human Services, Centers for Disease Control and Prevention, National Center for Health Statistics.

Woolhandler, S., Campbell, T., & Himmelstein, D. U. (2003). Costs of health care administration in the United States and Canada. *New England Journal of Medicine, 349*(8), 768–775.

World Health Organization (WHO). (2000). *World health report 2000—Health Systems: Improving Performance.* Geneva, Switzerland: Author.

Key Terms

Learning Objectives

- Describe the various types of inpatient settings and services.

- Discuss the factors that led to a dramatic decline in inpatient service utilization.

- Differentiate among various types of hospitals.

- Discuss the likely future role of inpatient care in the United States health care system.

- Describe and differentiate the types of health services provided in outpatient settings from those provided in inpatient and long-term care settings.

- Discuss the political, economic, social, and regulatory factors that led to dramatic growth in outpatient services.

▪ Health Care System

The organization of the health care system in the United States is complex. It is a pluralistic system—a "patchwork quilt" with a wide variety of components that interrelate in a variety of ways. There are three primary components of the health care system (Figure 4–1). First, patients need health services. Patients consume health care to relieve pain, prevent illness, cure illness, or help with disabilities. Patients comprise the first party in the health care system.

Second, providers seek to deliver the best care possible within the limits of their training and available technology, and in return they expect to be paid commensurate with the cost of their training and the level of their responsibilities. Providers make up the second party in the health care system.

Third, the social component, the health care system, encompasses the organization and delivery, financing, regulation, allocation of resources, planning, and policy, and focuses on reducing mortality and morbidity to the lowest level possible and ensuring access to high-quality care.

post-acute care

short-stay hospitals

skilled nursing facilities (SNFs)

solo practitioner

sub-acute care

teaching hospitals

terminally ill

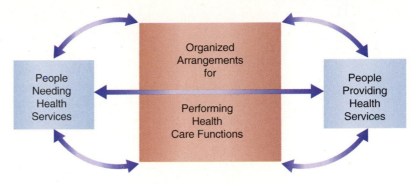

Figure 4–1 Primary components of the health care system.
© *Cengage Learning 2013*

▪ Social Components and the Roles They Play

The United States health care system is divided into various components based on the roles that each component plays within the system. First, the organization and delivery component includes the different organizations that deliver care to patients. These entities include private physician practices, hospitals, nursing homes, and hospice and home health care agencies, among many others. Second, the financing component determines how we pay for care. We call the organization that pays for care the "third party" in a health care transaction, because the payer is outside of the first- (patient) and second- (provider) party contract. Since the 1940s, the financing of health care has shifted from direct, or out-of-pocket, payment from the first party paying the second party, to third-party payers reimbursing providers for care. Under a third-party payer system, at the time patients use services, someone else is paying on their behalf.

There are many types of third-party payers. These payers include not-for-profit health insurers such as the many Blue Cross/Blue Shield plans; private for-profit commercial insurers such as Aetna U.S. Healthcare and United Health Care; government programs (Medicare, Medicaid, and Children's Health Insurance Programs [CHIP]); and regional not-for-profit managed care plans such as Kaiser Permanente (West Coast), Geisinger Health Plan (Pennsylvania), and Group Health Cooperative of Puget Sound (Northern West Coast). Many health insurers are for-profit. However, these companies must still set competitive prices, cover all costs, and reinvest profits into charity care and capital improvements.

Third, the regulation component includes such activities as state government licensure of hospitals and physicians and federal government oversight of the pharmaceutical industry, among many other examples. Most regulations involve the federal and state levels of government. In addition, health care quality is also "regulated" by nongovernmental, private accrediting bodies. Some may mimic the power of government in health care, because the government will often accept accreditation in place of independent certification for payment for Medicare and Medicaid. For example, the Joint Commission (JC), formerly called the Joint Commission on Accreditation of Healthcare Organizations (JCAHO), can have a great deal of influence on the success of a hospital. Hospital reimbursement by private insurers may be tied to accreditation. The Centers for Medicare and Medicaid Services (CMS) will accept JC accreditation in place of independent certification for Medicare and Medicaid reimbursement. Likewise, the certification of a physician by a private specialty board can have greater influence than government licensure, because all physicians must be licensed to practice, but not all physicians become board certified. It may enable physicians to negotiate better payments from insurance companies or to gain privileges (permission to practice) at a hospital sooner than or over a non–board certified provider. However, regulation imposes costs on the health care system. It has been estimated that one-quarter of all health care expenditures result from complying with regulations (Conover, 2004).

Allocation of resources and health planning should go hand in hand. Planning seeks to improve allocation and efficiency, reduce costs, and improve the quality of, access to, and distribution of resources. Allocation of resources in health care involves determining where to place training centers (medical schools, dental schools, teaching hospitals, universities with health professions, health administration and/or public health programs, pre-med, and nursing programs); how many seats should be offered; where and in what specialties residencies should be offered; and whether new hospital or nursing home beds should be added in an area. Planning in health care occurs at government and private levels.

▪ Ownership of Health Care Organizations

The U.S. health care system is a pluralistic/multifaceted system that is comprised of a variety of organizational types. Organizations can be classified as inpatient or outpatient/ambulatory care, and they can be classified by ownership type. The largest percentage of hospitals in the United States is nongovernmental and not-for-profit. If an organization has **not-for-profit** tax status, also called 501(c)(3), based on the section of the Internal Revenue Code that governs tax exemption, no profit can accrue to any shareholders. However, it is legal to show excess income, a "profit" or surplus in the hospital's balance sheet of profits and losses. Any excess income must be reinvested in the organization, and the organization must provide community benefits as part of its tax-exempt status. Community benefits include providing care to uninsured or indigent patients and to Medicaid patients, and providing some specialty care that is unprofitable to the organization (CBO, 2006).

Many organizations in health care are for-profit. Approximately 19 percent of community hospitals are for-profit enterprises. Some examples of national for-profit hospital corporations are Hospital Corporation of America (HCA) and Tenet Health Care Corporation (Tenet). HCA owns 163 hospitals in the United States and England and had profits of $28 billion in 2008 (HCA, 2010). HCA has a board of directors, and investors can buy shares in the company on the stock exchange. Other for-profit enterprises include insurance companies such as Aetna and United Healthcare, nursing homes (two-thirds of nursing homes are for-profit), as well as pharmaceutical companies, home health companies, durable medical equipment suppliers and private physician practices. Private professional practices include physicians, dentists, psychologists and psychiatrists, and chiropractors, among others. Most of these offices are operated for profit. Some people believe that the profit motive associated with these companies may interfere with the delivery of appropriate, high-quality, and equitable health care, although this issue is clearly debatable and will be discussed in the Your Opinion Matters segment. The percent of specific organization types that are for-profit is listed in Table 4–1.

Table 4–1: **Percentage of Selective Health Care Organizations That Are For-Profit**

Ownership of Health Care Organizations	Percentage Investor Owned
Community hospitals	19% (AHA, 2009)
Psychiatric hospitals	43% (Andersen, 2006)
Nursing homes	67% (AHCA, 2010)
Home health care agencies	52% (CMS, 2010)

© *Cengage Learning 2013*

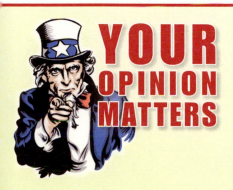

YOUR OPINION MATTERS

Should For-Profit Organizations Be Allowed to Provide Care for Patients in the United States?

Yes

Competition is an integral part of who we are as a nation. People have come to the United States to pursue new opportunities and follow the "American dream." Profit is an integral part of that dream: the ability to earn money, support a family, and make a name for oneself. Allowing people and organizations to earn profits promotes innovation, efficiency, and achievement. Most businesses in the United States are for-profit entities. In health care, some industry subtypes, such as the pharmaceutical industry and medical device manufacturers, are dominated by for-profit entities. Pharmaceutical companies and medical device companies contribute billions of their profits each year to conduct medical research. These profits enable advances such as better pharmaceuticals, better technological innovations, and better medical procedures and devices, which improve mortality and quality of life. We need to maintain profit in health care to keep our levels of innovation and discovery high.

In addition, careful study with appropriate case-mix controls has determined that quality of care in for-profit hospitals can be superior to not-for-profit hospitals. When hospital quality was compared within specific markets, for-profit ownership appears to be associated with better quality care (McClellan & Staiger, 2000). Finally, there is evidence that commercial or for-profit health plans are first to inculcate demonstrated cost-saving measures like chronic disease management, case management, and health promotion and wellness, which are also known to provide higher quality care for its members (Draper, 2007).

No

The profit motive does not belong in health care. **For-profit organizations** generate higher costs and produce lower quality. For-profit hospitals and home health agencies have higher costs than their not-for-profit counterparts.

For-profit hospitals spend more on administration than not-for-profit or public hospitals and less on patient care (Woolhandler et al., 2003). In addition to higher costs, for-profit organizations usually have lower quality than not-for-profit or public organizations. A majority of nursing homes are for-profit. Investor-owned nursing homes have more deficiencies overall (areas where they are not complying with federal law with regard to quality of care, quality of life, safety of patients, and other areas) than not-for-profit and public hospitals (Comondore et al., 2009; Harrington et al., 2001). They also generally have a larger percentage of Medicaid patients. For-profit HMOs have lower scores on process and outcomes quality indicators and lower patient satisfaction scores than not-for-profit HMOs (Himmelstein et al., 1999). Although many studies have indeterminate results concerning mortality rates associated with profit status, for-profit hospitals had the highest mortality rates in one study using Medicare data and may have more preventable errors and adverse events (Sloan et al., 2001; Taylor, Whellan, & Sloan, 1999; Woolhandler & Himmelstein, 1999). Higher cost and lower quality means the for-profit motive should be driven from health care.

You decide:

1. What kind of balance should be reached between the roles of for-profit and non-for-profit organizations?

2. Is it necessary that profit be made to assure investment in research and development?

3. What role do non-profits play in providing essential services?

4. What should non-profit organizations do with the "profits" they do make?

5. Do shareholders create the same pressure on non-profits as consumers places on for-profits?

Government's Role in Health Care

The government is one of the most important stakeholders in the U.S. health care system. It performs several important roles, including financing, delivering, and regulating the delivery of health care. The government—federal, state, and local combined—is the largest single payer of health care. Approximately 48 percent of health care was paid for by public dollars in 2008 (CMS, 2009). This expenditure includes Medicare, Medicaid, CHIP, Departments of Defense and Veterans Affairs, and state and local public health programs. The federal and federal/state insurance programs Medicare, Medicaid, and CHIP account for almost three-quarters of all governmental health care spending (CMS, 2009). State governments jointly fund the Medicaid program along with the federal government. Federal and state governments also provide funding for long-term mental health services, medical education, community health centers, and public health programs. Local governments subsidize public hospitals and local public health departments.

The government also delivers health care to patients. The federal government operates facilities for American Indians through the **Indian Health Service**; for military service personnel through Army, Navy, and Air Force hospitals; for veterans through the Department of Veterans Affairs hospitals and facilities; and for indigent or uninsured patients through federally qualified health care centers and rural health clinics. State governments operate mental hospitals, health departments, and medical schools. Local governments operate municipal/county hospitals and local health departments.

The government regulates the delivery of health care as well. From a political-economic perspective, government involvement in the health care marketplace is justified when the free market does not "work," meaning that there are market failures (discussed in Chapter 15) *and* when the health, safety, and welfare of its citizens are affected. The federal government is also involved in setting implementing regulations for Medicare and Medicaid providers, prohibiting discrimination by providers, and determining what drugs and devices are sold. The **Food and Drug Administration (FDA)** regulates drugs and medical devices. State governments regulate the insurance industry, license health care personnel and facilities, and establish health codes. Local governments also establish local health codes.

State governments have traditionally been the most involved of any level of government in health care. These governments, often in coordination with local health departments, perform the following functions:

- Regulation/licensing

- Mental health services

- Vital statistics (births, deaths, divorces, marriages)

- Public health laboratories

- Communicable disease control programs

- Environmental health

- Maternal and child health

- Health planning and health education

■ Ambulatory Care

Ambulatory care is often used synonymously with the term *outpatient care*. These services are personal health or health care services that are provided to a patient who is not institutionalized (the person does not need an overnight stay). The majority of physician–patient contacts in the United States occur in ambulatory settings such as private practice offices, such as physician office visits, dental office visits, mental health services, physical therapy, diagnostic testing, and ambulatory surgery.

Many types of clinicians provide ambulatory care in various settings. These clinicians include doctors, physician assistants, nurse practitioners, nurses, physical therapists, occupational therapists, and many others. The settings include physician offices, hospital outpatient clinics, freestanding outpatient specialty clinics, and freestanding laboratories and MRI or X-ray centers. A list of ambulatory care providers and settings is provided in Table 4–2.

Ambulatory care such as outpatient surgery is delivered in ambulatory surgery centers and **hospital outpatient centers**. Physical therapy is delivered in freestanding centers or outpatient hospital clinics. Mental health professionals deliver mental health services in community mental health centers, outpatient psychiatric treatment centers, or private offices, where they provide counseling and drug and alcohol treatment.

Other types of ambulatory services and settings include eye care, podiatry, home health care, family planning, neighborhood/community health centers, school clinics, and emergency care. Hospitals are not required to have an emergency department (ED). However, because of the **Emergency Medical Treatment and Labor Act of 1986 (EMTALA)**, if a hospital does have an ED, it must examine and stabilize all patients who seek care there, regardless of their willingness or ability to pay. EDs face difficulties surrounding the controversy over "patient dumping" (i.e., rejecting or inappropriately transferring patients who do not have insurance), and some hospitals have closed their EDs as a result. All hospitals must abide by the EMTALA provisions; however, public and not-for-profit hospitals receive funding and tax-exempt status to care for indigent patients, whereas for-profit hospitals do not. Nevertheless, patient dumping still occurs even in public and not-for-profit facilities (DHHS, 2010).

The ED is an important intake point for inpatients. Approximately 45 percent of all hospital admissions originate in the ED ("The Emergency Department," 2007). However, the ER can also be one of the primary sources of hospital "bad debt," especially for hospitals located in inner cities, where a higher percent of residents are without health insurance of any type. Sometimes the ER is the only source of primary care for the poor.

Another model for the delivery of ambulatory care is freestanding urgent care centers, often colloquially referred to as **"docs in a box,"** for non-life-threatening emergency care. These centers are usually open outside of normal office hours but may charge more than a standard physician office visit. These centers also originally operated on a cash-only basis, and although many now will take some forms of insurance, they will also still see uninsured patients who pay with cash or credit card.

The use of ambulatory surgical care has been increasing over the last three decades. In 2006, about 62 percent of surgeries were conducted on an outpatient basis (Cullen, Hall, & Golosinskiy, 2008). This trend is in contrast to the care that was provided before the early 1980s, when most surgeries were performed on an inpatient basis. From 1982–1992, outpatient surgeries increased by over 200 percent, and inpatient surgeries declined by 32 percent. From 1994–1998, outpatient surgeries increased another 16 percent, whereas inpatient surgeries declined slightly. From 1996–2006, ambulatory surgery increased another 300 percent (Cullen et al., 2008). Ambulatory surgery can be performed at a hospital outpatient department or a freestanding ambulatory surgery center (ASC). Currently, 42 percent of ambulatory surgical procedures are performed at ASCs (Cullen et al., 2008).

There are several reasons why the use of ambulatory care, especially ambulatory surgical care, has increased since the 1980s. First, new medical and diagnostic procedures and better technology have enabled providers to perform more procedures safely in an outpatient setting. The improved technology makes outpatient surgery safe and

Table 4–2: Types of Ambulatory Care Settings, Practitioners, and Level or Type of Service

Settings	Principal Practitioners	Level or Type of Service
Private office-based solo and group practice	Physicians, dentists, nurses, physician assistants, nurse practitioners, therapists	Primary and secondary care
Hospital clinics	Physicians, dentists, nurses, physician assistants, nurse practitioners, therapists	Primary and secondary care
Hospital emergency rooms	Physicians, nurses	All types
Ambulatory surgery centers (hospital-based and freestanding)	Surgeons, nurses, anesthesiologists	Surgical secondary care
Community wide emergency medical systems	Technicians, nurses, drivers	Emergency transportation, communications, and immediate care
Poison control centers, community hotlines	Physicians, technicians, nurses	Emergency advice
Neighborhood health centers, migrant health centers	Physicians, dentists, nurses	Primary care
Community mental health centers	Psychologists, social workers	Primary health services
Federal systems—Department of Veterans Affairs, Indian Health Service, Public Health Service military	All types	All types
Home health services	Nurses	Primary care
School health services	Nurses	Primary and preventive care
Prison health services	All types	Primary care
Public health services and clinics	Physicians, nurses	Targeted programs (e.g., family planning, immunization, inspections, screening programs, health education); primary care
Family planning and other specialized clinics (nongovernmental)	Physicians, nurses, aides	Specialized services; primary care
Industrial clinics	Physicians, nurses, environmental health specialists	Preventive, primary, and emergency care
Pharmacies	Pharmacists	Drugs and health education
Vision care	Opticians Optometrists Ophthalmologists	Examinations, screening, prescriptions filled
Medical laboratories	Technicians	Specialized laboratory services
Indigenous practices	Chiropractors, medicine men, naturopaths	Primary and supportive care

effective. Second, there is consumer demand for convenient and accessible services that do not necessitate an inpatient stay: people are usually more comfortable recovering at home than in a hospital.

Finally, changes in reimbursement, more than any other reason, have driven the shift from inpatient to outpatient care. Medicare changed hospital reimbursement from a cost-based system to the prospective payment system in 1983. Under the prospective payment system, using DRGs, hospitals reimbursed a set amount based on a predetermined formula driven by patient's diagnosis. It does not matter whether the patient stays 3 days or 6 days; the hospital receives the same amount. Hospital outpatient services did not begin to be paid prospectively until 2000. At the same time, other third-party payers gave providers and patients financial incentives to diagnose and treat on an outpatient basis. All else being equal, it is less expensive for the third-party payer to discharge the patient and leave the responsibility of care to individuals in the patient's home or home health care providers than to keep a patient in the inpatient setting.

▪ Inpatient Health Care

Inpatient care takes place in many settings. This section highlights the following types of inpatient and long-term care organizations: hospitals, nursing homes, assisted living, and home health and hospice care.

▪ Characteristics of Hospitals

Hospitals can be classified based on characteristics such as length of stay, size, ownership type, type of care delivered, and whether they have one or more approved residency programs, for instance in a teaching hospital.

First, hospitals may be either **short-stay hospitals** or **long-stay hospitals**. For short-stay hospitals, the **average length of stay (ALOS)** is less than 30 days. Short-stay hospitals are the most common type of hospital in the United States. A majority of short-stay hospitals are voluntary, not-for-profit, community, general hospitals. The ALOS was approximately 5.5 days in 2008 (AHA, 2010b). Of the approximately 5,800 hospitals in the United States in 2008, about 5,000 were short-stay hospitals (AHA, 2009). Long-term care hospitals (LTCHs) traditionally have stays longer than 30 days; however, the current average length of stay (ALOS) for these facilities is around 25 days. These facilities are designed to care for very complex patients with longer-term needs (mental patients, burn victims, patients on ventilators, etc).

Second, hospitals are classified according to size or the number of beds they have. Hospitals with fewer beds are gaining market share. Over half of the hospitals in the United States have 100 beds or less (AHA, 2010a). There are 2.7 beds per 1,000 people in the United States, and the average size of a hospital is approximately 164 beds (KFF, 2010). See Table 4–3 for the distribution of hospitals by bed size.

Third, hospitals have different forms of ownership, as discussed previously. Most (58% in 2008) hospitals are voluntary or not-for-profit (AHA, 2009). Not-for-profit hospitals may be stand-alone community hospitals, part of a hospital chain, part of a church affiliation or religious hospital group, or part of a not-for-profit managed care organization. New York-Presbyterian Hospital in New York City is the nation's largest not-for-profit, nonsectarian hospital. Proprietary hospitals are for-profit, are subject to taxes, and are often owned by shareholders, and many of these corporations are traded on the stock exchange. Over 19 percent of community hospitals are for-profit

Table 4–3: **Hospitals by Size (Number of Beds) and Percentage of Hospitals, 2008**	
Size (number of beds)	Percentage
Less than 50	30.7
50–99	19.9
100–199	21.3
200–299	11.9
300–499	10.8
500+	5.4

Source: AHA Hospital Statistics, 2010.

(AHA, 2009). HCA is the largest for-profit hospital corporation in the United States; however, for-profit hospitals may also be stand-alone facilities or provider-owned facilities. There has been a slight increase in for-profit hospitals and a corresponding decrease in not-for-profit hospitals over the last decade. Additionally, some states have much higher market penetration of for-profit hospitals than other states. For example, over 40 percent of hospitals in Florida and Nevada, and over one-third of hospitals in Texas, Utah, Tennessee, New Mexico, Louisiana, Alabama, and the District of Columbia are for-profit. On the other hand, no hospitals are for-profit in Delaware, Iowa, Hawaii, Minnesota, North Dakota, Rhode Island, and Vermont (AHA, 2009). Finally, hospitals may be owned by the government. The government owns approximately 25 percent of hospitals (AHA, 2009). Examples of hospitals that are owned or administered by the government include federal (armed forces hospitals, Department of Veterans Affairs, Department of Justice); state (long-term psychiatric hospitals, state university medical centers); and local (county hospital, city-county, hospital district or authority).

Hospitals are also classified based on the types of patients who receive care in a hospital. The most common type of hospital is a general medical/surgical allopathic hospital. Hospitals may have a special focus, depending on the types of patients received, such as the following:

- General medical or surgical

- Prison hospital

- Psychiatric

- Geriatric

- Women/maternity

- Eye

- Ear, nose, and throat

- Physical rehabilitation

> ### Table 4–4: Characteristics of Teaching Hospitals in the United States According to the Association of American Medical Colleges
>
> The AAMC represents the nation's nearly 400 major teaching hospitals and health systems and their associated clinical physicians. Comprising only 6 percent of all hospitals, AAMC members operate:
>
> - 40 percent of neonatal ICUs
> - 62 percent of pediatric ICUs
> - 61 percent of all Level 1 regional trauma centers
> - 75 percent of all burn care units
>
> These institutions also provide nearly half of all hospital charity care nationwide and a disproportionate share of care to patients who are severely ill or have rare conditions, including these:
>
> - 50 percent of the surgical transplant services
> - 41 percent of Alzheimer's centers
> - 22 percent of all cardiac surgeries

© Cengage Learning 2013

- Orthopedic

- Chronic/convalescent

- Institutions for mental retardation

- Epilepsy

- Alcoholism/substance abuse

- Children

- Allopathic or osteopathic

Finally, some hospitals are considered **teaching hospitals**. There are approximately 400 teaching hospitals in the United States (Association of American Medical Colleges [AAMC], 2010). A teaching hospital must have at least one approved residency program for medicine or dentistry. The American Medical Association (AMA) and specialty boards approve residency programs (non-governmental designation). The hospital does not have to be part of a medical school complex, but it must perform research. Teaching hospitals account for about 20 percent of hospital admissions, but only 6 percent of all hospitals in the United States (AAMC, 2010). Major teaching hospitals are more likely to offer cutting-edge services and tertiary care. See Table 4–4 for a list of tertiary services and the percentage of market share provided in teaching hospitals.

Hospital Summary Facts

- The most common type of community hospital is a voluntary, not-for-profit, short-stay, nonteaching, and acute/general allopathic hospital.

- The average size of these hospitals was 164 beds; the average length of stay (ALOS) is 5.5 days; and the average occupancy rate (percentage of beds filled in a day) was 64 percent in 2008 (AHA, 2009).

■ Long-Term Care

There are many types of long-term care providers and facilities. Some of the most common are nursing homes, assisted living, continuing care retirement communities, home health care, rehabilitation, and hospice. Chapter 7 provides more detail on various long-term care services.

Vignette

DECIDING THE APPROPRIATE LEVEL OF CARE

Michael is a 58-year-old man with multiple sclerosis (MS). He was diagnosed late in his 40s, and his condition quickly worsened from the point when he was diagnosed. Within a year, Michael had lost the use of his legs and was confined to a wheelchair. Michael underwent various treatments for multiple sclerosis, but his condition continued to relapse every 1 to 2 years. Usually, hospitalization helped him recover some of his functioning that was lost through each exacerbation. This year, Michael had an exacerbation of his MS that was worse than any of the others he had gone through in the past. He lost feeling in and the use of his nondominant hand. His MS doctor admitted him to the hospital for treatment for the acute exacerbation. Following treatment, his doctor wanted Michael to undergo inpatient post-acute care treatment at a rehabilitation hospital. There were no beds available when Michael was discharged, so he went home, and the doctor referred him to home health physical therapy and occupational therapy. After an evaluation session, the physical therapist did not think that Michael would benefit from outpatient therapy and felt that he needed to be admitted to the inpatient facility. A bed became available a week after Michael's discharge, and he was admitted to the rehabilitation hospital. Michael worked with the physical and occupational therapists at least 6 hours a day, as required by Medicare. He began very quickly to regain the function in his arm and hand. At the beginning of the second week, the physical therapist decided to try to help Michael walk again. At first, he just put Michael in a special sling to help him stand. Later that week, his caregivers started working on Michael taking steps with the sling supporting him. At the beginning of the next week, Michael started working with a walker. By the end of 3 weeks, when Michael was discharged, he was walking on his own with a walker for the first time in 10 years.

1. What are the various types of health care services that Michael received, and how did they differ based on his condition?

2. What would have happened to Michael if he had had no insurance to cover his health care bills?

3. Why would Michael's care have been covered by Medicare insurance if he had not been over 65 years of age?

4. If Michael's MS condition relapses or worsens, what are his best options for receiving therapy care?

5. Is there ever a point at which the cost of Michael's care would supersede the potential benefit from receiving care? And if so, what should Michael or his family do next to best meet his care needs?

▪ Nursing Homes

Nursing homes are establishments with three or more beds that provide nursing or personal care services to the senior, infirm, or chronically ill populations. Nursing homes or parts of nursing homes are classified as skilled nursing facilities (SNFs), nursing facilities, sub-acute care facilities and post-acute care facilities. **Skilled nursing facilities (SNFs)** provide short-term skilled nursing care on an inpatient basis, usually following hospitalization. These facilities provide the most intensive care available outside of a hospital. Most SNFs are in nursing homes, but many hospitals may also have SNF beds.

Nursing facilities provide health-related services on a regular basis to individuals who do not require the degree of care or treatment that a skilled nursing unit is designed to provide. This type of "nursing home" care comes to mind when thinking of people *residing* in nursing homes. This level used to be classified as intermediate care, but the Centers for Medicare and Medicaid Services now only use the SNF/NF designation for certification.

Sub-acute care is delivered in the inpatient setting to patients who are suffering from an injury or acute illness or an exacerbation of an existing condition. It may be used after a hospital stay or in place of an acute care hospital stay. The treatment is goal-oriented and is designed around one or more specific conditions or complex treatments. The patient will work with physical and occupational therapists at least 6 hours a day to regain as much functioning as possible. Sub-acute care can be provided in nursing homes and rehabilitation and long-term care hospitals.

Post-acute care is similar to sub-acute care but always occurs following an acute care hospitalization and does not have to be provided in an inpatient setting. It may be given in nursing homes, rehabilitation and long-term care hospitals, or through outpatient physical and occupational therapy. The treatment and rules for inpatient post-acute care are the same as for sub-acute care. The patient must undergo at least 6 hours of therapy per day if the patient is a Medicare beneficiary. Michael's story is an example of the provision of post-acute care.

There were 15,730 nursing homes in use in 2008. Approximately *67 percent* of nursing homes are proprietary or for-profit. About *52 percent* of nursing homes are part of a chain (American Health Care Association, 2010b). There were over 1.4 million nursing home residents in 2008, and the average occupancy rate was 82.9 percent (NCHS, 2010).

Certain types of patients require special needs above what is provided in a traditional nursing facility. Therefore, some nursing homes have created special care units. Special care units accounted for 7.2 percent of nursing home beds, and most were dedicated to Alzheimer's disease or related dementias in 2004 (American Health Care Association, 2010a).

▪ Assisted Living

Assisted living is another type of long-term care service for patients who have limitations in some activities of daily living or instrumental activities of daily living, but do not need full-time nursing care. People who choose assisted living contract with an assisted living facility to provide specific personal or health care services as stipulated in their rental contracts. They pay rent and an additional fee for those services. About 50 percent of assisted living facilities are for-profit. There are over 36,000 assisted living facilities in the United States, and over 1 million residents live in assisted living (Assisted Living Federation of America, 2009).

▪ Home Health Care

Home health care is care that is provided in a person's private residence. The person must be home bound and receive a prescription from a provider for home health services. Home health care is designed to promote, maintain, or restore health, or can be prescribed to minimize the effects of a disability and/or illness. The elderly are the primary consumers of home health care. As the baby boomers and their parents have aged, fewer people have wanted to enter nursing homes and instead prefer being cared for at home. Additionally, technological advances have helped to make more complex care possible within the home environment.

Until 1998, there was a substantial increase in the number and variety of services offered by home health care providers. This trend was sustained by an aging society and generous Medicare reimbursement. Home health care has been less expensive than inpatient care, so Medicare and other insurers have been willing to pay for home health care. *Medicare-certified home health care agencies increased from 1,700 in 1962 to 6,100 in 1992, to 10,027 in 1996.* After passage of the Balanced Budget Act of 1997, which changed payments from a cost basis to a very strict prospective payment system, the number of certified home health agencies (HHAs) had decreased to 6,861 by 2001. Due to further revisions to the Balanced Budget Act in 2000 and 2001, HHAs began re-entering the market after 2002. There were 9,284 certified home health agencies in 2007 (National Association for Home Care and Hospice, 2008).

▪ Hospice Care

Hospice care is palliative care to the **terminally ill** (those with a life expectancy of 6 months or less) and their families. This care involves the medical *relief of pain* and supportive services that can be provided in an inpatient setting, such as a hospital or nursing home or in a patient's home. These programs address the *emotional*, social, financial, and legal needs of patients and their families. It is frequently used for the treatment of terminal cancer and AIDS patients. Patients in hospice cannot receive curative care.

There has been substantial growth in the number of hospices, partially attributable to an increase in third-party reimbursement for hospice's lower costs in comparison to hospital or nursing home care. Medicare certifies hospices that can provide this type of care to Medicare patients. An increase in expenditures for hospice occurred shortly thereafter. The number of Medicare-certified hospices increased from 31 in 1984 to 3,346 in 2008 (see Table 4–5).

Table 4–5: Number of Medicare-Certified Hospices, 1984–2008	
Year	Total
1984	31
1985	158
1986	235
1987	389
1988	553
1989	701
1990	806
1991	1,011
1992	1,039
1993	1,288
1994	1,604
1995	1,857
1996	2,154
1997	2,274
1998	2,215
1999	2,274
2000	2,273
2001	2,265
2002	2,322
2003	2,444
2004	2,670
2005	2,884
2006	3,078
2007	3,257
2008	3,346

Source: *Centers for Medicare and Medicaid Services (CMS). Health Standards and Quality Bureau (February 2009)*

▪ Physician Practice Arrangements

Physician practices are the predominant mode of ambulatory care. Practice arrangements have many variations, but a shift has been taking place away from solo physician practices toward more group practices over the last 20 years. This shift has caused the number of solo physician practices to decline.

▪ Types of Physician Practice Arrangements

Solo Practice Physicians

A physician practicing independently without any partner is considered a **solo practitioner**. Before the 1980s, most physicians were in solo practice; since then, the number of group practices and physician associations has been increasing. The proportion of physicians in solo practice has declined from 50.8 percent in 1994 to 32.5 percent in 2004 (Liebhaber & Grossman, 2007).

There are several important advantages to solo practice for physicians. Physicians delivering services in their own practice have more autonomy. Solo practitioners have more discretion about what office hours they keep during the week, the location of their offices, their choice of office staff, and what insurance companies they will accept. Finally, solo practitioners report better personal relationships with patients and a lower level of bureaucracy.

There are also several important disadvantages for physicians practicing in a solo practice. Solo practitioners have to compete with group physician practices. Groups can compete on prices and services better than solo practitioners. Solo practitioners bear the full financial risk for their practices. Group practices are more likely to be incorporated or to spread the risk among several partners. Further, private practice physicians may need to be on-call more often for their patients than physicians who practice in a group. Solo practitioners need to make arrangements for other physicians to cover their patients when they are on vacation or otherwise unavailable to their patients, whereas group practice physicians rotate on call schedules. Third, solo practitioners have more administrative responsibilities. Solo practice physicians are required to perform more of the billing, documentation, and any other administrative tasks that are required in their private offices. Group practices more often can afford trained health administrators and other ancillary personnel to deal with the nonclinical aspects of the practice (see following section).

Group Practice

A **group practice** may be a single-specialty practice or a multi-specialty practice. Three or more physicians constitute a group practice. Most group practices are single-specialty and have less than eight physicians. Physicians may own the practice jointly, or there may be a mixture of owners (partners) and employed physicians. Figure 4–2 shows the distribution of physicians by group size.

There is a wide range of partnership agreements for group practices, from associations to limited partnerships, to incorporating practices. Associations are agreements where physicians simply share office space, equipment, and personnel. However, they do not share patients or income and do not operate under a legal partnership structure.

There also may be other loose physician partnerships with other cost and patient sharing agreements. Some group practices are also owned by the physicians with full-cost and income-allocation arrangements spelled out in the contract or incorporation documents. Older and larger group practices will have a mix of founding "partners" and physician employees, similar to the way that a law firm operates. The partners employ physicians on a salary basis and may offer bonuses based on productivity, but

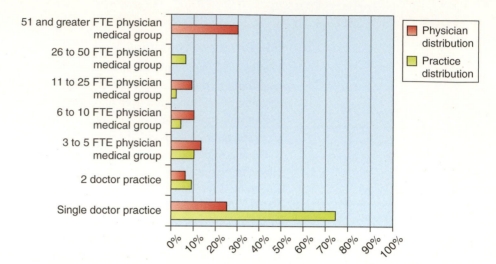

Figure 4–2 Distribution of medical groups and physicians in the United States.

Source: Data extracted from American Medical Association (2007). Physician Characteristics and Distribution in the U.S. 2006. Chicago; and Medical Group Management Association (MGMA) (2007). Cost Survey for Multispecialty Group Practices 2006. Englewood, CO.

the partners keep the profit. The partners also generally have fewer hours in the office and less on-call time.

There are numerous advantages to providers to practicing in a group practice setting. First, physicians who enter established group practices do not have any overhead costs. Physicians who establish group practices share overhead and start-up expenses among each other, which reduces the cost to the individual physician. Group practices have better leverage and ability to negotiate contracts with insurers and suppliers due to patient volume and the ability to hire professional staff. Group practices offer economies of scale that solo practitioners do not have, allowing group practices to obtain better value on their purchases and receive lower reimbursement than a solo practitioner can afford. Physicians working in group practices also have more flexible work schedules than solo practitioners. They are usually able to share on-call time with other physicians and have less responsibility for administrative tasks and more opportunities for continuing education credits within the group practice structure. Additionally, physicians in group practices have less financial risk than solo practitioners. They either share the risk with the other physicians or incorporate to protect themselves from personal risk or are employees of a group practice with no financial risk. Physicians in group practices experience more interaction with their peers. They can consult other physicians in their practice for second opinions, refer easily within the group in the case of a multi-specialty group practice, and they have more opportunities for continuing education in a group setting. Group practices are also more likely to hire professional management and personnel to work on billing and reimbursement. Therefore, the physicians have no direct financial interaction with the patient and can rely on professional management for scheduling, pre-certification, referrals, billing, and other administrative tasks. A group practice also gives physicians marketing power and prestige if it is a well-known local, regional, or even national group practice, for example, the Permanente Medical Group of Kaiser-Permanente and Geisinger Health System.

However, there are several disadvantages to providers who choose to practice in a group practice setting. Physicians have less individual freedom, in that they must work with others including administrators. In fact, many physicians have reduced autonomy as a result of working in a group practice setting. Administrators may set patient and on-call schedules in a way that the solo provider would not. Shared risk can also be a disadvantage from a malpractice or litigation standpoint. All physician owners of a group practice are likely to be named in a lawsuit and are at financial risk if a suit is lost or settled. The potential for higher incomes is also reduced in a group practice setting. In exchange for less on-call time, fewer office hours, and better peer interaction, physicians in group practice settings face higher patient loads, which may inhibit the physician–patient relationship, and physicians in a group practice may receive less money than a solo practitioner due to the income distribution arrangements.

Group practice arrangements offer many advantages to their patients seeking care. In many offices, patients can receive all or most of their care under one roof, particularly in large multi-specialty group practices. Patients can have laboratory work completed, obtain records and second opinions, and be referred to specialists within the same practice. Even in a single-specialty group practice, patients will experience better emergency coverage and an easier referrals process, and will benefit from behind-the-scenes peer interaction among providers. Group practices have personnel and administrators that have better knowledge of costs and billing and may accept more forms of insurance than solo practices. These attributes may result in better quality of care. However, some patients dislike the group practice atmosphere. They believe that they have less of a relationship with their physicians and may feel rushed during their appointments. Physicians in group practices usually have higher patient loads and heavier schedules than solo practitioners, resulting in an "assembly line" atmosphere for patients, longer waits to see their providers, and more bureaucracy. Group practices may also have high provider turnover, leading to less continuity of care for patients.

Trends in Types of Practices

There has been an increase in the number of group practices, as well as the average size of group practices. The average number of physicians per group has grown. However, relatively small groups are still the most common. Approximately 70 percent of group practice physicians are in groups with less than eight physicians (Liebhaber & Grossman, 2007).

The legal form of group practices has also changed. In the past, group practices were investor-owned and un-incorporated. Now, they are increasingly forming corporations because it provides physicians with more financial protection by limiting their legal liability. Many physicians are also selling their practices to hospitals. Almost two-thirds of physicians worked in hospital-owned practices in 2009 (Medical Group Management Association, 2010).

The proportion of physicians as employees has increased in most health care settings over the last decade. The more years of practice physicians have, the less likely they are to be an employee. However, the curve is shifting upward, meaning that more physicians overall are becoming employees regardless of their years of practice. In 2008, 44 percent of physicians were employed in various settings including small group practices, large group practices, group or staff model HMOs, community health centers, medical schools, and hospitals.

Physicians may be employed by a group that then contracts with a hospital, or they may be employed as individuals by hospitals. Traditionally, hospitals employed practitioners such as radiologists, pathologists, and emergency providers. However, hospitalists, or physicians who only treat patients within the hospital, are becoming more common in the hospital setting. See Figure 4–3 for the percentages of physicians by practice setting.

Throughout the 1990s, practice composition, ownership, and relationships with hospitals changed as providers started to come to terms with prospective payment and reduced payments from managed care providers. For example, many physicians sold their practices to hospitals and became employees of hospitals. Although a large percentage of physicians are still employees of hospital-based practices, hospitals were divesting themselves of these practices by 2001 because they were not effective at improving access to care or controlling costs. Some physicians also entered into physician hospital organizations (PHOs) to be able to better contract with managed care organizations. PHOs are legal entities generally formed by physicians and one or more hospitals with the intention of negotiating contracts with payers and sharing in the financial rewards of controlling costs while delivering high-quality care. Many of these arrangements no longer exist because they were not successful at developing the infrastructure needed to manage utilization cost-effectively, and they failed to sign many contracts with health plans. In addition, the Federal Trade Commission (FTC) found fault with the way most PHOs negotiated fees for doctors, finding that in practice they amounted to price fixing, a violation of antitrust laws. However, health

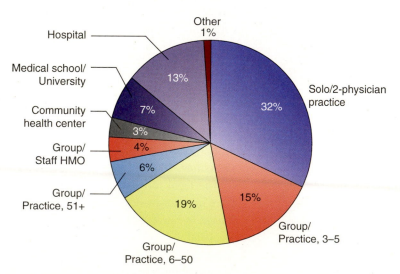

Figure 4–3 Percent of physicians by employment or office setting.

Source: Boukus, Ellyn, Alwyn Cassil and Ann S. O'Malley, A Snapshot of U.S. Physicians: Key Findings from the 2008 Health Tracking Physician Survey, Data Bulletin No.35, Center for Studying Health System Change, Washington, D.C. (September 2009).

care reform is encouraging the bundling of payments and formation of **accountable care organizations (ACOs)**. An ACO is a network of doctors and hospitals that shares responsibility for providing care to patients. In the new law, an ACO would agree to manage all of the health care needs of a minimum of 5,000 Medicare beneficiaries for at least 3 years. These new Medicare and Medicaid payment models require hospital physician cooperation, such as global payments, bundled payments, episode-based payments, and reductions of readmissions. ACOs would make providers jointly accountable for the health of their patients, giving them strong incentives to cooperate and save money by avoiding unnecessary tests and procedures. For ACOs to work, they would have to seamlessly share information. Those that save money while also meeting quality targets would keep a portion of the savings. But some providers could also be at risk of losing money. More details on what comprises accountable care organizations will emerge as rules and regulations for the Patient Protection and Affordable Care Act of 2010 are promulgated.

▪ Summary

In this chapter, we surveyed the organization of the U.S. health care system. The system is a complex set of stakeholders who have different priorities and incentives. Although the primary players may be providers, patients, payers, and the government, they rarely have the same goals and objectives. We identified three primary components of the health care system, including patients, providers, and the social component that is responsible for delivery and reimbursing care to improve health.

We further explored the social components of the health care system and identified the roles that they play. First, the organization and delivery component includes the different organizations that deliver care to patients. Second, the financing component determines how we pay for care. Third, the regulation component includes such activities as state government licensure of hospitals and physicians and federal government oversight of the pharmaceutical industry and medical device manufacturers, among many examples. Fourth, there is the role of allocation of resources and health planning of health care services. Planning seeks to improve allocation and efficiency; lower costs; and improve the quality of, access to, and distribution of health care resources.

The United States is unique among other economically developed countries in that a larger percentage of the health care system is privately owned. Organizations can be classified as inpatient or outpatient/ambulatory care, and they can be classified by ownership type. The largest percentage of hospitals in the United States is nongovernmental and not-for-profit. If an organization has not-for-profit tax status, or 501(c)(3), based on the section of the Internal Revenue Code that governs tax-exemption, no profit can accrue to any shareholders.

Many organizations in the health care system are operated for-profit or they are owned by shareholders. Examples of for-profit enterprises include insurance companies such as Aetna and United Healthcare, specialty hospitals, rehabilitation hospitals, nursing homes, pharmaceutical companies, home health companies, durable medical equipment suppliers, and private physician practices.

The government is one of the most important stakeholders in the U.S. health care system. It performs several important roles, including financing, delivering, and regulating the delivery of health care. The government—federal, state, and local combined—is the largest single payer of health care. Government has an enormous stake in the quality of care and the efficiency of its delivery. Therefore, it regulates the delivery of health because the health, safety, and welfare of its citizens are affected. At the federal level, the Department of Health and Human Services (DHHS), the Centers for Medicare and Medicaid Services (CMS), and the Food and Drug Administration (FDA) are key sources and enforcers of government regulation. At the state level, the Department of Insurance and Department of Health are key to enforcing state health regulations.

Delivery of care takes place in many forms, including ambulatory care such as private practice offices, physician office visits, dental office visits, mental health services, physical therapy, diagnostic testing, and ambulatory surgery centers. Inpatient care can take place in many settings such as inpatient and long-term care organizations, for example, hospitals, nursing homes, assisted living, and home health and hospice care.

Hospitals may be either short-stay hospitals or long-stay hospitals. For short-stay hospitals, the average length of stay (ALOS) is less than 30 days. Hospitals can also be classified based on their bed size and their ownership status, or whether they are for-profit or not-for-profit. Not-for-profit hospitals may be stand-alone community hospitals, part of a hospital chain, part of a church affiliation or religious hospital group, or part of a not-for-profit managed care organization. Proprietary hospitals are for-profit, are subject to taxes, and are often owned by shareholders, and many of these corporations are traded on the stock exchange. Teaching hospitals provide training for residents and interns and must have at least one approved residency program for medicine or dentistry.

Care is also delivered by many types of long-term care providers and facilities. The most common are nursing homes, assisted living, continuing care retirement communities, home health care, rehabilitation and hospice.

Physician practices are the predominant mode of ambulatory care. Practice arrangements have many variations, but a shift has been taking place away from solo physician practices toward more group practices over the last 20 years. This change has caused the number of solo physician practices to decline. We assessed the advantages and the disadvantages of solo and group physician practices. The overall trend due to reimbursement and the debt load carried by new graduates is toward practice in a group. The trend is for new physician graduates who carry a heavy debt load to be employed in a group practice. They are able to share the risks and financial rewards of the group practice with their colleagues and also have a convenient source for referrals and professional consultation. Group practice arrangements offer many advantages to their patients seeking care. In many offices, patients can receive all or most of their care under one roof, particularly in large multi-specialty group practices. Patients can have laboratory work completed, obtain records and second opinions, and be referred to specialists within the same practice.

■ Review Questions

1. What are the social components of the health care system, and what roles do they play?

2. Describe the different types of ownership in health care, and give examples of each.

3. Explain the various government roles in health care.

4. Explain the different ways that hospitals can be classified. What is the most common type in each category?

5. Discuss the differences between skilled nursing, nursing facility, sub-acute, and post-acute care.

6. Define home health, assisted living, and hospice in your own words and describe the trends in the use of or provision of these services.

7. Explain the shift in physician practice arrangements over time.

8. Describe the benefits and disadvantages of solo physician practice.

9. Describe the benefits and disadvantages of group physician practice (to both patient and provider).

■ Additional Resources

Ambulatory Surgery Center Association www.ascassociation.org/

American Health Care Association www.ahcancal.org/Pages/Default.aspx

Americas Health Insurance Plans www.ahip.org/

American Hospital Association www.aha.org/

American Medical Association www.ama-assn.org/

Assisted Living Federation of America www.alfa.org/alfa/Default.asp

Association of American Medical Colleges www.aamc.org/

Centers for Medicare and Medicaid Services www.cms.gov

Joint Commission www.jointcommission.org/

Medical Group Management Association www.mgma.com/

National Association for Home Care and Hospice www.nahc.org/

■ References

American Association of Medical Colleges (AAMC). (2010). What roles do teaching hospitals fulfill? Retrieved July 15, 2010, from www.aamc.org/about/teachhosp_facts1.pdf.

American Health Care Association. (2010a). Nursing facility beds in dedicated special care units. Retrieved July 15, 2010, from http://www.ahcancal.org/research_data/oscar_data/**Nursing Facility** Operational Characteristics/HIST_OPERATION_OscarDataReport_2009Q4.pdf.

American Health Care Association. (2010b). Nursing facility ownership. June 2010. Retrieved July 15, 2010, from http://www.ahcancal.org/research_data/oscar_data/**Nursing Facility** Operational Characteristics/HIST_OPERATION_OscarDataReport_2010Q2.pdf.

American Hospital Association (AHA). (2009, November 11, 2009). Fast facts on U.S. hospitals. Retrieved July 15, 2010, from www.aha.org/aha/resource-center/Statistics-and-Studies/fast-facts.html.

American Hospital Association (AHA). (2010a). *American hospital statistics*. Chicago: American Hospital Association.

American Hospital Association (AHA). (2010b). *Trendwatch chartbook 2010: Trends affecting hospitals and health systems*. Chicago: Author.

Assisted Living Federation of America. (2009). What is assisted living? Retrieved July 15, 2010, from www.alfa.org/alfa/Assisted_Living_Information.asp?SnID=1892690743.

Centers for Medicare and Medicaid Services (CMS). (2009). The nation's health dollar, calendar year 2008: Where it came from, where it went. Retrieved July 6, 2010, from https://www.cms.gov/NationalHealthExpendData/03_NationalHealthAccountsProjected.asp#TopOfPages.

Comondore, V. R., Devereaux, P. J., Zhou, Q., Stone, S. B., Busse, J. W., Ravindran, N. C., et al. (2009). Quality of care in for-profit and not-for-profit nursing homes: Systematic review and meta-analysis. *British Medical Journal, 339* (August 4), b2732.

Congressional Budget Office (CBO). (2006). *Nonprofit hospitals and the provision of community benefits*. Retrieved June 30, 2010, from http://www.cbo.gov/ftpdocs/76xx/doc7695/12-06-Nonprofit.pdf.

Conover, C. J. (2004). *Health care regulation: A $169 billion hidden tax.* (Washington, DC: The Cato Institute).

Cullen, K. A., Hall, M. J., & Golosinskiy, A. (2008). *Ambulatory surgery in the United States, 2006* (No. 11). Centers for Disease Control and Prevention.

Department of Health and Human Services (DHHS). (2010). Patient dumping: Emergency medical treatment and active labor act. Retrieved July 15, 2010, from http://oig.hhs.gov/fraud/enforcement/cmp/patient_dumping.asp.

Draper, D. (2007). Commercial health plans' care management activities and the impact on costs, quality and outcomes. Congressional testimony before the U.S. Senate Committee on finance hearing on the Medicare Advantage program, Associate Director, Center for Studying Health System Change, April 11.

The emergency department as admission source. (2007). *Healthcare Financial Management*, November 1.

Harrington, C., Woolhandler, S., Mullan, J., Carrillo, H., & Himmelstein, D. U. (2001). Does investor ownership of nursing homes compromise the quality of care? *American Journal of Public Health, 91*(9), 1452–1455.

Himmelstein, D. U., Woolhandler, S., Hellander, I., & Wolfe, S. M. (1999). Quality of care in investor-owned vs. not-for-profit HMOs. *Journal of the American Medical Association, 282*(2), 159–163.

Hospital Corporation of America (HCA). (2010). HCA Fact Sheet. Retrieved July 15, 2010, from http://hcahealthcare.com/util/documents/HCA-Fact-Sheet.pdf.

Kaiser Family Foundation (KFF). (2010). Hospital beds per 1,000 population, 2008. Retrieved July 15, 2010, from www.statehealthfacts.org/comparemaptable.jsp?ind=384&cat=8.

Liebhaber, A., & Grossman, J. M. (2007). *Physicians moving to mid-sized, single-specialty practices* (No. 18). Center for Studying Health Systems Change.

McClellan, M., & Staiger, D. (2000). Comparing hospital quality at for-profit and not-for-profit hospitals. In *The changing hospital industry: Comparing for-profit and not-for-profit institutions*, David M. Cutler, ed. Chicago: University of Chicago Press.

Medical Group Management Association (MGMA). (2010). MGMA physician placement report; 65 percent of established physicians placed in hospital-owned practices. June 3. Retrieved July 15, 2010, from www.mgma.com/press/default.aspx?id=33777.

National Association for Home Care and Hospice. (2008). Basic statistics about home care. Retrieved July 15, 2010, from http://www.nahc.org/facts/08hc_stats.pdf.

NCHS. (2010). *Health, United States, 2009: With special feature on medical technology*. Hyattsville, MD: U.S. Government Printing Office.

Sloan, F. A., Picone, G. A., Taylor, D. H., & Chou, S.-Y. (2001). Hospital ownership and cost and quality of care: Is there a dime's worth of difference? *Journal of Health Economics, 20*(1), 1–21.

Taylor, D. H., Whellan, D. J., & Sloan, F. A. (1999). Effects of admission to a teaching hospital on the cost and quality of care for medicare beneficiaries. *New England Journal of Medicine, 340*(4), 293–299.

Woolhandler, S., Campbell, T., & Himmelstein, D. U. (2003). Costs of health care administration in the United States and Canada. *New England Journal of Medicine, 349*(8), 768–775.

Woolhandler, S., & Himmelstein, D. U. (1999). When money is the mission: The high costs of investor-owned care. *New England Journal of Medicine, 341*(6), 444–446.

5 Health Manpower

Key Terms

certified nurse midwife (CNM)

certified nursing assistant (CNA)

certified registered nurse anesthetist (CRNA)

chiropractor

clinical nurse specialist (CNS)

dentist

licensed practical nurse (LPN)

nurse practitioner (NP)

physician

physician assistant (PA)

single-specialty group

Learning Objectives

- Analyze the roles and responsibilities of clinicians in the health care industry.

- Explain the relationships between reimbursement and practice patterns of clinicians.

- Describe the training and education required of clinicians in the health care industry.

- Discuss the changing roles of clinicians as health care costs increase and focus on primary care increases.

- Describe the responsibilities of allied health professionals.

■ Introduction

The labor force in the health care industry is highly trained, motivated, and compassionate, but it is stressed by changing reimbursement patterns, liability risk, and consumer demands. Throughout the history of the U.S. health care system, the physician has been the hub of the delivery of care for patients. **Physicians** are responsible for referring patients to hospitals, performing tests and procedures, and coordinating the care of their patients. Health care costs have continued to rise, reimbursement practices have changed, and consumers have become more demanding of their caregivers. Payers influence care providers by reimbursing them more for performing tests and procedures than for spending time with patients in counseling or listening to patients discuss their symptoms.

Clinicians operate within a dynamic and demanding environment. Many providers are pressured to see a defined number of patients per hour to meet performance goals as well as income targets. Caregivers also face the rising costs of protection from the risk of patient lawsuits, which influence their choices in delivering care to patients, practicing defensive medicine, or focusing on specialty rather than primary care medicine.

Providers other than physicians must also operate in a challenging environment because they are often the first contact for patients. Rising delivery costs have directed many hospitals and clinics to rely on nurses, **nurse practitioners**, and **physician assistants** to deliver primary care. Nurse practitioners have been given increasing responsibility for diagnosing and prescribing medications for patients. Licensure and liability standards vary by state regarding the power delegated to nurse practitioners to independently prescribe medications and diagnose diseases.

Rising costs also have led health care delivery systems to rely more heavily on nurses to assume an increased role in delivering primary care to patients. The shortage of nurses will exacerbate as the population ages and the supply of trained faculty in nursing schools remains low. Hospitals have resorted to recruiting nurses from second- and third-world English-speaking countries while subsidizing the training and recruitment of nurses in the United States.

■ Physicians

After World War II, the United States enjoyed a booming economy, and the 1950s were a time of plenty. During the late 1950s, U.S. social policy began to focus on assuring that the poor and elderly had adequate access to "the good life," including high-quality health care. In the 1960s, Congress and President Lyndon Johnson gave the poor and elderly the buying power to obtain adequate access to health care through the enactment of Medicare and Medicaid legislation.

The passage of Medicare and Medicaid increased the demand for health services and led to the perception by many that physician supply was inadequate (Fein, 1967). The federal government addressed this perceived shortage by funding medical school construction, providing grants to medical schools for training physicians, increasing research funding for medical schools through the National Institutes of Health, and loosening immigration regulations to encourage more graduates of medical schools outside the United States to practice here.

■ The Rising Costs of the Health Care System

The 1970s saw a significant increase in the number of physicians. Ironically, a decade after the federal government attempted to increase the supply of physicians, many policy makers expressed concerns that growth would overshoot the target and create an oversupply of physicians (Graduate Medical Education National Advisory Committee [GMENAC], 1981). Therefore, in the late 1970s, the federal government withdrew financial support to build medical schools and increase physician "output." However, public strategies to increase the supply of physicians in the United States could not be easily undone and continues even today. It is difficult to close medical schools and relieve medical school faculty of their jobs; hence, medical schools continue to produce physicians faster than population growth, thus increasing the physician-to-population ratio.

Along with concerns over a surplus of physicians is the issue of a surplus of physicians in certain specialties and a shortage of primary care physicians, particularly in poor inner city and rural areas. At the same time, the physician workforce is aging, average hours worked are falling, and many physicians are nearing retirement just as growth and aging of the population and advances in technology contribute to a growing demand for physician services.

Physicians are one of the most invested stakeholders in the health care industry. Physicians control the majority of health care spending and are able to generate their own demand for services. This phenomenon is referred to as "physician-induced demand" or "supplier-induced demand," and occurs because health care delivery is *not* determined from a medical "cook book" with which all experts agree. Physicians often practice medicine in a gray area where some doctors will agree with a particular diagnostic or treatment strategy and others will not. Many procedures and treatments have not been empirically tested or generally accepted as the preferred approach.

Thus, physicians often exercise a fair amount of variability in their approach in a particular clinical situation. When there is a large concentration of physicians in an area, they can induce their own demand, and that area is likely to have more health care provided per capita, regardless of the demographics of the area or the actual need for health care services, than those areas with fewer doctors (Wennberg, 2002).

Vignette

Recruitment and Retention of Physicians to Rural Settings. Memorial Hospital is an acute care community hospital located in a rural county in Pennsylvania. The hospital uses 45 swing beds as either acute-care or skilled nursing facility beds for patients in recovery. It provides an array of services, including surgery, inpatient care, pain management, wound care, labor and delivery, and renal dialysis. The hospital serves a community that is primarily composed of Medicare and Medicaid patients. Due to the slumping economy, many primary employers have left the area or been forced out of business by their competitors. Unemployment has been in the double digits throughout the past 5 years, but is slowing decreasing as people move away from the area in search of employment. Most of the patients who remain have lived in the area all their lives and will remain for the near future.

Memorial Hospital has staff privileges for 13 physicians, who primarily practice as solo practitioners in the area. Due to the loss of privately insured patients in the area, several physicians have moved their practice to areas near Philadelphia, Pennsylvania. Several primary care physicians and two surgeons have relocated to increase their volume of patients and revenue. They also moved to take advantage of the better school systems and cultural attractions of the metropolitan centers. The nearby city also provided more opportunities for revenue generation with a higher percentage of privately insured patients. The urban settings offered the physicians an opportunity to join group practices that were in the networks of commercial payers who provided reimbursement that is more generous. The surgeons were able to join a group practice and see an increase in the referrals they received from other physicians.

However, the primary reason that physicians moved was concern about their families. None of the physicians had ever lived in a rural setting, and they did not have family connections in the area. The city was much more familiar and provided many of the amenities that seemed to be lacking. The physicians were concerned that their children were advancing through school without many of the classes and activities that were offered in schools nearer the city. Their spouses did not have family or friends in the area, and their own career opportunities were limited in the rural area. Their previous careers were in areas such as computer science, consulting, and financial services, which the rural area lacked.

After the physicians moved from the area, Memorial Hospital immediately experienced a drop in inpatients, surgical procedures, and patient days. Patients began to travel to larger hospitals an hour away to undergo surgical procedures, complete diagnostic imaging tests, have biopsies, and obtain second opinions. One of the primary drivers of revenue and financial health for a community hospital is local physicians referring patients for inpatient and outpatient care. Local physicians are the main drivers of inpatient care, outpatient care, and diagnostic volume, and therefore reimbursement for hospitals. Local physicians provide referrals to the local community hospital for inpatient and outpatient surgical procedures, diagnostic tests, cancer treatment, and to specialists for procedures. Referrals to the specialists who provide tests and procedures represent substantial revenue opportunities for the local hospital. Therefore, the financial health of the hospital may be determined by the strategic relationships that are developed with local physicians.

Hospitals have faced significant challenges in recruiting and retaining physicians in rural markets because of hostile liability risks, low reimbursement rates, and the unattractiveness of isolated rural markets. Hospital costs for recruitment and retention are substantial for a physician to enter the market, establish a practice, and begin referring patients to the local community hospital. Many months or several years may pass before a physician builds a stable and high volume of patients to refer patients to the hospital. Whenever a physician informs patients of his or her departure, there is an immediate drop in patient volume. Overall, rural community hospitals typically lose money employing physicians or subsidizing their practice. Once a physician announces his or her departure from a market, there is a continual loss of revenue for the hospital as patients leave the physician's practice and transfer to other providers in the market.

The relationship between physician access and rural community hospital financial health is crucial to understand. Many rural community hospitals are in a state of financial crisis, and administrators should appreciate the factors that generate revenue for the hospital. Key sources of revenue, such as physician referral, can be identified and developed to ensure the long-term viability of the organization. Policy makers should be educated regarding the critical role that local physicians play in care delivery, the health of the local population, and the financial performance of the local hospital. The critical contribution of local physicians to the revenue streams for hospitals provides a policy justification for increasing the state and federal reimbursement for providers. Hospitals could also be financially subsidized for their efforts to recruit and retain physicians in their market. However, any of these subsidies would come at the expense of the taxpayer, and most do not live in rural areas.

From the physician practice perspective, primary care physicians provide critical services to many underserved rural populations. Primary care specialists are the lifeblood of many local community hospitals. Specialists in many services are rare in many rural markets. Patients in rural markets may be required to travel 2 to 3 hours for specialty care. Out-migration of such patients represents lost revenue generation opportunities for the local hospital, which further limits the resources available to recruit additional physicians.

1. What new strategies do rural hospitals need to implement to successfully attract and retain physicians in their markets?

2. What is the primary barrier for physicians to locate and practice long-term in a rural setting?

3. What can medical schools do to encourage their students to practice in rural underserved locations?

4. What can federal, state, and local governments do to encourage medical students to practice in rural underserved locations?

5. Do the benefits of government intervention in the health manpower marketplace exceed their cost?

▪ Physician Training and Practice Requirements

Physicians must obtain extensive training to practice medicine in the United States. Future clinicians must have a solid educational foundation to enter medical school, with a high school diploma and an earned undergraduate college degree in a well-rounded program that meets all standard pre-medical requirements. Then students must complete 4 years of medical training at an accredited allopathic or osteopathic medical school; the first 2 years are usually nonclinical and focused on the medical sciences, with limited patient contact and responsibility. Years 3 and 4 consist of clinical clerkships where students rotate through various medical specialty areas with more patient contact.

After the 2 nonclinical years, students must pass Step 1 of the U.S. Medical Licensure Exam (USMLE). Medical school students take Step 2 of the USMLE at the end of year 4. Upon graduation, students are awarded an MD or DO degree. However, graduation from allopathic or osteopathic medical school alone does not grant individuals the right to practice medicine.

Physicians must complete a general residency for 1 year, formerly known as an internship. After completion of year 1 of the residency, students take Step 3 of the USMLE. After passing Step 3, individuals are licensed in the state of practice location. States may have different passing scores, and physicians are licensed to practice medicine only in the state in which the exam was taken. Some states recognize other states licensures, also called reciprocity, but they are not required to do so. Ultimately, the power to license physicians is the responsibility of the state government.

If physicians decide to complete a specialty residency after 1 year of post-graduate training, depending on the specialty, another 3 to more than 5 years of training is required. The American Medical Association (AMA) and the respective specialty associations approve/accredit these programs. Upon completion of a specialty residency program, such physicians are considered "board eligible." After passing the specialty exam, which is composed of both written and oral sections, physicians are "board certified." For many medical specialties, physicians are required to complete an additional fellowship of a year or more after residency. Today, all specialties require periodic retesting of specialists for renewal of certification.

Board certification is not required by states and is not a federal or state administrative activity. Board certification is required to obtain hospital staff privileges and for participation with third-party payer programs. Two-thirds of all physicians who consider themselves specialists are board certified. The number is lower for physicians who were trained in medical schools outside of the United States.

After physicians complete residency or fellowship training, they apply for hospital privileges near their practice location. Application for hospital privileges is a separate credentialing process that takes place directly between the hospital and the physician. Figure 5–1 provides a summary of the steps required for physicians to practice medicine.

---

1. **The Road to Graduation from Medical School—MD or DO**
   - Four years of medical school
   - Degree awarded
     No right to practice

2. **Post-Graduate Training**
   - General residency—1 year
   - Medical examination by state board—license to practice
   - Specialty fellowship—3 to 5+ years

3. **Specially Board Certification***
   - Oral and written exam
   - Not required by states
   - Often required for hospital staff privileges or for participation in third-party payer programs

4. **Continuing Education Credits**
   - Hospital privileges
   - Continued certification
   - Third-party payers

* All specialties now require periodic retesting for renewal of certification.

Figure 5–1 Summary of steps to physician practice.
© *Cengage Learning 2013*

▪ Medical School Applicants

The number of graduates from U.S. allopathic medical schools has been relatively stable in recent years, at approximately 15,000 to 16,000 graduates per year. This steady flow of graduates reflects the relatively constant number of individuals accepted to medical school. In recent years, applicants to U.S. medical schools have fluctuated between approximately 25,000 and 45,000, whereas only 17,000 to 18,000 individuals are accepted in a typical year. The relatively constant number of individuals accepted, despite wide fluctuations in the number of applicants, reflects that the number of physicians trained is determined largely by the current capacity of the educational system (Association of American Medical Colleges [AAMC], 2009b).

Historically, white males have dominated medical school admissions. However, the representation of women has grown substantially, to nearly 50 percent of graduates today. The number of female doctors doubled since the 1970s, increasing the number of women physicians to nearly one in four. Recent trends suggest that within the next 2 decades, women will constitute nearly half the physician workforce (Health Resources and Services Administration, Bureau of Health Professions [HRSA, BHPr], 2008b). Women tend to gravitate to certain specialties such as obstetrics and gynecology, dermatology, and pediatrics, but not to others such as surgery.

On the other hand, the representation of historically underrepresented minorities (African Americans and Hispanics) has not grown appreciably and does not approach the current and growing fraction of the U.S. population that these groups represent. The imperative to increase the enrollment of underrepresented minorities has been based largely on considerations of social equity, cultural competence, and access to health care by underserved populations (Cooper, 2003).

▪ Physician Training Economics

Most physicians are heavily indebted upon graduation and completion of medical training. Upon completion of their training, and not including their undergraduate education, the average physician is over $150,000 in debt. According to the Association of American Medical Colleges (AAMC), 79 percent of graduates have debt of at least $100,000; 58 percent of graduates have debt of at least $150,000; and 87 percent of graduating medical students have outstanding loans (AAMC, 2009a). The amount of debt is increasing each year, driven by increases in tuition and inflation. A physician's training is very costly, and more than 80 percent of medical students borrow money to cover their expenses. Private school tuition, such as at Johns Hopkins, was almost $40,000 in 2009 (AAMC, 2010).

Throughout residency training, physicians earn a relatively small salary; in 2009, the average stipend for first-year residents was approximately $47,000 (AAMC, 2009c). Traditionally, the more prestigious residencies had lower pay. During residency, it is unlikely that physicians will be able to pay anything but the interest on their medical education debt. Salaries for residents are typically so low that they are unable to make debt reduction payments on the principle of their educational loans.

To address both the debt concerns of graduates and the geographic maldistribution of physicians, the Congress enacted legislation to establish the National Health Service Corps. In exchange for either scholarships to medical school or repayment of educational loans, graduates must agree to practice for a commensurate number of years in a health professions shortage area (DHHS, n.d.).

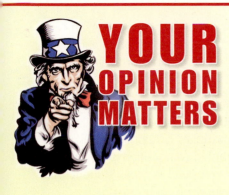

Should More Be Done to Alleviate Medical School Financial Debt?

Background

Most medical school students borrow money to pay for tuition and living expenses. Over time, the cost of living, books, and tuition has increased faster than their income. As a result, many medical school students graduate with a substantial burden of debt (Rosenblatt & Andrilla, 2005). Financial indebtedness influences decisions regarding which area of practice students pursue in their internship and residency (Rosenblatt & Andrilla, 2005). These decisions have consequences for the health care industry, which focuses on curative rather than preventive care.

Here are the facts. When the class of 2008 entered medical school, about a third of students had debt from their premedical education. By the time the class of 2008 graduated, 87 percent carried debt; the median debt load, including pre-medical debts, was $145,000 for students at public medical schools and $180,000 for those at private medical schools (Steinbrook, 2008). Another record set in 2008 was that 23 percent of the class of 2008 carried a debt load of $200,000 or more (Steinbrook, 2008). By 2033, the debt of both public and private medical school graduates is projected to be approximately $750,000 (AAMC, 2007).

In the 2009–10 academic year, the average tuition and student fees for medical school students in public medical schools was $25,209 for residents and $45,858 for nonresidents (AAMC, 2010). During the same time, the average tuition and student fees for medical school students in private medical schools was $42,906 for residents and $43,431 for nonresidents (AAMC, 2010). When these tuition and fees are multiplied over 4 years, not adjusted for inflation, they average between $100,938 for residents attending a public medical school to $183,423 for nonresidents attending a public medical school.

For public medical schools, average tuition and fees increased by 6.8 percent for residents and by 5.0 percent for nonresidents from 2008–09 to 2009–10 (AAMC, 2010). The average tuition and fees for private schools increased by 4 percent for residents, and by 4.2 percent for nonresidents during the same period (AAMC, 2010). The percentage increases are higher than the rates of inflation throughout these periods. These numbers include only the expenses and tuition for medical school and do not include debt for undergraduate education, living expenses, or consumer loans.

The modern medical school curriculum supports students who choose to pursue specialized careers in medicine (Chen, 2009). When the academic environment and financial pressures combine, they produce powerful

(*Continued*)

forces that influence medical students in their practice choices. As an example, there has been a rapid decline in the number of physicians choosing areas of primary care, particularly its most general form, family medicine (Rosenblatt, 2005).

Medical debt is rising faster than the rate of inflation. As debt repayment becomes an increasingly heavy burden for graduates, the impact on the choice to pursue primary care may increase (Rosenblatt & Andrilla, 2005). Increasing debt load may also impact the demographic composition of physicians. For instance, as more disposable income is required to repay student debt, students who lack such resources may be influenced to choose practice areas with higher salaries. Medically underserved areas may continue to lack physicians who are unable or unwilling to serve in an area where it would be burdensome to repay their loans with the offered salary.

Perhaps due to student indebtedness and future salary expectations, medical school graduates are increasingly choosing to specialize in other areas than primary care medicine. For instance, in the 2009 Main Residency Match, 3,703 U.S. allopathic senior students matched to an internal or family medicine residency program, compared with 4,617 in 2000 and 5,020 in 1996 (Harris, 2010). According to the AAMC data, all primary care practitioners entering general practice after residency are down from 8,162 in 2000 to an estimated low of 6,757 in 2007 (Harris, 2010). Primary care physicians currently comprise approximately 35 percent of practicing physicians, but that amount is rapidly declining because of physicians leaving the profession and fewer new doctors to replace them (Harris, 2010). Recent data show that fewer than 20 percent of all U.S. medical students are choosing primary care specialties (Harris, 2010).

The current payment system in health care rewards physicians for performing tests and procedures over spending time with patients. Even an office visit by a patient is a separate service to reimburse. Listening to patients describing their health care, family, and recovery history is not reimbursed generously. So-called "cognitive services" such as patient consultations are not reimbursed as highly as procedures physicians perform (Harris, 2010). Low reimbursement in primary care hampers the ability to repay debt, which now averages about $150,000 for each medical school graduate.

Yes

Medical school students do not enter graduate medical education with the expectation of carrying a heavy debt load for the rest of their lives. They expect to possess adequate earning power to pay off their debt within a reasonable time. Specializing in an area of medicine enables that goal, whereas focusing on primary care hampers their ability to repay their debt.

Medical training also contributes to students deciding to specialize in areas other than primary care. Factors such as who provides the training and where the academic medical center is located influence students' decisions. Academic and other medical centers are typically located in urban areas and staffed by specialists providing secondary and tertiary care (Harris, 2010). As a result, many physicians do not train in rural areas where primary care is in most demand. This trend leads to more physicians practicing in urban areas among patient populations that can support their practice.

Mentors play an important role in the decisions of graduates. According to data from the AAMC, role model influence was the top factor affecting specialty choice (Harris, 2010). Therefore, primary care physicians may have less influence on students during critical decision-making periods when they are underrepresented in these training settings (Harris, 2010).

One of the goals of the Patient Protection and Affordable Care Act passed in March 2010 is to provide more access to health care by persons who were previously uninsured. By 2014, many new people will have access to health care insurance and will demand primary health care; however, it is unclear whether there will be enough physicians and nurses to meet the demand. Hence, additional resources should be dedicated to facilitating physicians specializing in primary care through loan forgiveness and grants.

The more indebted that young physicians become, the higher the percentage of after-tax income is required to repay their loans. A repayment commitment of more than 15 percent of after-tax income may be burdensome for the average physician who practices primary care to bear.

No

There will always be a strong applicant pool of potential medical school students despite the high indebtedness that awaits them. In spite of the challenge of paying off debt over many years, on average, future physicians will be earning more than the average American, while enjoying stable positions, and will eventually have the income with which to pay off their loans (Steinbrook, 2008).

Further, in the near future physician services will be in high demand due to more patients being covered by health insurance plans. As a result, physicians will be able to secure positions upon graduation and generate higher salaries through increasing their patient volume. There will always be demand for physician services, and although physicians may not be as wealthy as in the past, they are certainly not going to be in poverty from medical indebtedness.

Lastly, the states and federal government have many programs whereby new physicians can serve in exchange for debt forgiveness. Typically, such

(Continued)

positions are in medically underserved areas. Therefore, it is a win–win endeavor: patients living in rural underserved areas have access to primary care, and physicians are able reduce a percentage of the medical school debt burden.

You decide:

1. What should be the top three important factors for graduates from medical school to evaluate when deciding which area of medicine in which to specialize?

2. Should there be more financial support given to physicians who decide to practice primary care?

3. How do the differences in reimbursement for primary care and secondary or tertiary care differ, and how does this impact the income of physicians?

Cost of Training New Physicians

One of the challenges for medical schools is they must be affiliated with a hospital to provide training for medical school students. Medical school hospitals have additional social responsibilities that increase their costs of operation. Additional responsibilities include teaching medical students and residents as well as the costs of performing medical research. However, in the highly competitive health care marketplace, purchasers of health care frequently do not wish to pay more for these "non–patient care" activities, such as teaching and research.

Medical Licensing

The USMLE became the standard medical licensure exam in 1994. Medical licensure is still a state-level responsibility. Medical licensure is a necessary prerequisite to practice because it helps protect the consumer from unqualified individuals practicing medicine. In addition to licensure, the following mechanisms aim to help protect the consumer from unqualified physicians: verification by a state of the physician's credentials, such as medical school graduation and specialty board certification; malpractice liability incurred by hospitals, HMOs, and PPOs if they permit incompetent physicians to practice; and utilization review and quality assurance programs.

International Medical Graduates

About 25 percent of physicians are trained outside of the United States (AMA, 2010). The infusion of international medical graduates (IMGs) into the U.S. health care delivery system has been a controversial topic for decades because there is a perception that these physicians have had a lower quality education and have inferior clinical skills. These allegations are unsupported by empirical data. The continued influx of IMGs has been problematic because many medical school applicants in the United States are not accepted to medical school, and there is the perception that there is an overall surplus of physicians in many areas.

In addition, the flow of IMGs from third-world countries who practice in the United States creates a "brain drain" from these developing nations. This phenomenon presents a moral or ethical dilemma for the United States when it is seen as taking valuable resources, such as physicians, away from less developed countries.

Many IMGs do not return to their home after training in the United States, even though it is unlawful. They marry or have children while in the United States. IMGs are also often willing to practice in areas that are not desirable to U.S. medical graduates such as rural and inner-city areas.

Criteria for IMG Licensure

There are several important criteria for licensure of international medical graduates (IMGs). IMGs must have (1) a sponsor, such as an employer or individual citizen, and must have graduated from a World Health Organization (WHO)–approved medical school; (2) an Educational Commission for Foreign Medical Graduates (ECFMG) certificate to demonstrate that they passed Steps 1 and 2 of the USMLE and must pass an English comprehension exam; (3) an approved residency (it is important to emphasize that rural or inner-city positions are usually the only available residencies, are often in medically underserved areas, and are rejected by U.S. medical school graduates); and (4) after the general residency, a passing grade on Step 3 of USMLE. A graduate of a Canadian medical school is not considered an IMG, as these schools are recognized by the AAMC. However, an individual born in the United States who does not graduate from a U.S. or Canadian medical school is considered an IMG.

The Maldistribution of Physicians

The physician workforce in the U.S. health care system has often been labeled maldistributed because the tendency is to practice in affluent urban and suburban areas (Council on Graduate Medical Education [COGME], 2001). Concern about a shortage is based on the adverse impact on access to care for patients who are not located near a physician's practice. Physicians may be unable to establish a practice in their area of specialization, which may depress their income.

A maldistribution may result in physicians being unable to practice in their preferred city or state. However, physicians can affect the demand for their services. Roemer's law says that wherever physicians are, they will be providing health care regardless of actual need. Physicians can "prescribe" return visits even for limited symptoms and minor illnesses. When physicians induce demand, costs continue to rise.

Primary Care Practitioners

Primary care physicians are general practitioners (GPs), family practitioners, general pediatricians, general obstetricians/gynecologists (OB/GYNs), and general internists. Surgeons, pathologists, and many other specialists are not considered primary care practitioners because they are usually not the regular and usual source of care for most patients, and they generally do not treat patients outside of their specialty area.

Figure 5–2 illustrates the shortage of primary care physicians and their distribution throughout the United States. The shortage is most severe in those areas that are darkly shaded and are predominately located in the south and the west.

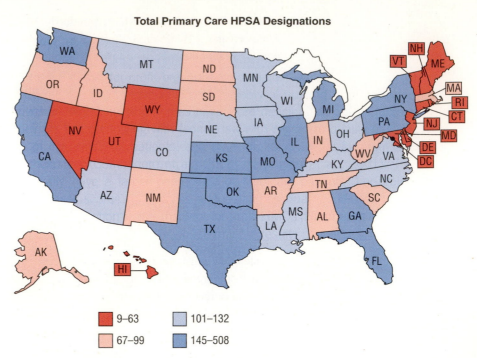

Figure 5–2 The shortage of primary care physicians and their distribution throughout the United States.

*Source: The Henry J. Kaiser Family Foundation, statehealthfacts.org **"Estimated Underserved Population Living in Primary Care Health Professional Shortage Areas (HPSAs), as of February 1, 2012"***; Data Source: State Population and Health Professional Shortage Areas Designation Population Statistics, Health Resources and Services Administration (HRSA), February 1, 2012.

Practice Trends

Group Practice versus Solo Practice

More physicians are working for other physicians or physician-management companies. Fewer physicians are self-employed or own their own physician office. More physicians are working as employees for hospitals as hospitalists and intensivists.

Less experienced or younger physicians are more likely to be employees, because new graduates of medical school carry heavy debt loads. Beginning a new medical practice is very expensive, requiring office space, information technology systems, lab equipment, trained staff, supplies, and marketing. Starting a new solo practice is prohibitive for many new physicians in areas where they must rely on lower reimbursement rates from Medicare and Medicaid and referrals from other physicians.

The proportion of physicians in solo and two-physician practices has decreased significantly over the last 10 years (Liebhaber & Grossman, 2007). More specialists and older physicians now practice as employees of a practice or in a group practice (Liebhaber & Grossman, 2007). This trend also applies to hospitals that have been hiring physicians at a much higher rate as hospitalists or attending physicians (Sharamitaro, 2010). In contrast, the percentage of primary care physicians that remain in solo or two-physician practices has remained stable from 1996 through 2005. For specialists, the trend is toward practicing in mid-sized, **single-specialty groups** of 6 to 50 physicians (Liebhaber & Grossman, 2007). Although there has been a shift away from solo practice for physicians, they have not been joining practices composed of many specialists in the large, multi-specialty practice model (Liebhaber & Grossman, 2007).

There are several forces operating behind this trend toward joining a group practice or becoming a physician employee. Financial pressures and the desire for work–life balance drives physicians to a more secure setting in a group practice. As a member of a group, physicians do not need to be on call every night and every weekend as in a solo practice. Call responsibilities are typically shared among the physicians in the group. They also do not have the sole responsibility for the administration and business side of their practice (Sharamitaro, 2010). Physicians have incentive to join mid-size practices to take advantage of economies of scale in distributing fixed costs (e.g., equipment, personnel) of the practice over more physicians (Liebhaber & Grossman, 2007). Physician-owned outpatient facilities provide opportunities for physicians to generate revenue from procedures and diagnosis services. Such services are reimbursed at a higher level than physician visits that would typically take place in a primary care physician office. Larger physician groups also have the advantage of more bargaining power with managed care plans.

There are important implications associated with physicians moving away from solo practice and joining group practices. Growth in group practice size could drive up prices in some markets for physician services. Health plans must first contract with physician practices in a market area before offering them in their networks to their health plan members. Perhaps large group practices will have enough bargaining power to drive up the price of their services. In addition, costs of care could be driven up and services could be over-used if physicians refer to colleagues within their own practice (Liebhaber & Grossman, 2007). When physician practices have multiple specialties, physicians have incentive to refer to their own colleagues rather than other specialists with whom they do not share profits and losses.

Physicians will continue to experience incentives to join larger practices. New physicians are saddled with significant debt. This debt most likely has been deferred for several years during internship and residency, with interest accumulating. Group practices offer an existing pool of patients, a salary, referral sources, and administrative support in the practice of medicine for new physicians.

Physicians are also faced with pay-for-performance incentives that require adoption of information technology (IT) to capture data regarding the care management of patients. Implementation of such IT requires significant capital investment, and larger practices have more access to implementation resources. Larger practices are also better able to collect quality data and implement process improvements to improve clinical outcomes for patients (Liebhaber & Grossman, 2007).

■ Physician–Patient Communication

Physicians who communicate with patients via email experienced a drop in office visits, according to a recent Kaiser Permanente study (Dolan, 2007). A decrease in patient visits may clear the office schedule for patients who have critical needs. However, a potential downside of this scenario is that in a system without capitation, a reduction in the number office visits may have a negative impact on the revenue for the physician office (Dolan, 2007).

When physicians communicate with patients via email, they can control when they write the message and manage how much time they spend on communicating with patients. However, insurers do not reimburse physicians for the time that they spend reading and composing their messages with their patients. Some physicians are still reimbursed for their time and effort through a special email system that requires patients first to enter a credit card before their message is sent. The cost of the e-mail is typically the cost of copay by the patient (Dolan, 2007).

Physicians have expressed concern that they may "drown" in the number of email messages from patients. But a Kaiser Permanente study indicated otherwise, as physicians typically answered two messages per day (Dolan, 2007). Many older patients with chronic conditions could benefit from email communication with their physicians as questions arise regarding how to manage their care.

According to a national study, during a typical office visit by older patients, on average, six problems are presented for the physician to assess and ask questions of the patient (Tai-Seal, McGuire, & Zhang, 2007). The physician and patient addressed the main issue for approximately 5 minutes, leaving the rest of the 16 minutes to address the other issues. Older patients who have one or more chronic conditions require more time with a physician to ask questions and address issues (Tai-Seal et al., 2007). However, physicians have a tightly regulated schedule and many times do not have significant time to address each question that a patient may present during the visit. Physician reimbursement does not reward for dedicating extra time to patients with comorbidities. Many physicians are reimbursed for performing procedures and making diagnoses, and therefore do not dedicate more of their time for evaluation and treatment (Tai-Seal et al., 2007). Experts recommend that when patients visit their physician's office, they bring a list of concerns with them and then work with their doctor to address the three or four most important ones.

The ultimate goal of all communication is to assure that patients understand and comply with or adhere to the plan for treatment to which both physician and patient have agreed. For effective treatment to have an impact on health, patients must follow instructions for prescriptions and suggested behavioral strategies. There is evidence that patients often do not find instructions clear and therefore do not adhere to regimens (Di Matteo et al., 2002). It is conceivable that the introduction of electronic communications will improve compliance and thus improve treatment outcomes.

Medical Malpractice

Physicians are required to be insured against medical malpractice cases that may be brought by patients or their representatives. Patients may sue a physician for many reasons, including injury acquired while receiving care or complications that arise later during recovery from treatment. Hospitals require physicians to be insured against medical malpractice as a condition of receiving admitting privileges. There has been an increase in the number of patients who have sued their physician for medical malpractice as well as an increase in the amount of damages that have been awarded by juries to patients who have sued their physician. Medical malpractice tort costs have risen an average of 11.7 percent annually since 1975 (Hellinger et al., 2003).

Throughout the last decade, the malpractice premiums that some physicians and specialists must pay have been steadily increasing. According to the Congressional Budget Office (CBO) (2006) insurance premiums for all physicians increased an average of 15 percent from 2000 to 2002. Specialists in obstetrics, gynecology, general surgery, and internists experienced higher increases. There is much speculation regarding the causes of these rate increases. Premium increases may be the result of investment losses that insurers have experienced, decreasing number of companies offering malpractice insurance, increases in jury awards to patients who have been injured, and rising health care costs for patients who have successfully sued their physician (KFF, 2007).

There are many sides to the medical malpractice debate regarding the reasons for the increase in malpractice suits and in monetary awards by juries. Trial lawyers argue that there are many incompetent physicians who practice medicine, injure patients through negligence, and should be sued for medical malpractice. They argue that the justice system is designed to compensate patients who are injured due to the negligence of physicians. Injured patients should be compensated for the economic damages, such as health care costs, lost wages, future health care expenses, and emotional pain and suffering due to incompetent physicians. According to trial lawyers, victims have no other recourse but the legal system, which brings physicians to justice. Lawyers are usually paid in these matters through a contingency fee. They argue that this method of payment is necessary in that only wealthy individuals could afford to sue a hospital or insurance company by paying the lawyer an hourly rate.

Physicians argue that many trial lawyers sue physicians for medical malpractice to achieve a monetary reward regardless of whether the suit has merit. The goal of a suit is to settle the case with the malpractice insurer, from which the trial attorney will take 30–40 percent for legal fees. This practice results in rising medical malpractice insurance premiums for physicians and financial rewards for trial attorneys. Physicians may also engage in unnecessary defensive medicine in order to lessen their risk of being sued by patients and to mitigate their liability if the case goes to trial.

The Bush Administration addressed the medical malpractice crisis by proposing caps on noneconomic monetary rewards for pain and suffering during its second term. Malpractice award caps are very controversial, with arguments in their favor and evidence that indicates that they are ineffective. The argument in favor of caps is that it lowers malpractice premiums, reduces overall health care costs, deters "defensive medicine" practices by physicians, and lowers the incentives for trial attorneys to bring unjustified lawsuits (KFF, 2007). However, others argue that caps on pain and suffering would be ineffective in dealing with the medical malpractice crisis. This side contends that caps would not decrease malpractice insurance premiums or overall health care spending, and it would limit those patients who have experienced damages from being compensated fairly for their suffering (KFF, 2007).

■ Cost, Access, and Quality

Medical malpractice affects cost and access to health care. It has been estimated that expenditures associated with increases in malpractice premiums are only a small portion of the national spending on health care (CBO, 2006). There are also concerns about the costs associated with physicians practicing unnecessary defensive medicine in response to increases in malpractice liability. However, the CBO has estimated that malpractice caps would be ineffective in reducing such costs (CBO, 2006).

Regarding access to care, there are concerns that physicians may leave the health care profession or relocate to states with lower malpractice premiums. Such trends may decrease access for patients residing in states that experience significant decreases in their physician population (KFF, 2007). However, there is no solid evidence that reductions in malpractice premiums would reverse such decreases in access to physicians, assuming that they did exist (KFF, 2007).

Current State of Medical Liability Rates

Medical malpractice premiums have continued to increase over the past 5 years, but may be leveling off. Medical liability insurers have reported that 70 percent of their premium rates have leveled off or decreased in some areas of the country (Weiss, 2009). Many states that have passed caps on pain and suffering are still waiting for the impact of the legislation in their states.

Many malpractice insurance companies wait until the cap is challenged in the state supreme court and its constitutionality upheld. Once the cap has been approved, companies may then adjust their premiums to lower levels for physicians. For instance, in 2003, the citizens of Texas passed a $250,000 cap on pain and suffering as a constitutional amendment. Since the amendment has taken effect, rates have decreased an average of 29.5 percent, and more physicians are entering the state to provide services (Sorrel, 2008).

Medical malpractice rates vary from state to state. According to the AMA, certain states are in a crisis where medical liability insurance rates force physicians to retire early, eliminate high-risk procedures, or leave the state (Sorrel, 2007). The number of states in crisis stood at 17 in 2007. Crisis states included Connecticut, Florida, Illinois, Kentucky, Massachusetts, Missouri, New Jersey, Nevada, New York, North Carolina, Ohio, Oregon, Pennsylvania, Rhode Island, Tennessee, Washington, and Wyoming. Since then, some states have tried to enact tort reform only to be struck down as unconstitutional. Moving out of crisis can be a protracted process (Sorrel, 2009).

Specialty Time Line

The first organized specialty was ophthalmology, or medical doctors specializing in the treatment of the eyes and vision. In the 1930s, specialists constituted one-fifth of physicians, and their numbers started to increase after World War II. During the war, specialists were assigned a higher military rank. In the 1950s, specialists increasingly dominated hospitals and medical schools. By the 1960s, specialists accounted for about half of all physicians. Today, only 10 percent of physicians are general practitioners, physicians with no more than 1 year of postgraduate training, and 90 percent are specialists.

There are several reasons for the increase in specialists. Specialists tend to have higher incomes and are also viewed as having more prestige. Expansion of health care knowledge "forces" the study of a specific area versus all possible areas to provide optimal quality (i.e., "*you can't possibly know it all*"). This compartmentalization is exacerbated by the growth of health care technology at a seemingly geometric rate. Furthermore, medical school role models and medical training are geared toward specialties. Finally, many physicians believe there is greater intellectual challenge in treating uncommon and/or serious illnesses or diseases than dealing with the self-limiting minor illnesses with which primary care physicians frequently deal.

There is concern about overutilization by specialists for several reasons. When there is high demand for health care services, specialists take on primary care functions, but they may not perform these generalist tasks as well as primary care physicians. For instance, specialists are reimbursed primarily on the number of procedures and diagnoses that they perform. They have incentive to perform these procedures more than primary care physicians. Specialist care is therefore higher and increases health care cost inflation throughout the industry.

As physicians become overly specialized, some argue they lose the ability to judge and do well in other areas of medicine. When practicing in their own field, they perform better than generalists treating the same problem. This specialization trend is not unique to the health care industry (e.g., professors, lawyers, and engineers also specialize).

With a shortage of primary care physicians, many policy makers have expressed concerns about what should be done about the excess supply of specialists. Solutions include cutting residencies, alerting medical school students about the difficulty they may have in finding a job, reducing Medicare funding for specialty residencies, controlling board certification, or reducing the influx of IMGs.

Physician Distribution and Supply

Maldistribution by Location

Physicians tend to locate in densely populated areas. Per capita, there are more physicians in urban areas than in rural areas. There are many reasons for this maldistribution. First, as the per capita income of a state increases, the number of physicians per capita increases. Physicians typically desire to locate and raise their own families in safe areas with the best educational opportunities, abundant cultural activities, and a high standard of living. The richest states have the most physicians, but the poor states have the sickest populations. Physicians are not appropriately located based on need; however, general practitioners and family physicians are distributed relatively more evenly with population than are other specialists.

Second, specialists tend to reside in higher income areas and areas where the population density is the greatest. Some specialists require a high population density for a clientele base that would support their practices. Family physicians typically see 1,500–2,000 patients per year (Murry et al., 2007) compared to neurosurgeons, who see fewer than 500 patients per year (American Association of Neurological Surgeons [AANS], 2005). In fact, the trend toward specialization has exacerbated the maldistribution of physicians, although market forces (a surplus of some specialties) have forced physicians into some undeserved areas.

Third, patients living in urban areas usually have access to better health care equipment and technologically advanced hospitals. Cost justification of equipment and services requires a higher patient use rate and therefore a larger population base. In addition, physicians often feel professionally isolated in rural areas. Family physicians and general practitioners are equally distributed between metropolitan and nonmetropolitan areas. Although general internists, general pediatrics, and general OB/GYNs are less evenly distributed by population density, the distribution of specialists such as cardiologists, neurologists, neurosurgeons, and oncologists is the most skewed toward metropolitan areas (Goodman & Wennberg, 2010).

There are consequences of the lack of primary care physicians in underserved areas. Places that are underserved have a higher infant mortality rate, more heart disease, and lower child immunization levels.

■ Future Surplus or Shortage of Physicians

By 2020, there may be a physician shortage in the United States, anywhere from 24,000 to 200,000 physicians (Commins, 2007). This shortage is the result of many factors such as the current levels of medical education and training, the aging population of physicians, the aging of the U.S. population, and the unwillingness of younger physicians to work 80-hour workweeks (Commins, 2007; Salsberg & Grover, 2006). This shortage is expected to appear by 2020, when the baby boomer generation will be over 70 years of age. Experts argue that a shortage will occur despite substantial increases in medical education and training of interns and residents (Salsberg & Grover, 2006) and in spite of the growing numbers of physicians who arrive from overseas programs and from osteopathic and off-shore schools.

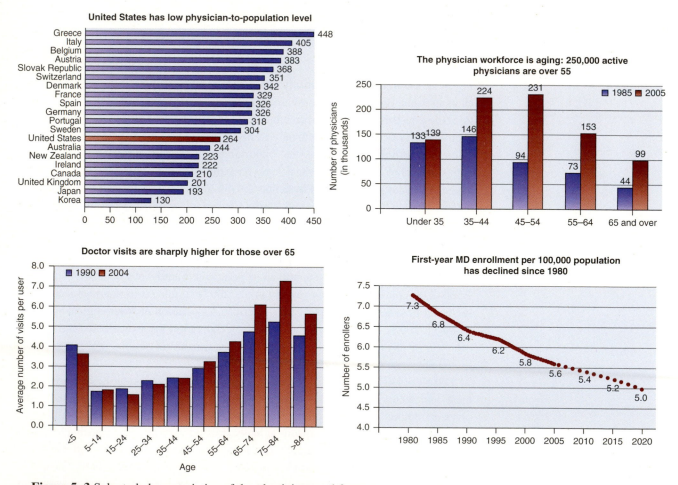

Figure 5–3 Selected characteristics of the physician workforce.

Source: MargaretAnn Cross, What the primary care physician shortage means for health plans. Managed Care, June 2007. Retrieved September 1, 2011, from http://www.managedcaremag.com/archives/0706/0706.shortage.html.

A physician shortage is expected by 2020, primarily driven by the demand for physician services. The number of persons over the age of 65 will double by 2030. However, first-year enrollment in medical schools has declined every year since 1980 (Salsberg & Grover, 2006). The first of the baby boomers will turn 65 in 2010, and according to the U.S. Census Bureau, the number of persons over the age of 62 will almost double by 2030 (Commins, 2007). The older population may also present with comorbidities that demand more physician services. Of the 83 million people over age 62, 14 million will have diabetes, and 21 million will be obese (Commins, 2007). Other conditions among the elderly that will drive demand for physician services include rates of heart disease and cancer, two of the leading causes of death in the United States.

The health industry will need to prepare for this oncoming physician shortage. It is projected that the shortage will most affect the primary care sector of physician services (Commins, 2007). Physicians who practice primary care are among the lowest paid specialties among physicians. Therefore, it is very difficult to convince new physicians to go into primary care when they earn a lower salary, work longer hours, and are exposed to higher risks for liability (Commins, 2007). There will not be sufficient physicians for hospitals and physician practices to meet the patient demand. Decision makers will need to determine how to best utilize nurses, technicians, and other professionals to close the gap in providing services to patients.

Figure 5–3 illustrates the relationships among the number of physicians, doctor visits, physician demographics, and the decline in the number of physicians over time.

Physician Income

Between 1995 and 2003, physician income decreased by an inflation-adjusted 7 percent (Tu & Ginsberg, 2006). Decreases in income occurred for surgeons and primary care physicians. Primary care physicians saw their income drop by 10.2 percent, whereas surgeons' income decreased by 8.2 percent (Tu & Ginsberg, 2006). Real income for medical specialists remained approximately the same throughout this period. By 2008, physicians were feeling the effects of the recession, with income dropping as well as productivity. In 1998, physicians collected an average of 68.4 percent of their stated charges after fees were discounted by insurers and other third-party payers. Collection amounts declined to 59.5 percent in 2008 (Medical Group Management Association [MGMA], 2009).

Although physicians report that their income has decreased, time spent providing direct patient care has not decreased (MGMA, 2009). Physicians are spending more time now than in the past caring for patients. More patient-centered time reflects the trend of physicians away from solo practices and into larger group practices or as employees of hospitals. When physicians practice in a group setting, many of the administrative responsibilities for billing and other administrative tasks are handled by non-physician staff members (Tu & Ginsberg, 2006).

This decrease in physician income is primarily derived from lower reimbursement from private and government payers for physician services (MGMA, 2009; Tu & Ginsberg, 2006). Health insurance plans are reimbursing physicians at lower rates than in previous years, partly due to annual increases in inflation since 1995 that reduce the value of physician reimbursement levels every year. Physicians would need

	Median Physician Compensation		
	2010	**2009**	**Percent Change**
Medical Specialities			
Allergy	$249,674	$241,138	3.54
Cardiology	$402,000	$398,034	1
Cardiology-Cath lab	**$484,092**	**$471,746**	**2.62**
Dermatology	$375,176	$350,627	7
Endocrinology	$218,855	$212,281	3.1
Family Medicine	$208,861	$197,655	5.67
Gastroenterology	$405,000	$389,385	4.01
Hematology/Medical Oncology	$320,907	$315,133	1.83
Hospitalist	$215,716	$211,835	1.83
Hypertension & Nephrology	$259,677	$246,049	5.54
Infectious Disease	$227,750	$222,094	2.55
Internal Medicine	$214,307	$205,441	4.32
Neurology	$236,500	$236,500	0
Pediatrics & Adolescent–General	$209,873	$202,832	3.47
Psychiatry	$214,740	$208,462	3.01
Pulmonary Disease	$306,829	$278,000	10.37
Rheumatologic Disease	$224,000	$219,411	2.09
Urgent Care	$222,920	$215,625	3.38
Surgical Specialities			
Cardiac & Thoracic Surgery	**$533,084**	**$507,143**	**5.12**
Emergency Medicine	$268,787	$267,293	0.56
General Surgery	$357,091	$340,000	5.03
OB/GYN—General	$295,761	$294,190	0.53
Opthalmology	$343,945	$325,384	5.7
Orthopedic Surgery	**$500,672**	**$476,083**	**5.16**
Otolaryngology	$368,777	$365,171	0.99
Urology	$413,941	$389,198	6.36
Radiology/Anesthesia/Pathology			
Anesthesiology	$370,500	$366,640	1.05
Diagnostic Radiology (M.D. Intv.*)	**$478,000**	**$478,000**	**0**
Diagnostic Radiology (M.D. Non-Intv.)	$454,205	$438,115	3.67
Pathology—Combined (M.D. only)	$354,750	$344,195	3.07

Figure 5–4 Median physician compensation.*

*The highest paid specialties are listed in bold.

Source: Who's making what? More than three-quarters of physician specialties saw increased compensation in 2009. Practice Link: The Online Physician and Job Bank Magazine, Spring 2011. Retrieved September 1, 2011, from http://www.practicelink.com/magazine/departments/vital-stats/.

to be reimbursed at levels higher than inflation each year for their income to increase, all else constant.

The median salary of physicians is approximately $180,000. Although seemingly high, physicians spend more time and incur more debt as a result of their education than do most workers. Cardiovascular surgery generates an income of approximately $600,000 per year and is one of the highest paid compared to family practice, which generates only $140,000 per year (DOL, 2009).

Historically, the reimbursement system has rewarded procedural and diagnostic skills rather than cognitive skills. Self-employed physicians earn more than employed physicians, and those in groups make more than solo practitioners. Managed care has brought decreased physician salaries; however, in some cases, that trend is now reversing.

Figure 5–4 illustrates the median physician compensation and the change from 2009 through 2010. The graphic illustrates the disparities in earning power between physicians practicing in primary care and specialists.

▪ Dentists

Dentists are responsible for the prevention, diagnosis, and treatment, both surgical and nonsurgical, of the problems in the mouth and maxillofacial area and associated structures (American Dental Association [ADA], 2010a). Most dentists practice as solo practitioners and practice general dentistry, treating a variety of dental conditions (DOL, 2010b). They also employ a variety of assistants such as dental hygienists, dental assistants, dental laboratory technicians, and receptionists.

▪ Dental Specialties

Approximately 15 percent of dentists practice in one of the nine dental specialties (DOL, 2010b):

- *Orthodontics*, the largest dental specialty, consists of the diagnosing, preventing, and treating of dental and facial irregularities, known as malocclusions. The irregularities may be treated by straightening the teeth, among other treatments.

- *Endodontics* focuses on treatments such as root canals and endodontic surgery.

- *Oral and maxillofacial pathology* is the identification and management of oral diseases.

- *Oral and maxillofacial radiology* is the treatment of dental conditions by using imaging techniques.

- *Oral and maxillofacial surgery* is the treatment of diseases, injuries, and defects of the oral and maxillofacial region.

- *Pediatric dentistry* provides oral health services for children through adolescence, including those with special health care needs.

- *Periodontics* focuses on the treatments for diseases of the gums and surrounding tissues, while maintaining healthy gums and their surrounding tissues.

- *Prosthodontics* restores natural teeth or replaces them with artificial teeth or dentures.

- *Dental public health* specialists promote good dental health and disease prevention in the community (ADA, 2010a).

Education and Training

General dentists complete 4 years of undergraduate training and then 4 years of dental school. Dentists graduate with either a Doctor of Dental Medicine (DMD) or a Doctor of Dental Surgery (DDS) degree. Most dentists obtain DDSs, but there is no difference in procedures performed among general dentists with either degree. Dentists who specialize must complete additional postgraduate work and training before practicing in their respective specialty (ADA, 2010b).

Dentists are more likely to locate in highly populated areas for the same reasons physicians do, but they are more evenly distributed with population than physicians. Dentists have become very efficient in their practices. They employ more ancillary personnel and have many techniques that have proven efficiency and effectiveness. In the United States, dentistry espouses preventive techniques such as brushing, flossing, and fluoridation.

Licensure

Dentists are required to obtain a license to practice. They must graduate from an accredited dental school and pass written and practical examinations. The written portion may be satisfied by passing the National Board of Dental Examiners Examinations (DOL, 2010b).

The Future of Dentistry

Employment in dentistry is projected to grow by at least 16 percent through 2018 (DOL, 2010b). The expansion of the profession is stimulated by the growing general population, but particularly by increases in the elderly population at an even faster pace. The demand for dental treatments will increase as the elderly are able to keep their own teeth for longer periods of time, necessitating complicated bridgework and prosthodontic services (DOL, 2010b).

Greater public awareness of oral health care may lead to higher demand for services. Younger patients will continue to require preventive checkups, and the demand for cosmetic procedures such as teeth whitening is increasing (DOL, 2010b).

Dental technology is projected to improve the effectiveness and efficiency of dental practices. New technologies such as digital radiography, laser systems, and informatics will enable future dentists to provide effective treatments and improve the efficiency of their practice (ADA, 2010a).

Nurses

Nurses represent the single largest group of health caregivers. Nurses practice where their patients require skilled care, including in hospitals, nursing homes, rehabilitation hospitals, schools, and their patients' homes. Most nurses work in hospitals in surgery, intensive care, neonatal intensive care, labor and delivery, and in outpatient services (American Nurses Association [ANA], 2010a). Advanced practice nurses, such as nurse practitioners, certified nurse midwives, and credentialed nurse anesthetists, earn higher salaries than registered nurses as these positions increasingly require a Masters of Science in Nursing (MSN) degrees.

The Nursing Shortage

The current nursing shortage in the United States is projected to reach between 340,000 and 1 million by 2020 (Kuehn, 2007). Nurses are subject to difficult and stressful working conditions, demanding supervisors, and very sick patients (Spence Laschinger & Finegan, 2005). The shortage of nurses is not limited to the United States. Germany, the Netherlands, France, Australia, Denmark, Canada, and countries in Africa are experiencing shortages of skilled nurses (Oulton, 2006).

Figure 5–5 illustrates the disparity between the demand for registered nurses and the supply of registered nurses through 2020.

The nursing shortage is driven by four primary factors. The nursing workforce is aging, retiring, and leaving the profession. Enrollment in nursing programs is declining as women find other career opportunities. The increased demand on nurses to provide care for sicker patients, using complex health care technology, while patients are staying in hospitals fewer days because of cost constraints, makes the nursing work environment less than optimal. Finally, the nursing profession suffers from historically negative stereotypes of women. Although nurses rank high in trust, they remain undervalued and underappreciated (Janiszewski Goodin, 2003).

Most significantly, there is a lack of qualified faculty in nursing schools to provide training for new nurses. Applicants have been turned away from nursing training who could otherwise fill job openings in hospitals (Kuehn, 2007). To meet the increasing demand for nurses, admissions to nursing schools would need to increase by 40 percent per year (Kuehn, 2007).

The nursing shortage affects access and quality of care in hospitals (Kuehn, 2007). According to researchers, communication between staff members, relationships with patients, bed availability, and patient-centered care are all negatively affected by the lack of

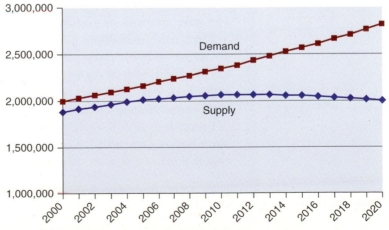

Figure 5–5 Registered nurse supply and demand projections.

Source: U.S. Department of Health and Human Services (DHHS), Health Resources and Services Administration, Health Professions. (2010b, March). The registered nurse population: Findings from the 2008 national sample survey of registered nurses. Retrieved September 1, 2011, from http://bhpr.hrsa.gov/healthworkforce/rnsurvey2008.html.

nurses (Kuehn, 2007). These issues are critical as hospitals focus on reducing medical errors and hospital-acquired infections, while preserving their quality of care and reimbursement.

In addition to the shortage of trained faculty in nursing schools, there is also a lack of training facilities, as fewer hospitals offer programs to train student nurses (Kuehn, 2007). Patients in the hospital are sicker and require direct attention by skilled staff; health care technology is more complex and demanding; and hospitals are more at risk for malpractice (Kuehn, 2007).

Nursing shortages have occurred several times throughout history. During the late 1980s and early 1990s, as the economy grew, there were fewer applicants to nursing schools because nursing salaries were not attractive (Janiszewski Goodin, 2003). Although nursing salaries have increased significantly since then, they plateaued quickly. Labor represents a significant portion of hospital expenses, so salaries of staff are often the first item to be limited. There are many other professional options and expanded opportunities in other fields such as law, medicine, and business for people who would have otherwise chosen nursing in the past (Janiszewski Goodin, 2003). Hospitals increasingly use lower-skilled workers, such as **licensed practical nurses (LPNs)** and **certified nursing assistants (CNAs)** to reduce costs under managed care.

The nursing shortage is being addressed by hospitals, employers, states, and training programs (Kuehn, 2007). Four strategies have shown promise for increasing nursing enrollment. First, recruitment by hospitals, schools of nursing, and nursing associations have expanded (Janiszewski Goodin, 2003). High school students are presented with opportunities to take summer courses and have hands-on experience in preparation of future nursing training (Janiszewski Goodin, 2003).

Second, nurse retention in the workforce is increasing with improved personnel policies, opportunities for career advancement, and flexible work schedules (Janiszewski Goodin, 2003). Nursing schools are partnering with foundations to subsidize graduate study in nursing to increase the numbers of trained faculty (Kuehn, 2007). Nurse training is also subsidized by hospitals who fund faculty and students who commit to a work agreement, and allow appropriately trained staff to teach part-time (Kuehn, 2007). States have funded increases in faculty salaries and loan forgiveness to nurses who agree to provide instruction to nursing students (Kuehn, 2007).

Third, nurse associations have worked to improve the image of nursing as a positive caring profession (Janiszewski Goodin, 2003). Strategies include providing high-school students with career information that depicts nursing realistically as a positive professional goal. Marketing has been expanded through television, print, and web-based content to enhance the image of nursing.

Fourth, legislators have passed and funded bills that provide scholarships, grants, career ladders, loan cancellation, and public service announcements advocating for the nursing profession (Janiszewski Goodin, 2003).

▪ Nurses and Hospital Quality

Nurses are critical to provide high-quality care in hospital or physicians offices (Draper et al., 2008). Hospitals are under increasing pressure to delivery high-quality, patient-centered care, and nurses play a critical role in their success. Physicians may deliver orders regarding care planning, but nurses have the most direct contact with patients

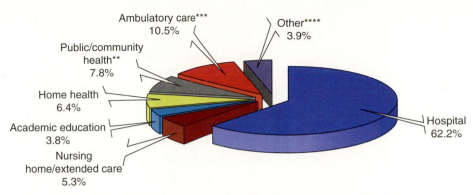

*The totals may not add to 100 percent due to the effect of rounding. Only RNs for whom we have setting information are included in the calculations used for this chart.
**Public/community health includes school and occupational health.
***Ambulatory care includes medical/physician practices, health centers and clinics, and other types of non-hospital clinical settings.
****Other includes insurance, benefits, and utilization review.

Figure 5–6 Registered nurse population by employment setting, 2008.*

Source: U.S. Department of Health and Human Services (DHHS), Health Resources and Services Administration, Bureau of Health Professions (HRSA, BHPr). (2010a, March). Chart 13: Registered nurse population by employment setting, 2008. Retrieved September 1, 2011, from http://bhpr.hrsa .gov/healthworkforce/rnsurveys/rnsurveyinitial2008.pdf.

and administer the care at their bedside (Draper et al., 2008). Nurses are uniquely positioned to detect medical errors, harmful drug interactions, patient slips and falls, and declining health status of their patients.

Figure 5–6 illustrates the large percentage of nurses who practice in a hospital setting (62.2%) as compared with other types of settings. They have a critical influence on the quality of care received by hospital patients.

Researchers indicate that nurses are critical to improving quality in organizations that have a culture of openness and support for nurses (Draper et al., 2008). A culture of quality is important for all staff to contribute to improvements (Draper et al., 2008). Successful hospitals have been champions for quality by establishing high standards for all hospital staff (Draper et al., 2008).

However, quality improvement efforts are challenging in an era of a nursing shortage (Draper et al., 2008). Nurses are already overworked, and many services are consistently short-staffed. Many hospitals depend on extra nurses from agencies who may not be as vested in the quality improvement efforts of the organization. Agency nurses are also very expensive and drive up staff expenses (Draper et al., 2008). This predicament requires hospitals to prioritize and optimize their resources while maintaining very thin profit margins.

■ Training for Nurses

Registered nurses graduate from accredited nursing schools and pass state licensing exams called the National Council Licensure Examination for Registered Nurses (NCLEX-RN) (ANA, 2010a). State boards are responsible for licensing, establishing educational and continuing educational requirements, and handling discipline issues. A state-accredited school of nursing can be a 4-year university program, a 2- to 3-year associate degree program, or a 3-year diploma program (ANA, 2010a, p. 1).

Programs that lead to a Bachelor of Science in Nursing (BSN) provide training in the biomedical sciences and leadership preparation. These programs comprise 4 to 5 years of college and include general studies and 2 years of clinical experience (ANA, 2010a). The BSN provides superior preparation for leadership positions and graduate study. The BSN serves as the foundation for advanced training programs for nurse practitioners, certified nurse midwives, and certified, registered nurse anesthetists.

An associate's degree program focuses on specific roles and technical skills. Associate degree nurses have completed 2 to 3 years at a community or junior college, with an intensive focus on clinical training. These programs represent a little over half of all nurse training programs (ANA, 2010a).

A diploma nursing program is typically completed in a hospital and includes both classroom and clinical instruction. Diploma programs comprise only a small percentage of the overall nursing training programs (ANA, 2010a).

Advanced Practice Nurses

Nurses have taken on expanded roles with advanced training and responsibility. Such nurses have met advanced educational and clinical training requirements, such as earning at least a Master's degree, and provide direct care to patients.

Nurse practitioners (NPs) work in many types of clinical settings, including hospitals, clinics, and physician offices. They provide primary, specialty, and preventive care to pediatric, adult, and geriatric patients. They prescribe medications, order tests, and diagnose and treat many common injuries and illnesses (ANA, 2010b).

Certified nurse-midwives (CNMs) deliver low-risk births and provide primary gynecological care for women. They deliver care in many settings, including hospital labor and delivery services, physician offices, homes, and clinics (ANA, 2010b).

Clinical nurse specialists (CNSs) provide specialized care for physical and mental health issues in hospitals and physician offices. They also may have training, management, or research responsibilities (ANA, 2010b).

Certified registered nurse anesthetists (CRNAs) earn a Master's of Science in Nursing (MSN) degree and are the oldest of the advanced practice nurse positions. They provide the majority of anesthetics to patients each year (ANA, 2010b).

Other Categories of Nursing Staff

The nurse's aide is the lowest skilled position in the nursing profession, and is often referred to as a CNA. The LPN is not a registered nurse. An LPN may have a high school diploma and has taken a year-long training course in basic nursing skills and passed a licensing exam, the NCLEX-PN.

Doctoral-Level Health Care Providers

Chiropractors

Chiropractors treat conditions related to the musculoskeletal system and their interconnectedness with the rest of the body as reflected in the central nervous system that travels through and emanates from the spine. According to the American Chiropractic

Association, chiropractic practice is the specific adjustment and manipulation of the articulations and adjacent tissues of the body, particularly of the spinal column, for the correction of nerve interference and includes the use of recognized diagnostic methods, as indicated. Patient care is conducted with due regard for environmental, nutritional, and psychotherapeutic factors as well as first aid, hygiene, sanitation, rehabilitation, and related procedures designed to restore or maintain normal nerve function (American Chiropractic Association [ACA], 2010). Chiropractors do not prescribe drugs or perform surgery. In 2009, the mean salary for chiropractors was $94,454 (DOL, 2010a).

There are 16 accredited chiropractic programs in the United States, and most students possess undergraduate degrees before entering the program. A typical program of study is 2 years of clinical sciences and 2 years focusing on manipulation of the musculoskeletal system to treat patients (DOL, 2010a).

States regulate the licensure of chiropractors, who must meet educational and examination requirements before they begin their practice. Most chiropractors work in a solo practice; many are self-employed. Demand for chiropractic services is expected to grow by at least 20 percent over the next decade. This increase stems from the overall increase in demand for alternative therapies and noninvasive health care practices (DOL, 2010a). Health insurance plans vary in their reimbursement of chiropractic services. Coverage for services is not universal, although more plans are covering care by chiropractors (DOL, 2010a).

▪ Podiatrists

Podiatrists diagnose and treat disorders, diseases, and injuries of the lower leg and foot. They provide services by prescribing drugs and physical therapy, setting fractures, and performing surgery. Most podiatrists are found in solo practice and may specialize in surgery, orthopedics, primary care, or public health services. Podiatrists are small business owners whose practices must function with the assistance of staff who order supplies, keep records, and schedule patients. A typical salary for a podiatrist is approximately $113,000–$114,000 annually (DOL, 2010c).

There are eight accredited colleges of podiatric medicine offering a 4-year program with a curriculum similar in structure to schools of medicine. Graduates of the program receive the degree of Doctor of Podiatric Medicine (DPM). A two to four year hospital residency follows where additional training is performed in podiatric medicine and surgery (DOL, 2010c).

States regulate the licensure of podiatrists, which requires graduation from an accredited program and passage of a written and oral examination. Although many podiatrists are self-employed and own their own practice, others may partner with other podiatrists or other health care professionals. The podiatry field is projected to expand as the population ages but remains active and requires treatment for foot injuries. Increasing rates of obesity and diabetes, with associated circulatory problems, are expected to increase demand for foot and ankle care (DOL, 2010c).

▪ Optometrists

Optometrists provide care by diagnosing vision problems and testing depth and color perception. They test for glaucoma and diagnose conditions caused by diabetes and high blood pressure. However, a patient diagnosed with these conditions is referred to other clinicians. Most optometrists practice general optometry, but some may specialize in areas such as contact lenses, vision therapy, or geriatrics.

▪ Pharmacists

The growth, diversity, and efficacy of prescription drugs has made pharmacists valuable members of the health care team. Pharmacy is the health profession that has the responsibility for ensuring the safe, effective, and rational use of medicines. However, there remain wide variations in the practice of pharmacy. In recent years, there has been significant convergence, driven by a number of key factors, including the pursuit by pharmacists themselves of the goals of medicines management and pharmaceutical care (Anderson, 2003). By the mid-1990s, nearly all of the 81 schools and colleges of pharmacy had converted their graduate degree from a Bachelor of Science to Doctor of Pharmacy (PharmD) as the entry-level degree for pharmacists. Not all

Table 5–1: Non-Physician Practitioners and Expertise

Area of Expertise	Positions
Administration	Health administrator, health administrative assistant, health program analyst, health program representative, health system analyst
Biomedical Engineering	Biomedical engineer, biomedical engineering technician, biomedical engineering aide
Complementary and Alternative Medicine (CAM)	Acupuncturist, chiropractor, homeopath, naturopath
Clinical Laboratory Services	Clinical laboratory scientist, clinical laboratory technologist, clinical laboratory assistant, clinical laboratory aide, radiology technologist
Dentistry and Allied Services	Dentist, dental hygienist, dental assistant, dental laboratory assistant, dental laboratory technician
Dietetic and Nutritional Services	Dietician, nutritionist, dietary technician, dietary aide, food service supervisor
Environment Control	Environmental scientist, environmental engineer, environmental technologist, environmental technician
Food and Drug Protection Services	Food technologist, food and drug inspector, food and drug analyst, food and drug technician
Health Education	Health educator, health education aide
Information and Communication	Health information specialist, health science writer, health technician writer, medical illustrator
Library Services	Medical librarian, medical library assistant, hospital library
Others	Psychologist, social worker, medical record technician, natural scientist, physical therapist, occupational therapist, counselor, optometrist, speech pathologist

schools undertook the conversion at the same time. All but 11 made the transition during the 1990s; of the remaining 11, two had converted prior to 1980, four completed the transition during the first half of the 1980s, and five during the second half (HRSA, BHPr, 2000). There are nearly a quarter of a million practicing pharmacists in the United States, and nearly 60 percent are women (HRSA, BHPr, 2008a).

Other Members of the Health Care Workforce

A greater percentage of our population works in the health care field than any other area. The health care workforce accounts for approximately 10 percent of the U.S. workforce (DOL, 2009). Physicians are critical decision makers in primary health care. However, nurses require less time to train, are less expensive to train, cost less to employ, and can increase the efficiency and productivity of physicians who provide care to patients. The increase in use of health care services as well as the increase in the number of venues where health care is provided has also increased the job opportunities for nurses and other members of the health care workforce.

See Table 5–1 for examples of various non-physician health professions.

Summary

The professionals who work in the health care delivery system represent the single largest component of the U.S. labor force. Headed by physicians, a quarter who are trained in medical schools outside of the United States and Canada, these workers provide essential primary and preventive services as well as specialty services to millions of Americans. With the aging of the population, there has been and will continue to be an ever-increasing demand for health care services. Federal programs, including Medicare and Medicaid, provide insurance coverage for the elderly and poor who would otherwise seek uncompensated care from hospitals.

Increasing student indebtedness has deterred many college graduates from entering the medical profession, and for those who do enter, has directed them away from primary care and into specialty practices. As a result, the nation suffers from a shortage of general or primary care physicians and an oversupply of specialists. Such an imbalance can drive up the cost of health care as physicians are able to induce their own demand for services in many areas.

The demand for primary care services has stimulated the training of nurse practitioners, physician assistants, and certified nurse midwives who can deliver basic primary care to patients without access to primary care physicians. However, nurse practitioners and certified nurse midwives must first become nurses, and with a shrinking nurse faculty and competition from other occupations, the nation is currently experiencing a shortage of nurses. Moreover, a shortage of nurses affects the quality and quantity of hospital and other facility services that employ nurses.

Americans also obtain services from practitioners other than physicians. They obtain their oral care from dentists, foot care from podiatrists, eye care from optometrists, and often seek alternative therapies from providers such as chiropractors. With the longevity of the growing aging U.S. population, it is expected that the services provided by these professionals will be in greater demand.

▪ Review Questions

1. What is the projected demand for workers in the health care field over the next 20 years?

2. How does the aging of the population, health insurance reimbursement, and consumer demand impact the practice patterns of health care clinicians?

3. How does the projected physician shortage affect the manner in which patients will receive primary care services?

4. What are your ideas for solutions to the heavy load of indebtedness that physicians carry upon graduation from medical school? Should this financial obligation influence their choice of practice?

5. Should the federal government have the authority to regulate physician selection of practice specialty?

6. What are your ideas for improving the image of nursing among high school students?

7. Should there be a limit on damages for pain and suffering in medical malpractice cases?

8. How has the risk from medical malpractice suits influenced the manner in which physicians practice medicine?

9. If you were the CEO of a hospital, how would you provide incentives to nurses to work at your hospital and, once they were there, remain?

10. How is patient demand for alternative therapies influencing the demand for care from non-physician practitioners such as podiatrists and chiropractors?

▪ Additional Resources

Academy of General Dentistry: www.agd.org

American Academy of Family Physicians: http://fmignet.aafp.org.

American Academy of Oral and Maxillofacial Radiology: www.aaomr.org

American Academy of Pediatric Dentistry: www.aapd.org

American Academy of Periodontology: www.perio.org

American Academy of Prosthodontists: www.prosthodontics.org

American Association of Colleges of Podiatric Medicine www.aacpm.org

American Association of Endodontists: www.aae.org

American Association of Oral and Maxillofacial Surgeons: www.aaoms.org

American Association of Orthodontists: www.braces.org

American Association of Public Health Dentistry: www.aaphd.org

American Board of Medical Specialties: www.abms.org

American Chiropractic Association: www.acatoday.org

American College of Healthcare Executives: www.ache.org

American College of Obstetricians and Gynecologists: www.acog.org

American College of Surgeons, Division of Education: www.facs.org

American Podiatric Medical Association www.apma.org

American Psychiatric Association: www.psych.org

American Society of Anesthesiologists: www.asahq.org/career/homepage.htm

International Chiropractors Association: www.chiropractic.org

References

American Association of Neurological Surgeons (2005 Fall). Behind Every Successful Practice: Sound Data—Neurosurgical Practice Survey Results. *Bulletin*: 14 (3). Retrieved March 24, 2012 from http://www.aans.org/Media/Article.aspx?ArticleId=37096

American Chiropractic Association (ACA). (2010). What is chiropractic? Retrieved September 1, 2011, from http://www.acatoday.org/level2_css.cfm?T1ID=13&T2ID=61.

American Dental Association (ADA). (2010a). Dentistry definitions. February 12. Retrieved February 12, 2010, from http://www.ada.org/495.aspx.

American Dental Association (ADA). (2010b). What can a career in dentistry offer you? Retrieved September 1, 2011, from www.ada.org/sections/educationAndCareers/pdfs/dentistry_fact.pdf.

American Medical Association (AMA). (2010). *Physician characteristics and distribution in the U.S., 2009.* (Dearborn, MI: Author).

American Nurses Association (ANA). (2010a). More about RNs and advanced practice RNs. Retrieved February 12, 2010, from http://nursingworld.org/EspeciallyForYou/AdvancedPracticeNurses.

American Nurses Association (ANA). (2010b). How to become a nurse. Retrieved February 12, 2010, from www.nursingworld.org/EspeciallyForYou/StudentNurses/Education.aspx.

Anderson, S. (2003). The state of the world's pharmacy: A portrait of the pharmacy profession. *Journal of Interprofessional Care*, 16(4), 391–404. Retrieved September 1, 2011, from http://informahealthcare.com/doi/abs/10.1080/1356182021000008337.

Association of American Medical Colleges (AAMC). (2007). *Medical school tuition and young physician indebtedness*. Washington: Author.

Association of American Medical Colleges (AAMC). (2009a). AAMC 2009 graduation questionnaire. Washington, DC: Author.

Association of American Medical Colleges (AAMC). (2009b). *Databook*. Washington, DC: Author.

Association of American Medical Colleges (AAMC). (2009c). Preliminary data from 2009 AAMC Survey of Resident/Fellow Stipends and Benefits. Washington, DC: Author.

Association of American Medical Colleges (AAMC). (2010). *Tuition and student fees reports*, August 9. Retrieved August 9, 2010, from https://services.aamc.org/tsfreports/report_median.cfm?year_of_study=2010.

Chen, P. (2009, January 29). The hidden curriculum of medical schools. *New York Times,* Doctor and Patient. Retrieved July 30, 2010, from www.nytimes.com/2009/01/30/health/29chen.html?_r=1&emc=tnt&tntemail1=y.

Commins, J. (2007). Will there be enough doctors? Retrieved September 1, 2010, from http://www.lawlorandassociates.com/October%20Cover%20Story%20Will%20There%20Be%20Enough%20Doctors.mht

Congressional Budget Office (CBO). (2006). Medical malpractice tort limits and health care spending. Background paper. Congressional Budget Office Pub No. 2668. April. 20. Retrieved September 1, 2010, from http://www.cbo.gov/ftpdocs/71xx/doc7174/04-28-MedicalMalpractice.pdf.

Cooper, R. (2003). Impact of trends in primary, secondary, and postsecondary education on applications to medical school II: Considerations of race, ethnicity, and income. *Academic Medicine, 78*(9), 864–876.

Cross, M. (2007). What the primary care physician shortage means for health plans, *Managed Care*, June. Retrieved September 1, 2011, from http://www.managedcaremag.com/archives/0706/0706.shortage.html.

Council on Graduate Medical Education (COGME). (2001, November 20). Tenth report of the council on graduate medical education. Rockville, MD.

Di Matteo R., Giordani P., Lepper H., & Croghan T. (2002). Patient adherence and medical treatment outcome: A meta analysis. *Medical Care, 40*(9), 794–811.

Dolan, P. (2007). E-mail means fewer patient calls and visits. *American Medical News*. Retrieved September 1, 2010, from http://www.ama-assn.org/amednews/2007/08/27/bil20827.htm.

Draper, D. A., Fell, L. E., Liebhaber, A., & Melichar, L. (2008). The role of nurses in hospital quality improvement. Washington, DC: Center for Studying Health System Change.

Fein, R. (1967). The doctor shortage—An economic diagnosis. Washington: The Brookings Institute.

Graduate Medical Education National Advisory Committee (GMENAC). (1981). Report of the Graduate Medical Education National Advisory Committee. Rockville, MD: Author.

Goodman, D., & Wennberg, J. (2010). *The Dartmouth atlas of health care*. Dartmouth Institute for Health Policy and Clinical Practice. Lebanon, NH.

Harris, S. (2010). Primary care in medical education: The problems, the solutions. Association of American Medical Colleges (AAMC). March 1. Retrieved August 9, 2010, from www.aamc.org/newsroom/reporter/march10/45548/primary_care_in_medical_education.html.

Hellinger, F., Encinosa, W., Hellinger, F. J., & Encinosa, W. E. (2003). Impact of state laws limiting malpractice awards on geographic distribution of physicians. July 2003. AHRQ, Rockville, MD: Author. www.ahrq.gov/research/tortcaps/tortcaps.htm.

Janiszewski Goodin, H. (2003). The nursing shortage in the United States of America: The Nursing Shortage—An integrative review of the literature. *Journal of Advanced Nursing, 43*(4), 335–350.

Kaiser Family Foundation (KFF). (2007). Medical malpractice policy. Retrieved September 1, 2010, from http://www.kaiseredu.org/Issue-Modules/Medical-Malpractice-Policy/Background-Brief.aspx.

Kuehn, B. M. (2007). No end in sight to nursing shortage. *Journal of the American Medical Association, 298*(14), 1623–1625.

Liebhaber, A., & Grossman, J. (2007). *Physicians moving to mid-sized.* Center for Studying Health System Change. Washington: Center for Studying Health System Change.

Medical Group Management Association (MGMA). (2009). Cost survey for multispecialty practices, 2009 report based on 2008 data.

Murry, M., Davies, M., & Boushon, B. (2007). Panel size: How many patients can one doctor manage? *Family Practice Management,14*(4), 44–51.

Oulton, J. A. (2006). The global nursing shortage: An overview of issues and actions. *Policy, Politics, & Nursing Practice, 7*(3), 34S–39S.

Rosenblatt, R., & Andrilla, C. (2005). The impact of U.S. medical students' debt on their choice of primary care careers: An analysis of data from the 2002 medical school graduation questionnaire. *Academic Medicine, 80*(9), 815–819.

Salsberg, E., & Grover, A. (2006, September). Physician workforce shortages: Implications and issues for academic health centers and policymakers. *Academic Medicine, 81*(9):782–787.

Sataline, S., & Wang, S. (2010). Medical schools can't keep up: As ranks of insured expand, nation faces shortage of 150,000 doctors in 15 years. *The Wall Street Journal*, April 12. Retrieved September 1, 2011, from http://online.wsj.com/article/SB10001424052702304506904575180331528424238.html.

Seaver, M. (2005). Behind every successful practice: Sound data—Neurosurgical practice survey results. *American Association of Neurological Surgeons Bulletin*, Fall; 14(3), 9–15.

Sharamitaro A, (2010). Trends in physician practice settings: Shift from independent private practice to hospital-centric. *Health Capital, 3*(2), February; http://www.healthcapital.com/hcc/newsletter/02_10/Shift.pdf

Sorrel, A. (2007, March 5). Tort reforms boost some states' liability outlook. *AMedNews*. Retrieved September 1, 2010, from http://www.ama-assn.org/amednews/2007/03/05/prsc0305.htm.

Sorrel, A. (2008, September 28). Texas liability reforms spur plunge in premiums and lawsuits. AMED News. Retrieved September 1, 2010, from http://www.ama-assn.org/amednews/2008/09/08/prl20908.htm.

Sorrel, A. (2009, November). Health reform bills light on medical liability reform. *AMNews*. Retrieved September 1, 2010, from http://www.ama-assn.org/amednews/2009/11/02/gvsb1102.htm.

Spence Laschinger, H. K., & Finegan, J. (2005). Using empowerment to build trust and respect in the workplace: A strategy for addressing the nursing shortage. *Nursing Economics, 23*(1), 6–13.

Steinbrook, R. (2008, December). Medical student debt—Is there a limit? *The New England Journal of Medicine, 359*(25), 2629–2632.

Tai-Seal, M., McGuire, T., & Zhang, W. (2007). Time allocation in primary care office visits. *Health Services Research, 42*(5), 1871–1894.

Tu, H., & Ginsberg, P. (2006, June). Losing ground: Physician income, 1995–2003. Tracking Report No. 15. Washington, DC: Center for Studying Health System Change.

U.S. Department of Health and Human Services, Health Resources and Services Administration, Bureau of Health Professions (HRSA, BHPr). (2000). A study of the supply and demand for pharmacists. Retrieved September 1, 2011, from http://bhpr.hrsa.gov/healthworkforce/reports/pharmaciststudy.pdf.

U.S. Department of Health and Human Services, Health Resources and Services Administration, Bureau of Health Professions (HRSA, BHPr). (2008a). Adequacy of the pharmacist supply: 2004 to 2030. Retrieved September 1, 2011, from http://bhpr.hrsa.gov/healthworkforce/reports/pharmsupply20042030.pdf.

U.S. Department of Health and Human Services (DHHS), Health Resources and Services Administration, Bureau of Health Professions (HRSA, BHPr). (2008b). The physician workforce: Projections and research into current issues affecting supply and demand. Retrieved September 1, 2011, from http://bhpr.hrsa.gov/healthworkforce/reports/physwfissues.pdf.

U.S. Department of Health and Human Services (DHHS), Health Resources and Services Administration, Bureau of Health Professions (HRSA, BHPr). (2010a, March). Chart 13: Registered nurse population by employment setting, 2008. Retrieved September 1, 2011, from http://bhpr.hrsa.gov/healthworkforce/rnsurveys/rnsurveyinitial2008.pdf.

U.S. Department of Health and Human Services (DHHS), Health Resources and Services Administration, Health Professions. (2010b, March). The registered nurse population: Findings from the 2008 national sample survey of registered nurses. Retrieved September 1, 2011, from http://bhpr.hrsa.gov/healthworkforce/rnsurvey2008.html.

U.S. Department of Health and Human Services (DHHS), National Health Service Corps. (n.d.) Building healthy communities in areas with limited access to care. Retrieved September 1, 2011, from http://nhsc.hrsa.gov/corpsexperience/index .html.

U.S. Department of Labor (DOL). (2009). *Occupational outlook handbook, 2008 edition.* Washington DC: Bureau of Labor Statistics.

U.S. Department of Labor (DOL). (2010a). *Occupational outlook handbook, 2010–11 edition: Chiropractors.* Washington, DC: Bureau of Labor Statistics. Retrieved February 12, 2010, from www.bls.gov/oco/ocos071.htm.

U.S. Department of Labor (DOL). (2010b). *Occupational outlook handbook, 2010–11 edition: Dentists.* Washington, DC: Bureau of Labor Statistics. Retrieved February 12, 2010, from www.bls.gov/oco/ocos072.htm.

U.S. Department of Labor (DOL). (2010c). *Occupational outlook handbook, 2010–11 edition: Podiatrists.* Washington, DC: Bureau of Labor Statistics. Retrieved February 12, 2010, from www.bls.gov/oco/ocos075.htm.

Weiss, G. (2009, November 20). Survey: Malpractice premiums. *Modern medicine: Medical economics.* Retrieved February 12, 2010, from http://www .modernmedicine.com/modernmedicine/article/articleDetail.jsp?id=643717.

Wennberg, J. (2002). Unwarranted variations in healthcare delivery: Implications for academic medical centers. *British Medical Journal, 325*(7370), 961.

Who's making what? More than three-quarters of physician specialties saw increased compensation in 2009. *Practice Link: The Online Physician and Job Bank Magazine*, Spring 2011. Retrieved September 1, 2011, from http://www .practicelink.com/magazine/departments/vital-stats/.

6 Public Health

Key Terms

- endemic
- epidemic
- epidemiology
- incidence
- pandemic
- prevalence
- primary prevention
- public health
- public health problems
- secondary prevention
- tertiary prevention

Learning Objectives

- Define public health, its current and traditional roles.
- Understand the differences among endemic, epidemic, and pandemic diseases.
- Describe the history of pandemics.
- Describe the history of the U.S. public health service.

■ What Is Public Health?

Public health is the term used to describe efforts made by communities to cope with health problems that arise when people live in groups. According to Dr. Winslow (1920), a pioneer in the field, "public health is the science and art of (1) preventing disease, (2) prolonging life, and (3) promoting health and efficiency through organized *community effort*" with the following initiatives (Winslow, 1920, p.30). Early public health strategies employed sanitation techniques to improve environmental conditions. Homeowners used to throw the "night sewage" out of their windows and then sweep it up in the morning. This practice ended once people realized that improper sewage disposal helped to spread disease. Within the last century, sewage treatment plants, drinking water filtration, enforcement of food-handling regulations, and other public health practices have helped to control the spread of disease through the separation of sewage and drinking water.

Later public health practices attempted to control the spread of communicable diseases. Diseases such as measles and scarlet fever used to occur frequently and affect most children. Many children would die or become hospitalized. Today, vaccines for many communicable diseases are required for school-aged children and have nearly eradicated these illnesses so that many fewer cases occur.

Public health officials are also responsible for collecting and analyzing data to determine the epidemiology of diseases. **Epidemiology** is the study of the distribution and determinants of diseases in a population (Coggon, Rose, & Barker, 1997). Public health also includes the education of individuals about personal hygiene. Many public restrooms in food-handling establishments (i.e., restaurants and grocery stores) have signs that require employees to wash their hands before returning to work. This strategy is a type of public health measure. Public health also includes the organization of medical and nursing services for early diagnosis and prevention of diseases. The Association of Schools of Public Health (ASPH), the U.S. Public Health Service, and agencies such as the Centers for Disease Control and Prevention (CDC) provide structure and training for the public health sector. Finally, public health is fostered through the development of social machinery to ensure everyone's health. Some programs can best benefit the public by implementation through social systems. For example, fluoridation of water has significantly reduced the number of dental caries in children. Pasteurization of milk and fortification with vitamins A and D are measures that should improve the health and longevity of the entire population.

Public health is a system designed to use community, state, and health care system resources to assure that conditions exist to promote a healthy society. Public health providers are trained to dispense scientific and technical knowledge to help prevent disease and promote health. Public health has a broad and global focus and includes environmental issues, injury prevention initiatives, screening for chronic diseases, and promotion of maternal and child health.

■ Traditional Aspects of Public Health

Historically, the primary responsibility of public health was the preservation of society and prevention of disease. In the nineteenth century, the rationale for this mission was driven by the fact that health care treatment at the time was hardly effective, while the separation of sewage from drinking water had a far greater impact on health. In fact, surgeons and public health professionals were the most prominent health care providers in the late 1800s and early 1900s.

Throughout history, public health activities directed at the nature, cause, and control or treatment of diseases reflected the state of knowledge at the time. Four tasks have traditionally been the purview of public health officials:

1. Identifying diseases that cause death or disability

2. Learning the causes of diseases and methods of transmission

3. Developing methods to prevent the occurrence of disease or minimize its impact

4. Organizing effective applications of prevention methods (applying this knowledge—for example, cleaning up garbage, making sure people are not bathing in and drinking the same water)

▪ Epidemiological Definitions

Definitions of several epidemiological terms are critical for the study of public health. **Endemic** is the usual, sustained occurrence of a disease in a population. For example, chicken pox had traditionally been endemic in children in the United States. Prior to the approval of the chicken pox vaccine in 1995, many children became ill with chicken pox early in elementary school. Even with the chicken pox vaccine, a small percentage of children still contract chicken pox each year. An **epidemic** is an unusual occurrence of disease in a population. Epidemics peak and ebb over time. Some epidemics have caused large numbers of deaths. Measles, cholera, and certain flu strains have become epidemic throughout the world and throughout history. A **pandemic** is an unusual occurrence of a disease that spreads around the world or in a large geographic area. For example, HIV/AIDS is now pandemic. There have been many pandemics recognized throughout history. Some of the major pandemics since the Peloponnesian War are listed in Figure 6–1.

- 430 B.C.—Peloponnesian War
- 165–180 A.D.—Antonine Plague
- 541 A.D.—Plague of Justinian (www.loyno.edu)
- 1300s—The Black Death
- Cholera (1816–1826) (1829–1851) (1852–1860) (1863–1875) (1899–1923)
- 1918–1919—Spanish Flu
- Modern day—AIDS
- Future—influenza, ebola, SARS, avian flu

Figure 6–1 History of pandemics.
© Cengage Learning 2013

▪ Levels of Public Health Prevention

Vignette

CHOOSING A CAREER IN PUBLIC HEALTH

Debbie is a student in a Master of Public Health (MPH) program. She knows that she wants to be involved in helping people live healthier lives but does not know whether she wants to focus on one specific area or on general disease prevention. Debbie has completed several papers on the Women, Infants and Children (WIC) program and believes that maternal and child health may be an interesting career to pursue, but she does not know what opportunities exist outside of WIC. She is also interested in how diseases spread and how prevalent chronic conditions are in certain populations, so she is considering an MPH in epidemiology. Debbie has a nutrition undergraduate degree and teaches aerobics at the local YMCA, so she is also interested in health promotion. She enrolls a survey class designed to address the areas of public health and decides that a specialization in health promotion would be the best fit for her interests and skills. After graduation, Debbie goes to work for a local not-for-profit health insurer, where she designs health and wellness programs and coordinates health fairs. She is able to use data from the health plan to decide which chronic conditions to target, and she establishes a healthy mother and baby program.

1. Based on your knowledge of the U.S. health care system, does the provision of care focus more on curative care or on primary care?

2. What classes in her master's degree program should Debbie consider to prepare her for working at the not-for-profit health insurer?

3. Based on your current knowledge, which chronic conditions should health insurance plans address to cut health care expenditures and promote healthy living among their members?

4. What types of services should the health plan provide to reach mothers in their market?

5. What stakeholders are potential partners for the health insurance plan in reaching mothers in the local market to promote healthy living?

There are three levels of public health prevention. **Primary prevention** focuses on preventing disease processes from ever getting started. Examples of these public health programs include immunizations, water and air purification, fluoridation of the water supply, and education such as diet and exercise programs. **Secondary prevention** emphasizes the early detection of diseases. Examples of these public health programs include high blood pressure screening, cholesterol screening, Pap smears, and mammograms. **Tertiary prevention** addresses the treatment of diseases once they are present, to avoid further complications. Examples of these programs include cardiac rehabilitation to prevent further heart attacks; stroke rehabilitation to limit permanent disability; disease management of diabetes or congestive heart failure, or treatment and management of HIV to prevent the transition to AIDS.

▪ Public Health Problems

Public health problems are diseases or issues that may be common or even increasing in incidence and prevalence in a community. **Incidence** is the number of new cases of a disease during a stated time. **Prevalence** is the existing number of cases of a disease during a stated time.

A problem may be deemed a public health problem if it involves socioeconomic or other exogenous factors or if it is beyond the individuals' control. A public health problem becomes a public health threat if the outcome of the event is very severe, as in causing death, or may affect many people. The threat can be actual or potential. A problem becomes a public responsibility if or when it is amenable to solution through systematized social action (Verweij & Dawson, 2007). An example of a public health problem amenable to a systematic solution would be the H1N1 vaccination program.

▪ Public Health versus Medical Care

Table 6–1 illustrates the traditional distinction between public health and medical care. The relationship between public health and private medicine should be symbiotic because both should function together for the greater good. In other words, prevention and treatment should complement each other. However, history reveals that this partnership has not always been complementary. Often, public health professionals and clinicians have had a contentious relationship. Those supporting public health programs directed at individuals have argued that any opposition from private practitioners is based on a concern over losing patients and income. On the other hand, some physicians have contended that some public health programs are duplicative of existing programs in the private sector and are an unwarranted intrusion into the doctor–patient relationship. Many clinicians, however, agree with a broader public health role and even receive additional training in public health. Today the roles between public health and medical care often overlap. For example, city health departments operate clinics where care is delivered. On the other hand, some medical care providers, particularly those in managed care arrangements, focus heavily on prevention. In fact, although 10 percent of all health care dollars are spent on health promotion and disease prevention, less than 3 percent of total dollars are spent in the public sector (Beitsch et al., 2006). More funding is devoted to reimbursing medical care providers for delivering preventive care than is spent on public health. This spending imbalance is explained by the fact that prevention is more costly to perform in the medical care sector.

Some private physicians associate public health physicians with government bureaucracy and the intrusion of government in the lives of individuals. Public health historically has been associated with the poor and "welfarism." Also, public health has not been considered as glamorous as medical care because it focuses on basic health monitoring, prevention, and primary care, whereas today much of private practice is devoted to specialization and the use of sophisticated technology.

Table 6–1 Traditional Difference between Public Health and Medical Care

	Public Health	Medical Care
Focus	Industry and environment Healthy individuals Populations Macro	Sick individuals Micro
Orientation	Preventive	Curative
Providers	Health departments	Physicians and hospitals
Sector	Public	Private

© Cengage Learning 2013

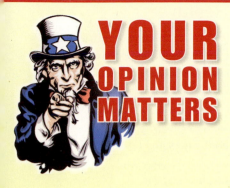

Can Private Clinicians Provide Preventive Care as Well as Public Health Providers Do?

Yes

Primary care clinicians are trained to provide preventive care as well as acute care and chronic disease management. For many preventive care tests, such as Pap smears, mammography, and colonoscopy, medical professionals have training that public health officials do not. They also are more likely to have newer and better technology now that insurance pays for many preventive diagnostic procedures. Primary care clinicians also have personal and continuous relationships with their patients that facilitate the treatment of patients over time and the tracking of when their preventive screenings are due. Clinicians are also able to both treat patients as well as screen for preventive care. The continuity of care that results from their ability to screen, treat, and refer when necessary is an advantage of receiving preventive care from clinicians in the private sector.

No

Clinicians may be able to provide secondary and tertiary preventive services, but their training and practice do not enable them to provide primary preventive care. Most primary preventive care must be provided at the population level. Large numbers of public health and other government officials are charged with maintaining the cleanliness of the water supply, ensuring air quality, keeping and maintaining vital statistics, controlling communicable diseases, and providing health education services. Public health providers are also better able to deliver these services to a large number of women and children through programs such as the Special Supplemental Nutrition Program for Women, Infants and Children (WIC). Private clinicians, with their one-on-one interaction with patients, do not have the time or the ability to reach people on a large scale. Public health professionals are trained to do so. Public health professionals can also provide screenings, immunizations, and other preventive measures at a much lower cost than private clinicians. Now that insurance covers many of these tests, the costs have increased in the private sector. Public health officials should be responsible for providing all primary and noninvasive secondary preventive services, which would result in more people being screened and lower costs to the health care system.

You decide:

1. Which health professional is best trained to provide primary preventive care?

2. If public health professionals are best trained to deliver primary prevention and receive funding to do so, then should they be held accoutable for the health of the population?

3. Can primary care providers who are trained to treat the individual address the problems of the population as a whole?

Evaluating Performance in Medical Care versus Public Health

There is a difference between the methods used to evaluate performance from a medical care as opposed to a public health perspective. The medical care perspective focuses on those who present for treatment, using those receiving good care in the numerator and all who sought care in the denominator. The public health focus is on those who receive care versus those who need the care.

$$\text{Performance in Medical Care} = \frac{\text{Those who received "good" care}}{\text{Those who sought care}}$$

$$\text{Performance in Public Health} = \frac{\text{Those who received care}}{\text{Those who need care}}$$

Approximately 10 percent of premature deaths are preventable with medical treatment alone, whereas 70 percent of premature deaths are preventable through population-wide public health approaches (DHHS, 2003). For example, smoking prevention and cessation programs have much greater potential for preventing lung cancer than medical treatment. Moreover, one of the best strategies to prevent contracting rabies is not by vaccinating people, but rather by vaccinating pets and thus creating a barrier between the common carriers of the disease and humans.

What Justifies the Federal Government's Involvement in Public Health?

The U.S. Constitution makes no reference to a federal or state role in the delivery of health care. Public health intervention derives its basis from the interpretation of the General Welfare Provision in the Preamble to the Constitution and the Interstate Commerce Clause. The General Welfare Provision of the Preamble to the Constitution says, "To promote the general welfare of its citizens …," which has been interpreted to include health care. The Interstate Commerce Clause is used as rationale for the federal government to regulate entities and processes that cross state boundaries such as air, water, and sanitation.

The Government's Role in Public Health

The government's role in public health historically has been critical to the viability of public health interventions. The federal government's primary role has been to fund public health strategies. The Department of Health and Human Services (DHHS) does not dictate the exact public health intervention or strategy that must be implemented, but rather influences what strategies are deployed through the control of funds distributed to state and local governments. However, the federal government does have some direct control over environmental issues through the Environmental Protection Agency (EPA).

State governments also assume a funding role. States often match federal dollars and disperse these total funds to local areas to implement public health services. State governments set public health standards and regulations. Local governments have traditionally played the "hands on" public health role. Local health departments interact directly with its citizens at the county, city, town, borough, and village levels.

History of Public Health

Before modern technology, much of what we knew about our environment came from what we could observe with our five senses. Thus, doctors knew that the urine of individuals with diabetes mellitus (which means "sweet urine") was in fact sweet because of its taste. The development of the microscope allowed scientists to study infectious diseases and observe the organisms responsible for their cause.

Public health strategies and interventions date as far back as early civilization. One distinctive feature about public health is that its efforts can have remarkable success, even when the exact root cause of a problem is unknown. Ancient civilizations such as the Minoans, Myceneans, and Egyptians used drainage and toilet systems thousands of years before the "germ theory" was postulated. The Romans were able to prevent many cases of malaria by teaching about the evil spirits ("miasmas") that lived around the swamps, without the knowledge that microscopic protozoa carried by mosquitoes were the root cause of the disease. Similarly, ancient Romans associated health with cleanliness and built aqueducts for clean water, sewers for waste disposal, and public baths (Pickett & Hanlon, 1990). Harmful behaviors have also been targeted by public health interventions for centuries. Ancient Grecians promoted exercise and healthy diets as well as cleanliness (Pickett & Hanlon, 1990). Since the 1600s, long before modern research demonstrated causality, many have known that smoking tabacco was a health hazard. The hazardous effects could be avoided simply by not using tobacco products.

▪ Major Highlights of Public Health in America

1639: First U.S. public health law

This first public health law, enacted in Massachusetts, required all births and deaths to be recorded (Public Health Museum in Massachusetts, n.d.).

1798: Marine Hospital Service

President John Adams signed into law an act providing for the care and relief of sick and disabled seamen. Such a law was enacted because healthy sailors were a valuable commodity to the shipping industry, and port cities did not want diseases contracted by sailors elsewhere spreading through their communities. The responsibility for the health of sailors fell under federal jurisdiction because port cities were responsible primarily for the health of their own citizens and not citizens of other cities.

1862: Founding of the Bureau of Chemistry in the Department of Agriculture

This organization was the forerunner of the Food and Drug Administration.

1865: Shattuck Report

Published by the New York City Council of Hygiene and Public Health, this report exposed the unsanitary conditions in the city and led to passage of a public health law that created a city board of health. This law was the first to create an administrative structure for local public health affairs.

1870: Marine Hospital Service

The Marine Hospital Service was reorganized as the national hospital system. The surgeon in charge was later given the title of Surgeon General. In 1902, the name changed to the Public Health and Marine Hospital Service, and in 1912 the name was again changed to The United States Public Health Service, which still exists today.

1887: First public laboratory for studying disease opened in Staten Island, N.Y.

This laboratory was the precursor to the National Institutes of Health.

1930: Creation of the National Institutes of Health
1933: Federal Emergency Relief Act

States and local governments were limited in their power to raise revenues from state and local taxes. This act provided federal aid to the states and authorized general medical care for acute and chronic illness, obstetrical services, emergency dental extractions, bedside nursing, drugs, and medical supplies. Not all states participated.

1935: Social Security Act of 1935

This act gave the Public Health Service the authority to assist states, counties and health districts to maintain public health services.

1939: Creation of the Federal Health Agency

President Roosevelt joined health, welfare, and education service programs to form a federal health agency. Public Health was removed from the Treasury Department, and a Federal Security Agency was created (health, education, and welfare services were consolidated).

1945: Emerson Report

According to the Emerson Report, there are six tasks of public health, which still prevail today (Turnock & Barnes, 2007):

1. Vital statistics—identifying problems and trends in births, deaths, marriages, divorces, morbidity, and other statistics.

2. Communicable disease control—establishing immunization programs, requirements for school entry, behavior modification strategies, and administering of CDC reportable disease programs.

3. Sanitation—ensuring the proper disposal of sewage and the purity of water, air, and food.

4. Laboratory services—testing water, air, and food quality; testing for diseases or pathogens with potential public health consequences.

5. Maternal and child health—ensuring appropriate prenatal care, nutrition for newborns, well baby care, and immunizations.

6. Health education—providing information about obtaining services; counseling for nutrition, smoking dangers/cessation, personal hygiene, and exercise.

(One additional task not included in this list is providing some outpatient care to poor people in clinics.)

1946: Federal Security Agency adds other public health agencies

The Federal Security Agency added the Children's Bureau and The Food and Drug Administration.

1946: Founding of the Centers for Disease Control and Prevention

Originally, this organization was named the Communicable Disease Center.

1953: Creation of the Department of Health, Education and Welfare

President Eisenhower created the Department of Health, Education and Welfare (HEW) as a cabinet-level position.

1964: First Surgeon General's Report on Smoking and Health published

1970: National Health Service Corps formed

Congress and the president established the National Health Service Corps to help offset the maldistribution of providers by financially rewarding prospective clinicians for their willingness to practice in needy areas.

1980: Department of Health and Human Services formed

After education was separated into its own cabinet-level department, HEW became the Department of Health and Human Services (DHHS, 2010a).

Public Health Agencies

Some notable public health agencies include the Department of Health and Human Services (DHHS), which encompasses the National Institutes of Health (NIH), Centers for Disease Control and Prevention (CDC), and Food and Drug Administration (FDA) (the agencies of the DHHS are listed in Figure 6–2), state departments of health, World Health Organization (WHO—part of the United Nations), Environmental Protection Agency (EPA), and many others.

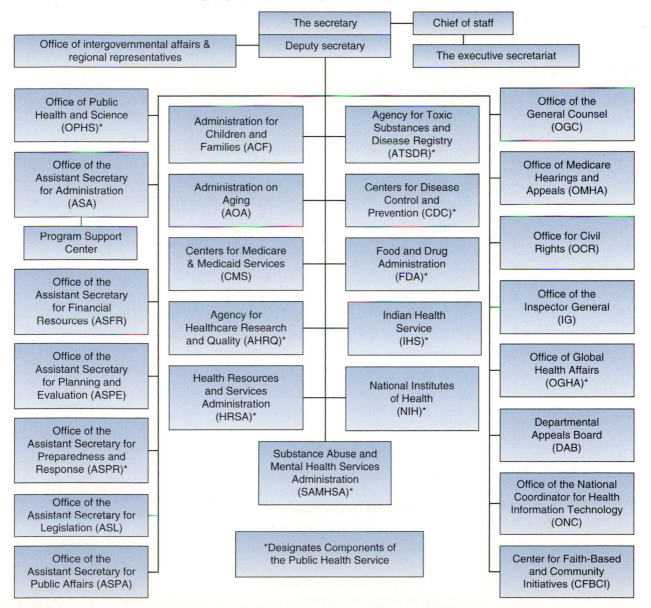

Figure 6–2 Agencies within the Department of Health and Human Services (DHHS)

Source: U.S. Department of Health and Human Services. Organizational Chart. (2010b). Retrieved September 2, 2011, from www.hhs.gov/about/orgchart/.

Review Questions

1. Define *public health* in your own words.

2. What are the roles of public health?

3. Explain the traditional aspects of public health.

4. Explain the terms *endemic, epidemic*, and *pandemic*, and give examples of each.

5. Explain the terms *primary, secondary*, and *tertiary prevention*, and give examples of each.

6. What are the differences between public health and medical care?

7. What are the state and federal government's roles in public health?

8. What do you believe are the major achievements in modern public health programs?

Additional Resources

Centers for Disease Control and Prevention (CDC) www.cdc.gov/.

Department of Health and Human Services (DHHS) www.hhs.gov/.

Environmental Protection Agency (EPA) www.epa.gov/.

Food and Drug Administration (FDA) www.fda.gov/.

National Center for Health Statistics (NCHS) www.cdc.gov/nchs.

National Institutes of Health (NIH) www.nih.gov/.

World Health Organization (WHO) www.who.org.

References

Beitsch, L. M., Brooks, R. G., Menachemi, N., & Libbey, P. M. (2006). Public health at center stage: New roles, old props. *Health Affairs, 25*(4), 911–922.

Coggon, D., Rose, G., & Barker, D. J. P. (1997). *Epidemiology for the uninitiated*, 4th ed. London: BMJ Publishing Group.

Pickett, G., & Hanlon, J. J. (1990). *Public health: Administration and practice*, 9th ed. St. Louis, MO: Times Mirror/Mosby College Publishing.

Public Health Museum in Massachusetts. (n.d.). Public health milestones in Massachusetts. Retrieved July 19, 2010, from www.publichealthmuseum.org/Milestones%20in%20Public%20Health.pdf.

Turnock, B. J., & Barnes, P. A. (2007). History will be kind. *Journal of Public Health Management and Practice, 13*(4), 337–341, 310.

U.S. Department of Health and Human Services (DHHS). (2003). *The power of prevention: Reducing the health and economic burden of chronic disease*. Washington, DC: Author.

U.S. Department of Health and Human Services (DHHS). (2010a). Historical highlights. Retrieved July 9, 2010, from www.hhs.gov/about/hhshist.html.

U.S. Department of Health and Human Services (DHHS). Organizational chart. (2010b). Retrieved September 2, 2011, from www.hhs.gov/about/orgchart/.

Verweij, M., & Dawson, A. (2007). The meaning of "public" in "public health." In A. Dawson & M. Verweij (eds.), *Ethics, prevention, and public health*. New York: Oxford University Press, Inc.

Winslow, C. E. (1920). The untilled fields of public health. *Science, 51*(1306), 23–33.

Long-Term Care

Written by Dr. Andrea S. Yesalis

Key Terms

acute care

adult day care

case management

chronic disease

continuing care retirement community (CCRC)

continuum of care

informal caregiver

palliative care

Program of All-Inclusive Care for the Elderly (PACE)

rehabilitation

residential care facilities

respite care

senior center

Learning Objectives

- Describe the domain of long-term care (LTC).

- Describe demographic and epidemiologic factors that will influence the demand for various LTC services.

- Identify institutional and community-based LTC providers.

- Describe the characteristics of the typical LTC recipient.

- Describe the regulatory environment of LTC facilities.

- Identify the reimbursement sources for LTC.

- Understand the main challenges for the LTC Industry.

- Describe typical mental health or disabled patients and their various sources of care.

- Describe key legal issues in LTC.

■ The Domain of Long-Term Care

Long-term care (LTC) encompasses a wide range of health care, as well as social and residential services, provided to people who have lost or never developed the capacity to care for themselves independently as a result of chronic illness or mental or physical disability. The main types of facilities that provide LTC and will be discussed in this chapter are nursing homes or skilled nursing facilities (SNFs), assisted living facilities (ALFs) or personal care homes (PCHs), and continuing care retirement communities (CCRCs). The main types of organizations that deliver LTC services are home health agencies (HHAs) and hospices.

Long-term care is more than just medical care and nursing care. It includes assistance needed for chronic illness or disability that leaves patients unable to care for themselves for an extended period of time (American Association of Health Plans, 2010).

According to the National Health Interview Survey of the National Center for Health Statistics a **chronic disease** is defined as a condition lasting 3 months or longer (CDC, 2009b). Many of the prevalent illnesses associated with aging, such as Alzheimer's disease and cardiac disease, are considered chronic—that is, they are incurable, albeit manageable and evolving, conditions. Once diagnosed, persons have these diseases until the end of their lives. Certain forms of cancer are now considered chronic illnesses; patients can be treated, but they will likely relapse.

LTC aids persons who do not necessarily need medical care but who do need assistance in order to survive. For example, although people with Alzheimer's may be physically healthy in regard to heart function and stamina, as their neurological disease progresses, they lose the ability to take care of themselves because of cognitive deficits. They may forget to eat and drink, or wander outside and become lost in the cold, or start a house fire when cooking or smoking. Physically, they may still be able to play tennis, but mentally they are disabled and in need of permanent assistance, usually in a special care dementia unit of a nursing home or assisted living facility. This type of care is discussed in more detail later in the chapter.

The goals of LTC are (1) to promote and maintain health and independence in functional abilities and to obtain optimal quality of life in individuals with decreased physical and or mental functioning; and (2) to help individuals with terminal illnesses to die in peace and with dignity. As an example, such care would include palliative care or hospice for the terminally ill, which can continue for months and years at times.

In contrast to **acute care**, which is hospital or clinic-based care for brief conditions, LTC is for the long haul. The recipient of LTC is referred to as a resident rather than a patient. Much of LTC care is given in a residence or a facility. Although acute care is crisis oriented and acute illnesses have a sudden onset, LTC focuses on managing conditions that often have a gradual onset. In contrast to acute care, LTC tends to use limited technology, focuses on nursing management, as opposed to medical treatment, and has a relatively long or indefinite duration. Acute care relies on sophisticated health care technology, and the duration of illness is usually short. The ICU, or intensive care unit, is an example of a setting where acute care is delivered. Whereas acute illnesses frequently respond to treatment, chronic illnesses and disabilities cannot be cured, but rehabilitation or optimization of function is considered possible. However, even persons who have hospice or palliative care may benefit from rehabilitation treatment modalities, such as physical, occupational, or speech therapy that can help with swallowing disorders often experienced by persons with certain chronic conditions. Just because a person is receiving LTC does not mean he or she cannot receive other treatment modalities. A key distinction between acute care and LTC is that acute care attempts to restore health or cure, whereas long-term care attempts to maintain health or slow the decline of functional abilities.

Persons receiving LTC may need acute care at certain times. For example, a person with Alzheimer's may suffer a hip fracture, pneumonia, or a heart attack and need to be hospitalized. Acute and sub-acute care, at the left side of the continuum (see Figure 7.1), focus on restoring health and include more skilled and technical care as well as rehabilitative services. A person recovering from a hip fracture, for example, will be discharged from the hospital usually after 3 to 4 days and sent to a rehabilitation facility, often part of a nursing home, for 1 to 2 months or however long it takes to regain the functional ability to return home and live independently again. However, a hip fracture or other significant negative health event can signal the initiation of permanent LTC, meaning that many people sent to rehabilitation never return home. It is very difficult for many older adults to accept the fact that they can no longer manage their home and live independently.

For many adult children, an acute hospitalization is often the opportunity to move parents into a safer environment such as an assisted living facility (ALF). The alternative to this environment is home health care from a home health agency (HHA). This service is covered after a hospital stay of 3 or more days, under Medicare Part A. It is also covered under Medicare B without a prior hospital stay (discussed in detail later). Home health services such as companion, custodial, and housekeeping can also be purchased out of pocket. Unfortunately, physicians must order these services if insurance coverage is needed, and many physicians are unaware of the benefits of these services. In addition, family members are often unaware of them, so many older adults who need assistance go to facilities rather than remaining in their home with necessary home health services.

The middle of the continuum of care includes nursing homes, assisted living facilities, adult day care, and home health care. Here the emphasis shifts toward maintaining health and functional abilities. The type of care provided tends to be less skilled and focuses on personal care. At the right end of the LTC continuum, the focus is on palliative care, which is provided through hospice programs. **Palliative care** provides care to individuals with a chronic incurable or terminal illness, and the focus is on ensuring that the end of life is filled with dignity and as little pain as possible.

The position statement of the American Academy of Hospice and Palliative Medicine (www.aahpm.org) reads:

> The goal of palliative care is to prevent and relieve suffering, and to support the best possible quality of life for patients and their families, regardless of their stage of disease or the need for other therapies, in accordance with their values and preferences. Palliative care is both a philosophy of care and an organized, highly structured system for delivering care. Palliative care expands traditional disease-model medical treatments to include the goals of enhancing quality of life for patient and family, optimizing function, and helping with decision-making and providing opportunities for personal growth. As such, it can be delivered concurrently with life-prolonging care or as the main focus of care.

Approximately 80 percent of elderly or disabled receive their LTC informally from friends and family. These family members and friends are referred to as **informal caregivers**, whereas those persons who work in nursing homes and other facilities and receive pay for their labor are referred to as "formal," or paid, caregivers. The Administration on Aging estimates that the economic value of our nation's informal caregivers exceeds $306 billion annually. Spector (2000) estimated that there are over 5.9 million informal caregivers of older adults (persons over age 65). The National Center on Caregiving, part of the Family Caregiver Alliance, has a wealth of statistics and helpful information for family or informal caregivers (www.caregiver.org/).

The continuum (Figure 7–1) measures service intensity on a spectrum from curative to palliative care. It does not reflect the pattern of any one individual's health care utilization trajectory. Some people may use no services other than palliative care at the end of their lives, whereas others may spend the majority of their aging in a nursing home or other facility. Other people may alternate between acute care and home health care. In fact, in our culture, where the emphasis is on avoidance of death and on

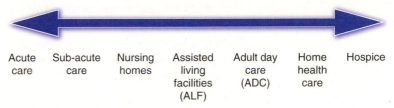

Figure 7–1 Long-term care continuum.
© Cengage Learning 2013

cure, numerous studies have found that most people wait too long to use hospice and palliative care services.

Physicians or other providers must order these services. Again, the main rate-limiting factor in utilization of these services is often the physician's and other providers' lack of knowledge of them. As a reflection of this lack of knowledge, the average length of hospice care is 2 months, whereas many patients would have benefitted from an earlier referral (NHPCO, 2005).

Demographic and Epidemiologic Factors That Influence Demand for LTC

Long-term care services can be provided to patients of any age and may be the result of diseases, disabling chronic conditions, accidents, or developmental disabilities (Tumlinson, Woods, & Avalere Health LLC, 2007). The elderly, the disabled, and the mentally ill primarily utilize services. Of these groups, the elderly are the largest consumers of LTC. For example, older adults may suffer a stroke that damages their ability to speak and to walk. These persons will need rehabilitation therapies such as speech, physical, and occupational therapy. They may also need what is called skilled nursing care for wounds and medications or cardiac monitoring. Skilled care can be provided by licensed skilled nursing facilities (SNFs), independent rehabilitation facilities, or home health agencies (HHAs).

In contrast, older adults who suffer from Alzheimer's disease and are unable to care for themselves, requiring ongoing assistance with dressing, bathing, and eating, need nonskilled, or "custodial," care. LTC takes many forms such as skilled nursing care in a nursing home or custodial care in an assisted living facility or nursing home with a special care unit (SCU) for dementia.

The need for LTC may result from chronic medical conditions such as diabetes, heart disease, pulmonary disease, or cancer. These conditions can lead to disability in mobility, endurance, sensory capacity, and cognition. Mobility limitations can also arise from arthritis, paralysis, and physical trauma. Asthma is a chronic pulmonary condition that decreases functional capacity and endurance. Persons with asthma may have full physical capacity for mobility, but their oxygen restriction has confined them to a wheelchair, and they lack the energy in some cases to even feed or dress themselves. Sensory disability includes blindness, hearing impairment, and communication disorders. Cognitive disability includes mental retardation and dementias or other cognitive impairment. The number of people with disabling chronic conditions is expected to increase because the prevalence of these conditions increases with age.

Most LTC patients are age 65 and over; however, almost 40 percent are under 65 years old (Tumlinson et al., 2007). The number of people needing LTC is expected to triple in the next 30 years, spurred by the growth in the aging population, increases in life expectancy, and increases in chronic illness with resultant disability. Advancement in health care technology and the emphasis on prevention have led to a longer life span and have resulted in individuals over 85 years of age becoming the fastest growing subset of the U.S. population. Roughly 19 percent of Americans aged 65 and older experience some degree of chronic physical illness. Among those who are 85 or older, 55 percent are impaired and require long-term care. By 2020, approximately 12 million older Americans are expected to need long-term care (American Association of Health Plans, 2010).

Chronic illnesses such as multiple sclerosis, paralysis, stroke, AIDS, birth defects, and accidents causing disability have increased the need and demand for LTC. The severely mentally ill of all ages require LTC. The majority of LTC users require assistance with three or more activities of daily living (ADL).

Consumers of LTC have chronic, complex health problems and functional disabilities. The criteria used to evaluate the need for care and to qualify for certain reimbursements includes whether an individual can perform activities of daily living (ADLs) and instrumental activities of daily living (IADLs). ADLs are the most basic tasks performed throughout the day and measure dependence on others for assistance with personal care functions. Examples of ADLs include bathing, dressing, eating, walking and mobility (which includes transferring from bed to wheelchair or from toilet to wheelchair), and toileting. IADLs measure a person's ability to perform household and social tasks. Examples of IADLs include preparing meals, heavy and light housework, using the telephone, managing finances, and shopping. The need for help with ADLs and IADLs increases with age.

Patients are prescribed LTC services based on the assistance that they require to perform ADLS and IADLS as well as the degree of "skilled" care they may need. Ratings on ADL and IADL scales are used as admission criteria to assisted living facilities as well as eligibility requirements for LTC insurance coverage. Naturally, otherwise healthy persons with dementia or Alzheimer's can usually physically perform all the ADLs. However, they forget to perform them and need prompting, which qualifies them as eligible for LTC. They lose ability to perform IADLs early on in their disease.

It would be helpful to clarify the main terms used for the cognitive problems seen in LTC. The majority of cognitive problems are dementias. Dementia is an umbrella term used to describe persons with memory and other cognitive deficits, including impaired language, emotional control, and reasoning or judgment abilities. These impairments usually progress over time to include motor losses such as decreased ability to walk and talk. Dementia is an umbrella term for memory loss and not a medical diagnosis. There are over 13 types of dementia, which represent specific medical diagnoses such as Alzheimer's, Parkinson's, Pick's or Lewy body dementia, and vascular dementia from stroke, as well as dementias related to HIV and alcoholism and those related to nutritional deficits and trauma.

The nosology, or classification, of dementia is constantly being revised. The DSM IV, or *Diagnostic and Statistical Manual of Mental Disorders*, published by the American Psychiatric Association (APA), is currently in its fourth edition. It is important to distinguish between delirium, which is cognitive impairment that is temporary and related to anesthesia, fever, and infection, versus dementia that is permanent cognitive impairment. The other main forms of cognitive impairment include congenital mental retardation and decreased cognitive ability due to trauma such as closed head injuries. The main dementias seen in LTC are Alzheimer's and the vascular dementias.

Institutional and Community-Based LTC Providers

Informal caregivers provide most LTC at home. The informal LTC system represents the care provided by family, friends, and relatives. Informal caregivers provide the majority of all LTC. Most informal caregivers are either spouses or a child of the person requiring the care. Among children, daughters and daughters-in-law provide the majority of care, at times relinquishing paid jobs in order to care for an aging family member.

The system of formal care includes institutional- and community-based services. Institutional-based services include skilled nursing facilities (SNFs); assisted living facilities (ALFs), also referred to as personal care homes (PCHs); and continuing care retirement communities (CCRCs). A home health agency (HHA) may provide community-based services in the home. Alternatively, services may be provided by local organizations such as adult day care centers that may be part of a SNF or ALF. A hospice may be either part of a hospital, SNF, or HHA, or it may be an independent organization. Hospice may provide services to patients at home or to patients in other SNFs or ALFs. Some hospitals with low occupancy have turned over some of their floor space to the creation of SNFs or rehabilitation services (Paone & Mullen, 2005).

Many patients will use a combination of care provided informally in their home and formal care with home care, adult day care, or brief admissions to SNFs. Typically, the mix of services utilized is determined by personal preferences and knowledge, availability of local services, and finances or resources to cover the services (Tumlinson et al., 2007).

Nursing Homes, or Skilled Nursing Facilities (SNFs)

Nursing homes, or skilled nursing facilities (SNFs), are an integral component of long-term care services (LTC). Nursing home admissions may be permanent or short term for **rehabilitation** (often referred to as post-acute care). Medicare covers 100 days of rehabilitation after a minimum 3-day hospital stay. A permanent nursing home admission is usually for permanent physical disability or loss of ADL functioning or for cognitive impairment. Persons are also admitted for hospice care at end of life.

Many nursing homes have a special care unit (SCU) for patients with Alzheimer's or other dementias. This facility is a locked unit that is designed to provide safety and security as well as recreation therapy. Demand for both permanent and long-term care has increased and is predicted to increase further as the baby boomers age. SNFs also provide technical care for persons needing ventilators or infusion therapy. A challenging younger group of long-term care residents is composed of persons too obese for gastric bypass surgery and who require ventilators to breathe due to their obesity. LTC residents are provided social services, counseling, dental care, podiatry services, pastoral care, and nutritional counseling (Evashwick, 2005).

Approximately 61.5 percent of nursing homes are proprietary, or for-profit, and are certified by both Medicare and Medicaid (NCHS, 2009). Most nursing homes are located in urban areas, in the Midwest, and in the South (NCHS, 2009). The average nursing home has approximately 100 beds.

Nursing homes are expanding their diversity of services to provide care for patients requiring adult day care, outpatient rehabilitation, and assisted living services (Evashwick, 2005). The trend in nursing home care is the provision of care for patients who are sicker, who have more dependence on care providers, (i.e., are more disabled), and who have a greater number of comorbidities.

The majority of nursing homes are overseen by licensed health care providers *and* are considered skilled nursing facilities (SNFs). But SNFs can also be comprised of 20 beds in a community hospital, a large facility owned by a corporation, or a 1,000-bed government operated institution (Paone & Mullen, 2005).

One of the core requirements for nursing homes is that they be licensed by the state. The home may be certified by both Medicare and Medicaid or by neither. Certified beds meet the criteria for reimbursement from Medicare and Medicaid for the care delivered to patients.

There are approximately 16,000 nursing homes and an average occupancy rate of 86 percent (CDC, 2009). Overall, the number of beds has been decreasing, but the average size of nursing homes has been increasing (CDC, 2009). From 2002 through 2007, the number of nursing home beds decreased from 1.875 million to 1.855 million (California Health Care Foundation, 2009).

Nursing homes come in all shapes and sizes. They may be freestanding facilities, located within a hospital, or part of continuous care retirement communities. (CDC, 2009). Providers such as hospitals, health systems, and other nursing home corporations have been purchasing and operating nursing home facilities. Finally, the demand for high-quality nursing home care is strong. Historically, abuses of this vulnerable population led to increased legislation and regulation. Currently, the federal government is undertaking several nursing home quality initiatives, including Medicare's Nursing Home Compare and Nursing Home Quality Initiative to mandate staffing ratios and monitor adverse events. Nursing homes are financially penalized for poor quality now.

■ Residential Care Facilities: Assisted Living Facilities (ALFs) or Personal Care Homes (PCHs) and Continuing Care Retirement Communities (CCRCs)

Residential care facilities refer to a category of facilities that are designed for residents who need minimal assistance with ADLs or who are in the early stages of dementia. In different parts of the country, these facilities may be referred to as ALFs or PCHs. They may still be referred to as board and care homes or rest homes in certain parts of the country. The regulations for these types of facilities are continuing to evolve, and an increasing number of states require certification and licensure for the managers of these facilities as well as for the facilities themselves. They are now part of the regulatory purview. In general, the cost of ALFs is paid for out of pocket. However, LTC insurance is becoming an increasing important payor for these services, although it is currently a small percentage overall (California Advocates for Nursing Home Reform, 2010). Medicare does not cover ALF care as it is not "skilled" care.

The costs of ALFs vary depending on the services provided for the resident. Typically, there is a base rate for a bundle of basic services provided for the resident. As services are added, the cost increases. In 2009, the monthly costs varied from roughly $2,700 as a basic rate to $3,500 for an all-inclusive package of services (Metlife Mature Market Institute, 2009).

Continuing care retirement communities (CCRCs) are unique entities that combine the insurance function with the residence and health provision. Both the state insurance board and the Board of Health must license these facilities, or campuses. In order to move into a CCRC, residents must pay a large entrance fee, which will then ensure that they will be taken care of as their needs evolve. The one-time entrance fee ranges from $60,000 to $120,000 on average (Metlife Mature Market Institute, 2009).

CCRCs provide an alternative to home care. When persons first enter a CCRC, they are at the level of independent living and may reside in a small home or condominium on the campus. In addition to the one-time entrance fee, residents pay a monthly fee, which varies depending on the level of services that are required. Usually, 1–3 meals per day are provided in a congregate dining hall (LeadingAge, 2011). Such services as light housekeeping, medication supervision, and personal care assistance with basic activities like hygiene, dressing, eating, bathing and transferring may be purchased as the need arises (California Advocates for Nursing Home Reform, 2010). As the individual's care needs progress, they can move into an ALF or SNF (with a rehab unit) on campus. CCRCs compete with each other to market their services to healthy, wealthy older adults. They offer educational programs, wellness and exercise facilities, computer rooms, field trips, and transportation services.

Medicare covers only the skilled nursing care provided in CCRCs, which is only a small part of the services received by residents. CCRCs are also a form of LTC insurance. Once individuals buy into a plan and secure a residence on the campus, their care will be provided for on the campus. If they need acute hospitalization and then rehab, Medicare will cover it. If they need to be moved to a SCU, the entrance fee will entitle them to those services. Individuals usually enter a CCRC when they need little or no assistance. The disadvantage of CCRCs is that the cost to buy into them is often very high and not affordable by all who would benefit. Many church organizations are starting CCRCs to provide this option at a more affordable cost.

▪ Rehabilitation Care

Rehabilitation, sub-acute, or post-acute care can be provided in different settings such as inpatient facilities, outpatient facilities, or in the patient's home. This type of care follows an acute illness such as a stroke or injury such as a hip fracture or total knee replacement. The goal is optimization of function, maintenance of health, or slowing the decline of the patient's health. Rehabilitation care can also be used to treat drug and alcohol addictions.

▪ Home Health Agencies

Home-based care is nursing, physical, occupational, and speech-language therapy, and other supportive services provided to patients in their own residences. Supportive services include companionship, assistance with ADLs, transportation, and light housekeeping. To receive home health care, patients must be "homebound" (meaning that they are physically unable to tolerate activity other than going out for doctor's office visits and an occasional trip to church); but within the home, they are capable of basic ADLs or just need assistance on an intermittent basis. Being homebound and needing skilled but intermittent care are the crucial qualifiers.

Home health care is the fastest growing segment in the health care industry. From 2003 through 2007, home health agencies increased by approximately 2,000 in the United States (California Health Care Foundation, 2009). Several factors contributed to this increase: The growth in the elderly population has increased demand for home health care; individuals prefer to remain in their homes whenever possible; and the number of informal caregivers has declined because of smaller families and more women working outside their homes.

Home health care is considered to be a cost-effective alternative to institution-based care. Technological advancements have enabled more diseases to be treated at home. Finally, changes in Medicare and Medicaid reimbursement led to expanded coverage for home health care.

▪ Adult Day Care

Some people who require LTC and who live at home or with family take advantage of services offered at **adult day care** centers. Adult day care can follow either a social or medical model, or be a combination model. The social model includes social activities and custodial care provided in **senior centers**. Medical model adult day care provides medical care and rehabilitation. Some adult day care programs provide both social and medical components.

The goals of adult day care are to prevent premature or inappropriate institution-alization and to provide respite care for informal caregivers. Most of the reimburse-ment for these services is through private pay or charitable or religious organizations. Medicare does not cover adult day care. Medicaid will only provide reimbursement for the medical model programs if the patient meets income eligibility criteria. The cost for adult day care services is about $56 per day, and many programs are not profitable (Tumlinson et al., 2007). Usually, a van or shuttle comes to the patient's home to pick up and drop off the patient.

▪ Hospice Care

Hospice care is typically provided in a person's own home when he or she is facing a life-limiting illness or injury, but hospice services can *also* be provided in SNFs and ALFs. Hospice services focus on supporting the primary family caregiver by manag-ing patient pain, providing drugs and supplies, and assisting the patient with many aspects of dying (Tumlinson et al., 2007). The goal of hospice is to improve quality of life and provide comfort. The focus is on relieving the symptoms of disease and pro-viding comfort and pain relief, but not attempting to cure. This type of care is known as palliative care.

Hospice also provides physical, psychological, emotional, social, and spiri-tual care for dying or terminally ill persons, their families, and other loved ones, including grief counseling and bereavement support. Physicians, nurses, home care aides, social workers, chaplains, therapists, and counselors work together as interdisciplinary teams to coordinate individualized plans of care for each patient and family (Hospice Facts, 2009). Overseeing all patient care is the hospice medical director, who may also serve as the attending physician for the patient (Naierman & Turner, 2010).

Historically, the majority of hospice patients have a primary diagnosis of cancer, but other diagnoses, including disorders related to normal aging such as debility, are increasingly being utilized by providers to obtain palliative care at end of life for their patients. Cancer, HIV/AIDS, and the end stages of emphysema, Alzheimer's, cardiovascular, and neuromuscular diseases are common conditions benefiting from hospice care (Naierman & Turner, 2010). Hospice care is provided to patients of all ages, and 20 percent of hospice patients are under the age of 65 (Naierman & Turner, 2010).

The average number of days that a patient receives care in a hospice ranges from 69.0 days in a freestanding facility to 53.6 days in a home-health agency based service (Hospice Facts, 2009).

From 1984 to 2009, Medicare-certified hospices increased from 31 to 3,346, a nearly 108-fold increase (Hospice Facts, 2009). Most hospices are freestanding; others are home health agency based, hospital based, or skilled nursing facility based. Many other hospice services are not Medicare-certified, but are staffed by volunteers who provide care for hospice patients.

Much of the growth in hospice care can be attributed to cost savings associated with providing efficient end-of-life care for patients in their own home, surrounded by loved ones. Hospice is a cost-effective service when compared to the inpatient costs of hospitals and skilled nursing facilities. Hospice charges per day are substantially lower than hospitals and skilled nursing facilities (Hospice Facts, 2009). Substantial cost savings for cancer patients receiving hospice during the last days of life care have been consistently shown.

Additional cost savings could be realized by patients who delay entering hospice care until they are just within a few days or weeks of dying. There is a strong reluctance among caregivers, patients, and their families to transfer a patient to hospice care as it is an acceptance of the inevitability of the patient's death (Hospice Facts, 2009). Most caregivers in the health care system are trained to treat and cure a patient with the goal being full recovery.

It has been estimated that 70 percent of terminal patients could benefit from hospice care, yet on average relatively few of those persons receive hospice care prior to their deaths (Paul et al., 2005). Hospice care is intended to alleviate some of the distress that patients typically face at the end of life (National Association of Homecare and Hospice, 2010). Hospice care allows patients and their families to remain together in familiar surroundings in the comfort and dignity of their homes. In addition, hospice care allows family members to take an active role in providing or complementing care by trained caregivers.

Trends indicate that hospice is growing as an attractive alternative to facing death in a clinical setting (National Association of Homecare and Hospice, 2010). It is recommended that more patients and families learn about its many benefits to plan ahead for end-of-life decisions. Unless physicians, nurses and families become more comfortable discussing death and the dying process, hospice will remain an under-used option for services during an extremely difficult time (Hospice Facts, 2009).

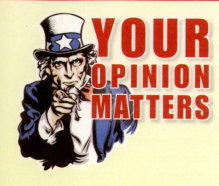

For-Profit Hospice Companies: Do They Focus on the Patient's Best Interest?

Background

Hospice services were added as an LTC benefit to Medicare in 1983 to control Medicare costs and to offer patients an alternative to inpatient care at the end of life. Patients prefer receiving care in their own home, surrounded by family and loved ones, and costs are contained by providing palliative care for patients. The hospice benefit is available for patients who have a life expectancy of 6 months or less and who relinquish Medicare reimbursement for curative treatment of their illness (Medicare Payment Advisory Commission, 2009). The Medicare beneficiary may receive a wide array of services, including social work services and pain and symptom management at minimal cost (Medicare Payment Advisory Commission, 2009).

Hospice patients suffer from a wide array of conditions, such as cancer, Alzheimer's disease, Parkinson's disease, and congestive heart failure. Medicare spending on hospice has quadrupled from $2.9 billion in 2000 to $11 billion in 2008 (Medicare Payment Advisory Commission, 2010). The number of patients taking advantage of the hospice benefit has increased dramatically as has their length of stay (Medicare Payment Advisory Commission, 2009). Medicare spending on hospice is expected to double over the next decade (Medicare Payment Advisory Commission, 2009).

Reimbursement for hospice care is based on the number of days the patient receives care, not the number of visits made or how severe the condition. Hospice organizations are able to maximize their profits by providing care for as long as possible. This payment scheme raises the concern that hospice organizations may desire to generate additional profits by extending the time they provide care for a hospice patient (Iglehart, 2009).

Recently, the hospice industry has experienced a surge in the number of free-standing hospices that are owned by for-profit companies, including Odyssey, Heartland, Vitas Healthcare Corporation, and VistaCare (McCue & Thompson, 2005). All of these companies have experienced substantial growth since the beginning of the Medicare benefit (McCue & Thompson, 2005).

The average stay of a patient in hospice has been increasing, and there is still a high level of variability in the quantity and quality of services delivered among hospice companies. Most of the care that is provided to hospice patients is not under the direction of the patients' physicians, but rather by the hospice's medical director. The medical director may continue to recertify the patient as eligible for hospice care if the patient's life expectancy remains 6 months or less (Medicare Payment Advisory Commission, 2009).

Yes

The U.S. economy is based on free-market capitalist principles. In such a market, the strongest competitors with the best product or service should profit and grow. Creating this environment means that more patients will seek the highest quality of care at the most successful for-profit hospices.

The for-profit status of the hospice is important because only successful enterprises survive, and such success provides a strong incentive to lure staff who are dedicated and of the highest quality. Thus, successful for-profit hospices will continue to provide the highest quality care by continuing to attract the most effective staff. In a free-market economy, operating profits are generated by increasing census, and hospices will compete based on their popularity. For instance, competition is based on satisfying patients and their families by offering more frequent visits; covering more supplies, equipment, and medications; and providing more services such as massage therapy or home visits from the medical director. For-profit hospices must remain profitable to stay in business, and when competition is present, organizations have incentives to provide higher quality of care.

For-profit hospices must operate more efficiently and effectively because they do not have access to additional funding through grants from sources that exist for their non-profit counterparts. These grants often provide incentives for non-profits to provide services that are not profitable, which often produces organizations that ultimately suffer from inefficiency, top-heavy administration, and resistance to new ideas. Often, these organizations do not survive, thus reducing access to hospice care for the increasing number of patients and families who desire such end-of-life care.

No

For-profit hospices do not focus on the best interests of their patients. In one study assessing the impact of ownership status on care provided to patients, researchers found that patients receiving care from for-profit hospices received a narrower range of services than patients from non-profit hospices (Carlson, Gallo, & Bradley, 2004). The narrower range of services meant that patients with for-profit hospices were not receiving as much counseling services, medications, and personal care (Carlson, Gallo, & Bradley, 2004).

Another study found that for-profit hospices that were publically traded earned substantially higher profits than non-profit hospices (McCue & Thompson, 2005). Specifically, the large publicly traded hospices enjoyed profit margins nine times higher than those of large nonprofits and three times higher than privately owned for-profit hospices of similar size (McCue & Thompson, 2005). Therefore, there is evidence that for-profit hospices are earning higher profits, may not be

(Continued)

providing as many services, and are extending the stay of patients to generate revenue. Profit may be compromising the quality of care patients are receiving.

Non-profit hospices are typically operated by independent community-based organizations, staffed by paid and volunteer staff, and generate less profit but offer more core services such as counseling, personal care, and bereavement support for the families. The fundamental principal of hospice is to support and comfort patients and families during the final months of life (McCue & Thompson, 2005). Such services are time intensive, highly technical, and require dedicated medical staff and volunteers. Hospices are not reimbursed for intensive personal grief counseling for families who have lost a loved one or the counseling provided to children who have lost a parent.

You decide:

1. What role should profit motive play in quality and length of care to hospice patients?

2. Can the free market and reimbursement provide an environment for expanding the number of hospices and therefore services to patients?

3. What are the unintended consequences of establishing a reimbursement method that enables companies to profit from continuing to provide services to hospice patients?

4. Are there any downsides to reimbursing hospice care so that for-profit companies generate profit if patients are receiving the care that they need?

▪ Respite Care

Respite care is designed to give informal caregivers a break by providing care for their loved one who requires LTC. Respite care is highly variable and may range from part of a day to several weeks. Respite encompasses a wide variety of services including traditional home-based care, as well as adult day care, skilled nursing, home health, and short-term institutional care. Respite care can be provided in-home, in adult day care, or in institutions. Coverage for respite care is very limited. Medicare and some private insurers provide limited coverage for respite care, but the majority is funded by out-of-pocket payments. Rehabilitation, hospice, and respite care can be institution or community based.

▪ Program of All-Inclusive Care for the Elderly

The **Program of All-Inclusive Care for the Elderly (PACE)** is a system of managed care serving frail elderly who are eligible for nursing home care. PACE provides case management and an all-inclusive set of acute and long-term care services under one umbrella, thereby ensuring coordination of care. Participation in PACE is associated with decreased or delayed nursing home placement and lower rates of hospitalization. Access and utilization vary by state.

▪ Long-Term Care Case Management

Case management is a care strategy that coordinates a combination of services that will allow for the most independent level of functioning within a supportive system. Case management involves joint decision making among the patient (whenever possible), the family, physicians, and social services, to determine the care plan most appropriate for the patient. The purpose of case management is to treat the whole patient and all of his or her health and health care needs rather than to treat only episodes requiring care. There is a new certification program for geriatric case management, a rapidly growing field. Payment is out-of-pocket usually. However, it is becoming popular for Medicare HMOs to utilize case managers to save on costs associated with unnecessary rehospitalization.

▪ Characteristics of LTC Recipients

Use of LTC services is influenced by social and economic status and social network as well as geographic factors and the "culture" of health care in an area that reflects provider beliefs and practices. Wealthier older adults are more likely to use home health services and to avoid SNFs. They may buy into continuing care retirement communities and use assisted living facilities. Married persons are less likely to be admitted to SNFs for long-term stays, although they do use respite care. Persons with larger social networks and family and friends to support them are more likely to stay at home than to be admitted into SNFs.

▪ Nursing Home Resident Characteristics

The most common characteristic of nursing home patients is that they are unable to continue to live at home independently due to physical or mental health problems or functional disabilities (Paone & Mullen, 2005). The majority of residents are provided assistance in all five ADL areas (CDC, 2009). More than one-half of residents require total assistance in all of these ADLs.

Most residents of nursing homes are over 65 years old, with almost half 85 years of age or older (NCHS, 2009). However, overall the percentage of persons over the age of 85 living in nursing homes has dropped from 21.1 percent in 1985 to 13.9 percent in 2004 (Tumlinson et al., 2007). Women generally outlive men by several years and are 50 percent more likely than men to enter a nursing home after age 65 (American Association of Health Plans, 2010).

The majority of residents are female across all racial groups including black, Latino, and Hispanic (NCHS, 2009). The median age of residents is 83.2 years (Metlife Mature Market Institute, 2009). Residents who are Hispanic or Latino tend to be younger than residents who are not Hispanic or Latino. A similar pattern exists, based on race, with black residents, who are twice as likely to be under age 65 as non-black residents (CDC, 2009).

Many residents are in nursing homes for an extended period of time. The average period of time since admission for residents is 835 days, or two and one-quarter years (NCHS, 2009).

A resident's stay in a nursing home is influenced by his or her social network. Residents who are not married, or who do not live with other family members or a companion, have a longer nursing home stay than those who reside with others. Family members and loved ones play an important role in providing care for the elderly, and on discharge from a nursing home they resume this important task (CDC, 2009). One of the primary causes of a nursing home stay is the decline in health of a primary caregiver (CDC, 2009). This stay is referred to as respite care if it is temporary and brief, and it is covered by many types of insurance.

Characteristics of ALF and PCH Residents

Residents of ALFs and PCHs, as well as CCRCs, tend to be wealthier and healthier initially.

The Regulatory Environment of LTC Facilites

SNF Regulations

It has been said by those in the industry that SNFs have more regulatory oversight than a nuclear power plant. Whether this statement is accurate or not, SNFs currently have a large paperwork burden. Residents must be assessed using a lengthy form called the Minimum Data Set, or MDS, within several days of admission, and this assessment is ongoing. Their scores on the MDS are used to determine a reimbursement level and to measure quality of care for the facility. There are specially trained staffed, referred to as registered nurse assessment coordinators (RNACs), who complete all these instruments and keep them updated for each resident.

As a state licensed health care facility, SNFs are inspected and accredited on a regular basis. The structure of the building must be safe and meet a large variety of requirements regarding safety in terms of evacuation, fire control, electricity, dietary services, and housekeeping. There are also staffing requirements.

ALF Regulations

Regulation of ALFs is not uniform across states and is nonexistent in some states. Staff members at residential care facilities have minimal training due to their nonmedical status. Staff is not permitted to treat open bed sores and feed residents through a tube (California Advocates for Nursing Home Reform, 2010). Administrators need to complete a certification program, pass a simple state test, and complete continuing education requirements. The regulations for their certification are becoming stricter quite rapidly. Staff need to complete 10 hours of training at the facility once they are employed (California Advocates for Nursing Home Reform, 2010).

State governments regulate assisted living facilities. In 2007, several states tightened the regulations for communities with residents with Alzheimer's disease. Increased training and disclosure requirements were added for communities that provided services to patients suffering from the condition (Metlife Mature Market Institute, 2009). Assisted living facilities may be voluntarily accredited through the Joint Commission or the Commission on Accreditation of Rehabilitation Facilities (CARF) (Evashwick, 2005). Unlike SNFs who are licensed through the Department of Health, ALFs are licensed through the Department of Social Welfare in most states. CCRCs that have both SNFs and ALFs must therefore seek licensure from these two distinct entities as well as the state board of insurance. This process is complex, costly, and time-consuming.

Reimbursement Sources for LTC Services by Facility

SNF Reimbursements

Medicare is not designed to cover LTC other than that required for rehabilitation and/or recovery from an acute hospitalization. However, because Medicare coverage is more generous than the daily Medicaid reimbursement rate, SNFs are eager to receive and compete for these Medicare hospital discharges. Medicare will pay for 100 days of skilled nursing care after a minimum 3-day hospitalization, provided that the patient is admitted to the SNF or rehabilitation facility within 30 days of discharge from the acute care hospital and that he or she does require skilled nursing services such as rehabilitation, wound dressing changes, tube feedings, or IVs, (Centers for Medicare and Medicaid Services [CMS], 2010).

There has been an increase in the numbers of residents paying for nursing home care through Medicare and a decrease in the numbers of residents covered under Medicaid (California Health Care Foundation, 2009), although the overall number of residents covered under Medicaid at any one time is much greater. In addition, some people under the age of 65, with disabilities, have LTC health coverage through Medicare.

Residents of nursing homes typically rely on evolving and multiple sources of payment throughout their stay. At the time of admission, the largest proportion of residents pay out of pocket, but the vast majority of SNF care is ultimately paid for by Medicaid. Medicare covers a relatively small percentage overall (NCHS, 2009). Medicaid is the ultimate payer for the majority of LTC as individuals either do not have or run out of private funds to pay for it, and do not meet the Medicare eligibility criteria.

Patients must qualify for coverage under Medicaid based on their level of poverty. Many elderly spend down, or liquidate their assets, so that they can qualify for Medicaid. There is typically a 6-year waiting period before one is qualified after liquidating assets and states have extensive regulations regarding eligiblity. The goal is to have older adults pay for their own care by liquidating all their assets. Relying on Medicaid coverage once meant impoverishing the spouse who remained at home as well as the spouse confined to a nursing home. However, the law now permits the at-home spouse to retain specified levels of assets and income (American Association of Health Plans, 2010).

The average yearly cost of nursing home care varies depending on the location and the level of service that the resident requires. National average rates for a private room were $219 daily or $79,935 annually in 2009. National average rates for a semi-private room were $198 daily or $72,270 annually in 2009 (Metlife Mature Market Institute, 2009). Because of the high cost of nursing home care, many residents exhaust their ability to self-pay after only 6 months.

The cost for care increases whenever a resident requires additional services such as wound care, physical therapy, or memory care. The national average daily rate for a private room in an Alzheimer's or special care unit (SCU) is $233, or $85,045 annually.

The national average daily rate for a semi-private room in an Alzheimer's unit or wing is $208, or $75,920 annually (Metlife Mature Market Institute, 2009).

Costs are affected by geographical location, type of facility, ADL and IADL assistance, and other factors (Paone & Mullen, 2005). Currently, Medicaid is a major payer for all SNF and SCU care. Medicaid pays almost half of all nursing home costs. Over the next 30 years Medicaid's portion is expected to increase to 70 percent. Long-term care insurance that will pay for nursing home care is available for purchase at younger ages and is expected to grow.

The heavy reliance on Medicaid, a cost-sharing state and federal program, as a primary source of payment for many residents represents a significant financial challenge for nursing homes (Paone & Mullen, 2005). Many states struggle to balance their budgets during economic downturns, at a time when Medicaid expenses tend to increase. Medicaid represents a very large percentage of state budgets, and therefore policy makers scrutinize the costs and quality of nursing home care closely (Paone & Mullen, 2005).

Most nursing homes operate with small profit margins. High occupancy is critical for nursing homes to maximize their revenue and utilize the benefits of their fixed operational costs. Due to the high percentage of reimbursement from Medicaid, nursing homes must maintain their occupancy rates at around 90 percent to maintain their long-term viability (Paone & Mullen, 2005).

Long-term care insurance covers for SNFs and ALFs. It provides a means to protect the family and the resident's assets from being spent on expensive nursing home services. Many residents require long-term stays at facilities and the expenses can quickly consume a life-time of savings and resources. However LTC insurance will cover SNF or assisted living care depending on the type of policy purchased. The LTC insurance industry is relatively new. There are many caveats regarding whether one should purchase this coverage. A thorough investigation of the company is warranted as several companies have closed and left buyers without any coverage.

Medicare supplement insurance, called Medigap or MedSupp, is private insurance that covers the gaps in Medicare coverage. Although these policies help pay the deductible for hospitals and doctors, coinsurance payments, or what Medicare considers excess physician charges, they do not cover long-term care (American Association of Health Plans, 2010).

Residential Care Homes: ALFs, PCHs, and CCRCs

Another option for LTC coverage is long-term care insurance. Costs of LTC insurance vary widely. For example, inflation adjustments can add between 40 to more than 100 percent to premiums. However, this option can keep benefits in line with the current cost of care. The actual premium depends on factors including age, the level of benefits, and the length of time before benefits are used (American Association of Health Plans, 2010).

The cost of LTC insurance is heavily dependent on the age of the beneficiary and when they enroll in the plan. For instance, on average a policy offering a $150 per day long-term care benefit for 4 years, with a 90-day deductible, cost a 50-year-old $564 per year. For someone who was 65 years old, the national average cost was $1,337, and for a 79-year-old, the national average cost was $5,330. The same policy with an inflation protection feature cost, on average nationally, $1,134 at age 50, $2,346 at age 65, and $7,572 at age 79 (American Association of Health Plans, 2010). Therefore, it pays for beneficaries to enroll in LTC insurance during their younger years when they are healthy.

Typically, LTC insurance policies require that the policy holder pay out of pocket for the first 90 days of care. This stipulation is referred to as the elimination period. There may also be specific exclusions such as mental and nervous disorders. Alcoholism and drug abuse are usually not covered, along with care needed after an intentionally self-inflicted injury (American Association of Health Plans, 2010).

LTC insurance policies can help to cover skilled, intermediate, and custodial care in state-licensed nursing homes (American Association of Health Plans, 2010), but their main focus is covering the type of care that Medicare does *not* cover for perons who do *not* qualify for Medicaid. LTC insurance is an option for older adults with discretion-ary income, who can afford to buy it and afford the risks associated with it, and who want to perserve inheritance for their children. LTC policies usually also cover skilled home care, physical therapy, and homemakers, and home health aides if they are con-sidered necessary for the skilled care plan. Usually, these services must be provided by a licensed and certified agency for reimbursement. They also cover assisted living, adult daycare and other care in the community, alternate care, and respite care for the caregiver (American Association of Health Plans, 2010).

LTC policies generally limit benefits to a maximum dollar amount or a maximum number of days and may have separate benefit limits for nursing home, assisted living facility, and home health care within the same policy (American Association of Health Plans, 2010). As an example, a policy may offer $100 per day for up to 5 years of nurs-ing home coverage. Other policies may offer only up to $80 per day for up to 5 years of assisted living and home health care coverage (American Association of Health Plans, 2010). Some polices will just have a cap on reimbursement and not cover more than $140,000 of any type of service for any one person, for example.

■ Home Health Reimbursement

The primary payer for home health services is Medicare. Medicare Part A covers home health care after a minimum 3-day hospitalization. Medicare Part B will cover home health care without a prior hospitalization. The length of time covered is 100 visits, and the patient must be recertified after 60 days to make sure he or she is still eligible in terms of needing skilled nursing care or physical therapy *and* being homebound. Home care is considered underutilized. It is not ordered by doctors as often as some feel it should be. Part B is especially underutilized, and many providers are unaware it exists.

Medicare-covered home care is intended to be intermittent. It is not for custodial care. Persons desiring custodial care can always purchase it out of pocket. Other payers of custodial care include private insurance and Medicaid.

The implementation of Medicare's prospective payment systems for hospitals led to shorter hospital stays and increased use of Medicare's home health coverage. Initially, Medicare reimbursed home health care on a fee-for-service basis. During this period, the number of home health agencies (HHAs) grew rapidly. Under the Balanced Budget Act of 1997, HHA reimbursement changed from fee-for-service to the prospective payment system (PPS). The PPS was based on severity scores captured on an admission and assessment tool referred to as the outcome and assessment information set (OASIS). This new PPS led many HHAs to close because of financial losses. As a result, the number of people receiving home health care and the amount of care received by patients decreased.

Home care is less expensive than nursing home care. But nurses aide services three times a week for 2 to 3 hours per visit to help with dressing, bathing, preparing meals, and similar household chores can cost approximately $1,000 a month, or $12,000 a year (American Association of Health Plans, 2010). When skilled services are required from physical and/or occupational therapists, these costs can be much greater (American Association of Health Plans, 2010).

▪ Hospice Care Reimbursement

The primary payer for hospice care is Medicare, followed by private insurance and Medicaid (California Health Care Foundation, 2009). Most people who use hospice are over age 65 and are entitled to the Medicare hospice benefit. As a result, Medicare covers the cost of more than 80 percent of hospice patients (Tumlinson et al., 2007). This benefit covers virtually all hospice services such as medications and durable medical equipment such as beds, commodes, and other assistive devices. Therapeutic modalities such as physical therapy (PT) can be covered if ordered for comfort as opposed to curative reasons. Acute end-of-life care can be very costly. It is estimated that an individual incurs the bulk of his or her lifetime health care expenditures in the last month or so of life (Scitovsky, 1984).

Hospice care is believed to not only provide a high quality of life at the end of life but to do to so at a lower cost for families and society (Naierman & Turner, 2010). Once enrolled under hospice care, the individual is no longer eligible to be covered for any curative services. He or she can, however, receive physical and occupational therapy with a palliative focus.

The number of Medicare-certified hospice programs has increased over the last 10 years and with it the spending on hospice care by Medicare. This sector of LTC services continues to grow as the cost advantages to providing end-of-life care in a hospice setting are preferred by patients and payers.

▪ Challenges for the LTC Industry

The nursing home industry faces challenges of access, cost, and quality. A shortage of nursing home beds creates access problems for Medicaid patients and patients who need aggressive care, particularly for the oldest old, the sick and the poor, and those without any social support. The costs associated with LTC have increased significanty. Although expenditures are rising, reimbursement is not keeping pace for Medicaid patients, which lessens access and creates quality-of-care concerns.

Demand for SNF care has changed over the years; although there is a decline in the percentage of older adults demanding care, the overall size of this population has increased so that demand overall has gone up and will continue to do so due to the aging of the baby boomer generation. The decline in the percentage of older adults demanding care has resulted from changes in the changes in the Medicare reimbursement policy, growth in demand for nursing home alternatives, and a higher rate of seniors living independently (Tumlinson et al., 2007).

The quality of SNF and ALF care has been under scrutiny since an Institute of Medicine Report on errors and abuses. This review led to the implementation of new federal and state regulations to monitor and improve the quality of care delivered to residents (CDC, 2009). The lengthy MDS mentioned above measures quality in terms of critical incidents that affect residents such as death, the incidence of pressure ulcers, the number and types of medications for residents, pain management, and the prevalence of falls (CDC, 2009). Uncontrolled pain clearly decreases the resident's quality of life (NCHS, 2009).

Unfortunately, the focus on improving the quality of LTC created a negative impression regarding the use of chemical restraints. Currently, many remain untreated because of biases against the use of antianxiety and antipsychotic medications in this population. Recent studies argue that the level of agitation is also a quality measure that should be decreased. The focus on decreasing chemical restraints has many residents over-agitated and undermedicated, posing a serious risk to their safety and that of other residents and staff. Agitated residents have been found to physically injure themselves and others more often than calm residents (Cohen-Mansfield, 2008).

Researchers have examined whether there are differences in quality between for-profit SNFs and not-for-profit SNFs (Hillmer et al., 2005). For-profit nursing homes have been found to provide lower quality of care in many important areas (Hillmer et al., 2005).

Long-term care facilities are experiencing staffing shortages, chiefly driven by an overall national nursing shortage (Castle, 2006). The American Health Care Association reported that in 2003 the yearly turnover rate (meaning the rate at which people quit a job) for nurses in long-term care facilities was 49 percent, whereas the turnover rate for certified nurse assistants (CNAs) was 71 percent (Pratt, 2010). Long-term care facilities must compete with hospitals for highly trained staff where the latter pay higher salaries and the care is less routine and therefore preferred. In addition, they must compete with the fast-food industry and retail sales industries that also pay higher wages. Moreover, these latter industries have fewer training requirements, and work schedules may be better. These issues raise concerns about staffing morale and place additional pressure on administrative personnel to retain nursing staff. Of course, dealing with incontinence and often disagreeable residents adds to the difficulties in staffing long-term care facilities.

Following are several questions that you may consider as a family member of a hospice patient, health care administrator, or clinician:

1. What role should the profit motive play in the quality and length of care that is provided to hospice patients?

2. Can the free market and reimbursement provide an environment for expanding the number of hospices and therefore services to patients?

3. What are the unintended consequences of establishing a reimbursement method that enables companies to profit from continuing to provide services to hospice patients?

4. Are there any downsides to reimbursing hospice care so that for-profit companies generate profit if patients are receiving the care that they need?

Innovations in LTC have taken place over recent years and have improved the care and quality of life of patients. Research has shown that when an individual is able to age in place at his or her own residence, the longevity and quality of life is enhanced. It is also less costly for an individual to remain in his or her residence rather than in an institution. High-tech home care such as IV therapies, vents, dialysis, and medic alerts have also helped in allowing individuals to age in place.

Vignette

WHEN THE GOLDEN YEARS ARE NOT SO GOLDEN

Mr. Andrews is a 75-year-old former teacher who spent his career teaching poetry in the Cook County school district. He was recently widowed as his wife passed away a year ago after a lengthy illness. She had suffered from breast cancer for the last 5 years of her life, and Mr. Andrews was her primary caregiver. He drove her to doctor's appointments, accompanied her at chemotherapy treatments, and dressed and bathed her as her health deteriorated. He was at her bedside to care for her when she became confined to bed due to frailty.

Mr. Andrews' wife was eventually unable to remain comfortable even with higher and higher dosages of morphine. She refused further hydration and nutrition and lapsed into a coma. She passed away while Mr. Andrews was holding her in his arms one evening. He was a patient and gentle caregiver for many years.

Now, Mr. Andrews is suffering from Alzheimer's disease, incontinence, and mild hypertension. He resides in a skilled nursing facility that provides specialized care for residents with memory loss. He requires assistance, in terms of prompting, with activities of daily living (ADLs) such as bathing, dressing, walking, and eating. Left to himself, he would forget to bathe and eat. He is confused as to where he is and anxious about what he "should" be doing. He spends the greater part of every day trying to find where he believes the staff has put his wife. At times, he becomes very agitated, accusing the staff of taking his wife away from him. This once gentle and patient man is now considered one of the most difficult residents on the dementia unit. He is still physically strong and has thrown objects at staff as well as pushed them and hit them on many occasions. Staff members are generally frightened of him, and it is difficult for them to work on his unit. He has also been violent toward other residents.

Mr. Andrews' immediate family is comprised of a sister and a son. His sister has been involved in his life and visits frequently. She has a good relationship with staff, and they have told her about his agitated and aggressive behavior. Because she visits often, she has witnessed several aggressive episodes. Mr. Andrew still recognizes his sister, and she is able to calm him down so far, but she is not always there.

His son lives across the country and has not been part of his father's life for many years. The last time he saw him was at his mother's funeral. He and his father are estranged and have also not spoken since the funeral of his mother. He talked via telephone with his aunt regarding his father's condition every other month. However, on hearing that his father's condition has dramatically worsened, he has taken a new interest. He calls the nursing home several times a week to ask how his father is doing. He sends books and asks the recreational therapist to spend time reading poetry with his father. He has visited several times and taken his father out, but he has not spent much time in the facility with his dad, so he has never seen his father's aggressive outbursts.

Prior to being admitted to the nursing home, Mr. Andrews had drawn up a will. Virtually all estate wills today must contain a section on advanced directives, or what are referred to as the person's wishes for end-of-life care in terms of the degree of aggressive resuscitation he or she would desire should he or she become incompetent. These "living wills," or advanced directives, are required prior to admission to a SNF or ALF facility. The other document that is required is durable power of attorney (DPOA). This role can be assigned to one person or divided between two persons, with one assigned responsibility for finances and the other for health care. The health care DPOA is often referred to as the health care proxy. Mr. Andrews stated that he did not want any invasive treatment were he to lapse into a coma or become "incompetent" (competency is a complex legal decision that we will not discuss at length here). Also, during his tenure as his wife's caregiver, he often remarked that he did not want to suffer and hoped that someone would help him avoid this outcome if the need arose. He authorized his son as his DPOA for finance and his sister as his DPOA for health care.

His sister has seen his agitation and feels it is indeed a form of pain and suffering. To watch her once intelligent and gentle brother abuse staff and constantly try to return back to his dead wife is almost more than she can bear. She has asked the nursing supervisor whether he can be mildly sedated. He seems to be worse in the afternoon, around 4 o'clock. This behavior is common among Alzheimer's and other demented persons and is referred to as sundowning. The nursing supervisor emphatically stated that the staff would not tranquilize Mr. Andrews. She indicated that this treatment would be somehow "wrong" but did not explain her rational. His sister has gone to Mr. Andrews' primary care provider and explained what has transpired. The provider has a background in geriatrics and recommended a small dose of an antipsychotic medication. When Mr. Andrews' son heard that his father had been medicated, he was furious. He remembers his father the way he used to be and feels that the staff is provoking this aggressive behavior. He ordered the nursing supervisor to stop the antipsychotic and requested that the staff to read more poetry to his father. He stated that if they continue to medicate his father, he will move him to another facility.

1. What are the legal issues here? Who is empowered to make decisions regarding the use of medications?

2. Why does the nursing supervisor think that medications to control agitation are wrong?

3. Does staff have any rights here? Should part of this job include being physically abused? What are the rules regarding occupational risks in this setting?

4. What do you think would be best for Mr. Andrews, and why?

Vignette

END-OF-LIFE CARE

Several weeks ago, Mrs. Jones, who has been a resident on the Dementia SCU for 2 years, contracted pneumonia and was admitted to the hospital for IV antibiotics. An X-ray found that she has advanced lung cancer. Her physician states that she is too weak for surgery. She has a long history of cardiac disease. After multiple courses of antibiotics, the infection was successfully treated. It left Mrs. Jones weaker and unable to walk, and she now refuses all food and liquid. She developed delirium in the hospital and was confused and agitated, constantly trying to get out of bed and constantly trying to remove her IV. She is now discharged back to the skilled nursing level of this facility, and the staff has contacted the family about feeding tube placement. She frequently moans and grimaces, which indicates she is in severe pain. An X-ray found metastatic bone cancer in her spine. She states that she wishes to die. She is refusing to eat and will not stop removing her IV.

There are very strict guidelines for the appropriate use of chemical and physical restraints in nursing homes. The staff is required to monitor the patient in physical restraints virtually non-stop, and the patient's bed is often moved into the nursing station for this purpose.

Mrs. Jones did complete advanced directives prior to admission. She stated that she did not want a feeding tube. Her DPOA for health care is her sister, who wishes to abide by the advanced directives. In contrast, Mrs. Jones's children are adamant that their mother should have a feeding tube placed.

1. What are your thoughts on providing feeding tubes for a person in this situation? Are there any benefits?

2. Who has the legal authority to make end-of-life decisions for Mrs. Jones?

3. What does the American Association of Hospice and Palliative Care Medicine have to say regarding the use of feeding tubes in persons with dementia?

4. Is hospice care covered in an SNF or SCU? How would you go about receiving hospice care? How is it paid for?

■ Mental Health in LTC

■ What Is Mental Health and Mental Illness?

An important type of LTC is care provided to mental health patients. Mental health is a state of successful performance of mental functioning resulting in productive activities, fulfilling relationships with other people (social health), and the ability to adapt to change and cope with adversity (key characteristic of mental health). Mental illnesses are health conditions that are characterized by alterations in mood and thinking; such behaviors are associated with distress and impaired functioning.

Mental illness is the collective term for all diagnosable mental disorders and brain diseases. Collectively, mental illnesses are the third leading cause of hospitalization. Some examples of mental illnesses include schizophrenia, antisocial personality disorder, mania, posttraumatic stress syndrome, panic disorders, major depression, and social phobia. About one-fifth, or 22 percent, of the population has a mental disorder, whether with or without addiction. Only 19 percent have just a mental disorder without an addictive disorder. Depending on the definition of mental disorder, 3–30 percent of the population can be considered to have a mental disorder.

▪ Who Are the Mentally Ill?

The mentally ill are old and young. Approximately 20 percent of those ages 9–17 years and 20 percent of those over age 65 are mentally ill. Mental illness does not affect one gender more than the other, but the prevalence of certain mental illnesses varies by gender. For example, women tend to be diagnosed more with depression, whereas men tend to be diagnosed more with schizophrenia. Mental illness is higher among racial and ethnic minorities. However, the results of studies that report differences in racial and ethnic groups may be muddied due to biased reporting.

▪ Mental Health Treatment

Mental health professionals provide the care in various settings. Such professionals include psychiatrists, psychologists, psychiatric nurses, and psychiatric social workers. Care is provided in settings such as clinician offices, community mental health centers, private psychiatric hospitals, general hospitals, and state mental health facilities. Less than 6 percent of adults in any given year will seek help from the specialty mental health sector. Approximately 8 percent of children will receive help from this sector.

Other providers also deliver mental health services as part of general health care in the primary care sector. These providers include general internists, pediatricians, and nurse practitioners. The benefit of this sector is that individuals are receiving help, but the providers do lack specialty training. The care is provided in settings such as physician offices and community health centers. Slightly more than 6 percent of the adult population and about 3 percent of children will receive help from this sector.

The human services sector provides mental health care through the following settings and their associated providers. These providers include social service agencies with help lines, schools, residential rehabilitation services, vocational rehabilitation, the criminal justice system, and religious and professional counselors. Approximately 5 percent of adults receive care from this sector. Approximately 16 percent of children receive care from the school-based system, and 3 percent through the juvenile welfare system.

Mental health services are also provided through volunteers. Individuals who provide care through this sector of the mental health system are not required to have any training because they are just providing support. The types of groups that provide this care include community organizations, support groups, and faith-based organizations.

▪ Summary

In this chapter, we discussed the many different settings in which LTC is provided and the professionals who deliver that care. We described the various types of LTC services and how they are reimbursed. In terms of primary settings for LTC, we identified nursing homes or skilled nursing facilities (SNFs), assisted living facilities (ALFs) or personal care homes (PCHs), and continuing care retirement communities (CCRCs).

The goals of LTC are (1) to promote and maintain health and independence in functional abilities and to obtain optimal quality of life in individuals with decreased physical and or mental functioning; and (2) to help individuals with terminal illnesses to die in peace and with dignity.

Most LTC patients are age 65 and over; however, almost 40 percent are under 65 years old (Tumlinson et al., 2007). The number of people needing LTC is expected to triple in the next 30 years due to our aging population, increases in life expectancy, and increases in chronic illness and resultant disability.

Informal caregivers provide the majority of all LTC. Most informal caregivers are either spouses or a child of the person requiring the care. Among children, daughters and daughters-in-law provide the majority of care, at times relinquishing paid jobs in order to care for an aging family member.

Hospice is a critical service delivered to patients with the goal of improving quality of life and providing comfort. Hospice care is provided in a person's own home when he or she is facing a life-limiting illness or injury. However, caregivers deliver hospice services in SNFs and ALFs as well. Hospice services focus on supporting the primary family caregiver by managing patient pain, providing drugs and supplies, and assisting the patient with many aspects of dying. Much of the growth in hospice care can be attributed to cost savings associated with providing efficient end-of-life care for patients in their own home, surrounded by loved ones. Hospice is a cost-effective service when compared to the inpatient costs of hospitals and skilled nursing facilities.

We identified sources of reimbursement for LTC services and emphasized the important role that self-pay or paying out of pocket plays for LTC services. Medicare does not cover many of the services, and therefore patients are required to pay for many of the services themselves. This burden emphasizes the importance of LTC insurance for patients and the role it plays in providing financial assistance to pay for critical services. Only a small portion of Americans is covered by LTC insurance; therefore, most people are required to cover the cost of many LTC services out of their own pocket, thus diminishing their savings and ability to pass on wealth to their heirs. It is estimated that an individual incurs the bulk of his or her lifetime health care expenditures in the last month or so of life.

Finally, we outlined the challenges faced by the nursing home industry in the areas of access, cost, and quality. A shortage of nursing home beds creates access problems for Medicaid patients and patients who need aggressive care, particularly for the oldest old, the sick and the poor, and those without any social support. Demand for SNF has changed over the years; although there is a decline in the percentage of older adults demanding care, the overall number of this population has increased so that demand overall has gone up and will continue to do so due to the aging of the baby boom generation.

▪ Review Questions

1. What are the major trends in the LTC industry?

2. What factors are the most influential in the increased demand for LTC services?

3. What is the difference between institutional and community-based providers of LTC services?

4. What is the primary source of reimbursement for each of these different types of LTC services?

   a. Skilled nursing home care

   b. Home health care

   c. Assisted living

   d. Adult day care

   e. Senior center

   f. Respite care

   g. Hospice care

   h. Palliative care

   i. Continuing care retirement community (CCRC)

5. Are there differences in the quality of care between privately owned and publicly owned nursing homes?

6. What is the benefit of having LTC insurance?

7. What LTC organization is the fastest growing segment in the health care industry, and why?

8. How is most LTC provided, informally or through a professional caregiver? Why is this the case?

9. Describe the typical mental health patient.

10. What is the extent of direct and indirect costs that are incurred from mental health illnesses?

▪ Additional Resources

Administration on Aging (AoA): www.aoa.gov/

American Health Care Association: www.ahca.org

California Health Care Foundation: www.chcf.org/

LeadingAge: www.leadingage.org/

National Adult Day Services Association: www.nadsa.org/

National Association of Home Care and Hospice: www.nahc.org/

National Association of Insurance Commissioners: www.naic.org

National Council on the Aging: www.ncoa.org

National Hospice and Palliative Care Organization: www.nhpco.org/templates/1/homepage.cfm

The American Geriatrics Society: www.americangeriatrics.org/

University of Minnesota Extension Service: www.financinglongtermcare.umn.edu

■ References

American Academy of Hospice and Palliative Medicine. Retrieved June 1, 2011, from www.aahpm.org/Practice/default/quality.html.

American Association of Health Plans. (2010). *Guide to long-term care insurance.* Washington: American Association of Health Plans.

California Advocates for Nursing Home Reform. (2010). What you need to know about residential care facilities. RCFE/Assisted Living Fact Sheet. Retrieved July 5, 2010, from www.canhr.org/factsheets/rcfe_fs/html/rcfe_needtoknow_fs.htm.

California Health Care Foundation. (2009). *California health care almanac.* Oakland, CA: Author.

Castle, N. (2006). Measuring staff turnover in nursing homes. *The Gerontologist* 46(2): 210–219.

Carlson, M., Gallo, W., & Bradley, E. (2004). Ownership status and patterns of care in hospice: Results from the National Home and Hospice Care Survey. *Medical Care*, *42*(5), 432–438.

Centers for Disease Control and Prevention (CDC). (2009a). *The National Nursing Home Survey: 2004 overview.* Washington, D.C. National Center for Health Statistics.

Centers fo Disease Control and Prevention (CDC) (2009b). *The 2008 National Health Interview Survey.* National Center for Health Statistics, Centers for Disease Control and Prevention, Hyattsville MD. Retrieved on March 24, 2012 from http://www.cdc.gov/nchs/nhis/nhis_2008_data_release.htm

Centers for Medicare and Medicaid Services (CMS). (2010). *Your Medicare benefits.* Washington: U.S. Department of Health and Human Services.

Chou, W., Cooney, L., Van Ness, P., Allore, H., & Gill, T. (2007). Access to primary care for Medicare beneficiaries. *Journal of the American Geriatrics Society*, *55*(5), 763–768.

Cohen-Mansfield, J. (2008). Agitated behavior in persons with dementia: The relationship between type of behavior, its frequency, and its disruptiveness. *Journal of Psychiatric Research, 43*(1), 64–69.

Cunningham, P., & O'Malley, A. (2009). Do reimbursement delays discourage Medicaid participation by physicians? *Health Affairs*, *28*(1), w17–w28.

Evashwick, C. (2005). The continuum of long-term care, 3rd ed. Clifton Park, NY: Thomson Delmar Learning.

Hillmer, M., Wodchis, W., Gill, S., Anderson, G., & Rochon, P. (2005). Nursing home profit status and quality of care: Is there any evidence of an association?. *Medical Care Research and Review*, *62*(2), 139–166.

Hospice Facts and Statistics. (2009, September). Hospice Association of America. Retrieved July 6, 2010, from www.nahc.org/facts/HospiceStats09.pdf.

Iglehart, J. (2009). A new era of for-profit hospice care—The Medicare benefit. *New England Journal of Medicine*, *360*(26), 2701–2703.

LeadingAge (2011). Aging Serivces: What You Need to Know about CCRCs; Washington, DC. Retreived on March 24, 2012 from http://www.leadingage.org/Article.aspx?id=205

McCue, M., & Thompson, J. (2005). Operational and financial performance of publicly traded hospice companies. *Journal of Palliative Medicine*, *8*(6), 1196–1206.

Medicare Payment Advisory Commission. (2009). *Report to the Congress: Medicare payment*. Washington, DC: Medicare Payment Advisory Commission.

Medicare Payment Advisory Commission. (2010). *Report to the Congress: Medicare payment*. Washington, DC: Medicare Payment Advisory Commission.

Metlife Mature Market Institute. (2009, October). Mature Market survey of long-term care costs. The Metlife Market Survey of Nursing Home, Assisted Living, Adult Day Services and Home Care Costs. Retrieved June 1, 2011, from http://www.metlife.com/assets/cao/mmi/publications/studies/mmi-market-survey-nursing-home-assisted-living.pdf.

Naierman, N., & Turner, J. (2010). Debunking the myths of hospice. American Hospice Foundation. Retrieved July 7, 2010, from www.americanhospice.org/articles-mainmenu-8/about-hospice-mainmenu-7/36-debunking-the-myths-of-hospice.

National Association of Homecare and Hospice (2010). Expert Panel Highlights Capacity of Home Care to Improve Health Systems; December 8; Washington DC. Retreived on March 24, 2012 from http://www.nahc.org/Media/mediaPR_120810.html

National Hospice and Palliative Care Organization (NHPCO) (2005). 2005 hospice and palliative care leadership survey. Retrieved on March 24, 2012 from http://www.nhpco.org/files/public/Furst-Group_Hospice_Exec_Survey_2005.pdf

Paone, D., & Mullen, D. (2005). Hospitals. In C. Evashwick, & C. Evashwick (Eds.), *The continuum of long-term care* (pp. 51–68). Clifton Park: Thomson Delmar.

Paul, B., Bartels, D., Abbot-Penny, A., Rawles, L., & Ward, A. (2005). *End of life care: Ethical overview*. Center for Bioethics University of Minnesota. Retrieved June 1, 2011, from www.ahc.umn.edu/img/assets/26104/End_of_Life.pdf.

Scitovsky, A. (1984). "The high cost of dying": What do the data show? *The Milbank Memorial Fund Quarterly: Health and Society*, *62*(4), 1984 (pp. 591–608).

Spector, W., Fleishman J., Pezzin L., & Spillman, B. (2000). The characteristics of long-term care users. AHRQ Publication No 00-0049. Rockville, MD: Agency for Healthcare Research and Quality.

Pratt, J. (2010). *Long-term care: Managing across the continuum*, 3rd ed. Sudbury, MA: Jones and Bartlett.

Tumlinson, A., Woods, S., & Avalere Health LLC. (2007). *Long-term care in America*. Washington, DC: Avalere Health LLC & National Commission for Quality Long-Term Care.

Key Terms

American Medical Association (AMA)

baby boomers

Balanced Budget Act of 1997

Centers for Medicare and Medicaid Services (CMS)

Children's Health Insurance Reauthorization Act of 2009 (CHIPRA)

donut hole

Dual eligibles

Great Society

Joint Commission

medical savings accounts

Medicare + Choice

Medicare Part A

Medicare Part B

Medicare Part C

Medicare Part D

Medicare Prescription Drug, Improvement and Modernization Act (MMA) of 2003

Continued

Learning Objectives

- Assess the importance of providing health care coverage to the elderly and to the poor and disabled.

- Describe the various parts of Medicare and what each one covers.

- Identify the cost and benefits of Medicare and Medicaid managed care plans.

- Identify the differences in the funding sources for both Medicare and Medicaid.

- Identify health care services covered by Medicare and Medicaid.

- Evaluate the long-term cost projections for Medicare and Medicaid.

- Review the costs and benefits of the State Children's Health Insurance Plan.

- Recognize health care services that are not covered by either Medicare or Medicaid.

■ Introduction

Together, Medicare, Medicaid, and the State Children's Health Insurance Program (SCHIP) financed $823.8 billion in health care services in 2008—slightly more than one-third of the country's total health care expenditures and almost three-fourths of all public spending on health care. Since their enactment, both Medicare and Medicaid have been subject to numerous legislative and administrative changes designed to make improvements in the provision of health care services to the elderly, disabled, and disadvantaged.

In 2009, Part A of Medicare covered almost 46 million enrollees (over 38 million aged and almost 8 million disabled enrollees), with benefit payments of $239.3 billion; Part B covered almost 43 million enrollees, with benefit payments of $202.6 billion; and Part D covered over 33 million enrollees, with benefit payments of $60.5 billion (CMS, 2010). Similarly, Medicaid benefit payments amounted to over $366 billion to more than 56 million enrollees (CMS, 2010).

The federal government's health insurance program for the elderly and disabled called Medicare was created in 1965 when **President Lyndon B. Johnson** signed into law the 18th Amendment to the **Social Security Act of 1935**. The Social Security Act was part of Roosevelt's "New Deal" social program. Medicare is administered by the U.S. **Centers for Medicare and Medicaid Services (CMS)**, which is a division of the Department of Health and Human Services. The Medicare program covers 95 percent of our nation's aged population, as well as many people who are on Social Security because of disability (CMS, 2010).

▪ Why Is Medicare Important?

Medicare covers a significant portion of the population with over 40 million Americans enrolled in Medicare. As the population ages, particularly as **baby boomers** age, there will be over 60 million Americans enrolled in Medicare by 2019 (CMS, 2010). Since its inception, actual expenditures for Medicare have always been higher than projected. In 2009, Medicare expenditures, at over $500 billion, grew 7.9 percent over the previous year, amounting to 20 percent of all national health expenditures. This figure is expected to reach $900 billion by 2019 (CMS, 2010).

In the mid 1930s, there were 30 wage earners to support one person on Social Security, now there are three workers paying into the program to support one. By the year 2025, it is projected that there will be two wage earners to support one Social Security recipient (CMS, 2010). Medicare outlays are expected to exceed revenues by 2019, and are projected to consume an increasing percentage of the federal budget (CMS, 2010). Increasing federal outlays for Medicare come from shifts in spending on other social programs. Most experts now agree that this trend is not sustainable, and if maintained in its current form, the Medicare tax burden on subsequent generations would be ruinous to the U.S. standard of living (CMS, 2010).

▪ What Is Medicare?

Medicare is the nation's largest health insurance program—beneficiaries number more than 40 million Americans, a 100 percent increase since 1967 when the enrollment was 19.5 million. Medicare is a social insurance program or an "entitlement" program; it is not a welfare program. To qualify for Medicare Part A (hospital insurance discussed later), beneficiaries have to pay Social Security taxes for 40 quarters, or quarter years, or for 10 years by way of a payroll tax.

Taxpayers through the federal government fund the program and use fiscal intermediaries, mainly Blue Cross/Blue Shield companies, to perform administrative tasks such as billing. Billing and administrative paperwork are efficient, accounting for only two cents of every $1 in Medicare spent.

▪ Background on Medicare

In 1945, **President Harry S. Truman** proposed a comprehensive, prepaid medical insurance plan for all people through the Social Security system. His proposal was referred to as National Health Insurance. The legislation failed to pass the Congress, but years later John F. Kennedy pledged in his presidential campaign of 1960 to offer legislation for health insurance for the aged. According to a national survey at the time, only 56 percent of individuals 65 and older had health insurance.

Within a month of taking office, **President John F. Kennedy** delivered a message to Congress calling for health insurance for the elderly. Proposed legislation to provide such insurance became the focus of debate throughout the early 1960s. President Kennedy was unable to pass health care coverage for the elderly during his presidency, but the bill was passed during the Johnson administration, and was a cornerstone of his **Great Society** program.

The **American Medical Association (AMA)** opposed Medicare, comparing it with socialized medicine. When it seemed that passage was inevitable, the AMA lobbied for the program to cover only the poor elderly.

Proponents of Medicare stressed the need for a plan that promised benefits for everyone over age 65 by highlighting the popularity of Social Security. President Johnson, with significant help from organized labor, was able to push Medicare and other Great Society legislation through Congress. The results of his efforts were the establishment of two programs, Medicare for the elderly and Medicaid for the poor of all ages. The overriding goal of Medicare was to assure access to health care for the elderly over the age of 65.

▪ Why Medicare Is Necessary

There were several reasons why Medicare was so important to the elderly when it was passed in 1965. The elderly were an underserved population because many were poor and could not afford care. During this time, nearly half of the elderly were uninsured and almost a quarter were in poverty.

Insurance coverage as part of retiree benefits was not common prior to the passage of Medicare. For higher-income elderly, only approximately one-half were insured. Private insurers were reluctant to offer insurance to the elderly because they are on average sicker.

Since its passage, Medicare has contributed to significant increases in access to care for America's oldest and most disabled citizens. It is also one of the fastest growing programs in the federal budget (CMS, 2010). The economic status of older Americans has improved substantially over the past three decades. The disposable income of older Americans does not differ substantially from their younger counterparts. The rate of poverty among the elderly is now lower than that for the rest of the population.

Experts anticipate the growth rate of the working-age population in United States to slow to a half percent per year by 2030, from about 1 percent per year today. In addition, the percentage of the population over 65 years of age will rise markedly, from less than 13 percent today to perhaps 20 percent by 2030. The aging of the population in the United States will have significant effects on the U.S. economy; in particular, it threatens the sustainability of both Social Security and Medicare programs. As a result, experts have suggested that the *only* way to ensure the sustainability of these programs is to increase immigration rates, accelerate productivity growth well beyond historical experience, increase the age of eligibility for benefits, decrease benefits, or use general revenues to fund benefits. Thus, there are no magic bullets, and most of these alternatives will face significant opposition from various stakeholders.

The utilization of Medicare benefits has increased. Between 2000 and 2008, the percentage of Medicare beneficiaries receiving physician services increased from just over 50 percent to nearly 60 percent, with a similar increase in the number of services provided per beneficiary (U.S. GAO, 2009). Medicare expands access to care for many individuals who would not be able to afford care without this program. Beneficiaries use health care services when services are made available, so utilization and costs will also increase.

Medicare can be considered a success because it created buying power for eligible individuals as it was intended. Medicare extended coverage to a large group of people, mainly the poor elderly, who previously lacked coverage. Supplying this buying power resulted in an increase in admissions, length of stay, and private physician visits. The largest percentage of Medicare spending has been on inpatient hospital services, followed by services rendered by physicians.

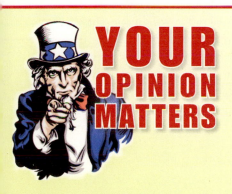

YOUR OPINION MATTERS

Should We Require That All Physicians Accept Medicare Patients and Medicare Payments?

Background

Providers choose whether to participate in the Medicare program during an open enrollment period. During this period, physicians can modify their status, and new physicians can elect to be participating providers. One of the key provisions of the Medicare program is that participants accept full assignment for their Medicare claims. In other words, providers agree that Medicare's allowed reimbursement is payment in full for their services. They further agree to submit all Medicare claims directly to Medicare and receive reimbursement from Medicare on behalf of the patient.

There are several incentives for physicians to participate in the Medicare program. Participating providers are reimbursed at a 5 percent higher rate than physicians who do not participate in the program. Medicare submits any insurance claims to a supplemental insurance carrier on behalf of the participating physician. Medicare then sends reimbursement from both Medicare and the supplemental insurance carrier directly to the physician. Participating physicians are included in Medicare's online directory, and therefore patients can identify which physicians accept Medicare reimbursement as payment in full. Participating primary care physicians who provide care in medically underserved areas receive a 10 percent bonus payment for covered Medicare services. Medicare permits physicians to bill their patients directly for services not covered by the program.

(Continued)

Providers who choose not to enroll entirely in the Medicare program (called opt out), must inform their patients in writing of their status. On agreement, their patients are then responsible for whatever the provider charges and patients cannot obtain any reimbursement from Medicare.

Yes

Medicare providers who do not accept Medicare payment require their patients to pay their full costs. Moreover, by agreeing to see these opt-out providers, these patients cannot bill Medicare for any of those costs. Physicians can require their patients to provide sufficient revenues to enable them to reach their target incomes.

Requiring providers to accept Medicare patients will improve senior's access to care at affordable prices. Many beneficiaries struggle to find providers who will take new patients and provide quality service. They face rising copayments and deductibles while on a fixed income.

If providers are allowed to set their own prices for Medicare patients and services, Medicare beneficiaries will find it increasingly difficult to obtain affordable services, as they must pay higher amounts for physician visits, tests, and procedures. Medicare patients will be required to budget increasing amounts of their fixed incomes for medical expenses, premiums for Medicare Parts B and D, and supplemental insurance. These increases are a considerable burden on their fixed incomes that often remain unchanged because of limited or no increases in Social Security and falling values of retirement funds invested in stocks and bonds.

No

Requiring providers to accept Medicare patients and payment is the same as mandating them to be employees of a government program as in other countries where there is a single-payer government health system. This insistence would also remove their freedom to choose whether to take new patients covered by Medicare or chose freely which new patients to accept. Requiring providers to accept Medicare would remove their choice of whether to participate only in private insurance plans or to not even participate in any third-party payer contracts. It would require providers to deliver a professional service to patients regardless of how much money they would lose in the process. The unintended consequence of this requirement would be that providers may leave markets where Medicare is the predominant source of reimbursement, which would result in an even more severe maldistribution of providers.

Medicare sets low reimbursement rates for various services and treatments, often at levels that may not even cover a provider's overhead. As a result, providers are caught in the middle of an endless cycle of spiraling costs for supplies, equipment, and staff and falling Medicare reimbursements. Providers also face obstacles to receiving reimbursement when insurers deliberately make the reimbursement process difficult, complicated and time-consuming. When reimbursement is approved, payments from insurers can take an extremely long times to reach physicians. Providers may need additional staff to handle the extra paperwork, phone calls, resubmissions, and negotiation with insurance companies.

Finally, the government should not interfere in a private business transaction between patients and their providers. Physicians provide critical professional services for their patients and should be reimbursed for the value delivered in the office. In a free market capitalist system, the consumer should be required to pay a fair price for the value of these services because they benefit with improved health status.

You decide:

1. Does requiring providers to accept Medicare patients go against the tenants of a free capitalist market economy?

2. How does the Patient Protection and Affordable Care Act (PPACA) (March 2010) affect the affordability of services for Medicare beneficiaries?

3. What are your recommendations for improving access to care for seniors who cannot find a physician who will agree to take new Medicare patients?

4. From a provider's perspective, do the costs outweigh the benefits for participating in the Medicare program given its requirements to accept assignment?

5. From a patient's perspective, do the costs outweigh the benefits for providers participating in the Medicare program given its requirements to accept assignment?

Medicare Benefits and Structure

Medicare provides health insurance to individuals who are 65 years of age and older and qualify for Social Security. To qualify for Social Security, an employee must pay into the system for 40 quarters. Medicare has covered such individuals since the inception of the Medicare program in 1965. Medicare also covers permanently disabled individuals regardless of age, as well as individuals with permanent kidney failure. Such individuals need renal dialysis because they have end stage renal disease or kidney transplants. Medicare coverage was extended to disabled individuals and those with end stage renal disease in 1972 through further amendments to the Social Security Act of 1935.

Medicare consists of four parts:

Medicare Part A—The hospital insurance program covers inpatient hospital, skilled nursing facility, hospice, and home health care. It is sustained through a payroll tax paid by employees and employers. Inpatient hospital services are subject to a deductible and daily coinsurance beginning after the 60th day of a hospital stay. Medicare covers up to 100 days of skilled nursing facility care after 3 days in the hospital, subject to coinsurance for days 21–100.

Medicare Part B—Supplementary medical insurance covers physician and outpatient hospital care, lab tests, medical supplies, and home health. Part B is financed by beneficiary premiums and general revenues. The monthly Part B premium is $112 in 2010. A 20 percent coinsurance payment is required for most Part B services after meeting a $100 Part B yearly deductible ($110 in 2005 and indexed to rise by the annual percentage increase in Part B expenditures thereafter) (CMS, 2010). Beneficiaries are not required to pay coinsurance for home health benefits received under Parts A or B.

Medicare Part C—Managed care plans provide Part A and Part B benefits, called Medicare Advantage (MA), to enrollees. Medicare Advantage plans contract with Medicare to provide both Part A and B services to enrolled beneficiaries. Due to changing payment rates and other factors, the number of participating plans has declined in the last several years, as have the supplemental benefits offered by the remaining plans. Experts estimate that such plans will decline 13 percent in 2011 (Johnson, 2010).

Medicare Part D—In 2006, under the Medicare Prescription Drug, Improvement and Modernization Act of 2003 (MMA). Beneficiary premiums and general revenues finance Part D and the premiums vary across plans.

Medicare and Prescription Drugs

Concerns about seniors lacking prescription drug coverage and the rising cost of drugs led to the enactment of the new Part D prescription drug benefit, which went into effect in 2006.

Through Part D private insurance plans offer drug benefits for a monthly premium. In 2006 when the legislation went into effect, under the standard benefit beneficiaries pay the first $250 in drug costs; 25 percent of the total drug costs between $250 and $2,250; and 100 percent of drug costs between $2,250 and $5,100 in total drug costs, or the **"donut hole."** This is coverage equivalent to a $3,600 out-of-pocket limit; the greater of $2 for generics, $5 for brand drugs, or 5 percent coinsurance after reaching the $3,600 out-of-pocket limit, $5,100 catastrophic threshold. The "donut hole" was included in the legislative package to make the overall benefit more affordable, or cost fewer tax dollars to fund.

President George W. Bush supported and signed the **Medicare Prescription Drug, Improvement and Modernization Act (MMA) of 2003**. This legislation made the most sweeping changes to Medicare since its inception by affording Medicare beneficiaries a prescription drug benefit.

Starting in 2006, individuals who are eligible for Medicare Part A or are enrolled in Medicare Part B were eligible to participate in Medicare Part D. Medicare Part D provides a voluntary drug benefit for beneficiaries through private companies. Private companies contract with the Department of Health and Human Services to either offer

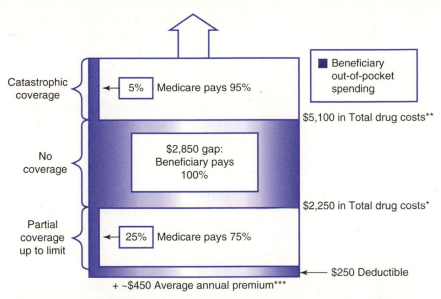

Note: *Equivalent to $750 in out-of-pocket spending. **Equivalent to $3,600 in out-of-pocket spending. ***Annual amount based on $37.37 monthly Part D premium estimate from 2005 Annual Report of the Medicare Boards of Trustees.

Figure 8–1 Standard Medicare prescription drug benefit, 2006.

Source: Kaiser Family Foundation illustration of standard Medicare drug benefit described in the Medicare Modernization Act of 2003.

a prescription drug–only plan or to offer a more comprehensive benefit package that includes prescription drugs. Figure 8–1 illustrates how the Medicare prescription drug benefit is administered with varying levels of coverage at different levels of prescription drug expenditure.

Medicare Expenditures and Financing

The components of the Medicare program are comprised of many sections, including inpatient hospital care, physician services, psychiatric hospital services, skilled nursing care, home health care, and hospice care.

Inpatient Hospital Care

Medicare pays up to 90 days for inpatient hospital care in a benefit period. During the first 60 days, Medicare pays all covered costs except for the $792 deductible; during the period of 61–90 days, Medicare covers all but copayment of $191 per day. Medicare covers medically necessary services such as a semi-private room, meals, regular nursing care, rehabilitation, drugs, medical supplies, lab tests, X-rays, operating and recovery room, intensive care unit (ICU), and critical care unit (CCU) services. Medicare does not cover personal convenience items such as telephone, television, or a private room. Medicare Part A is not comprehensive as it covers only short-term care.

Medicare Part B

Medicare Part B does not cover services unrelated to the treatment of an illness/injury, or outpatient prescription drugs. Over 96 percent of the elderly elect to take Part B coverage, and about 90 percent of disabled take Part B.

Premium payments and general federal revenues underwrite Medicare Part B expenditures. The monthly premium for Part B is deducted from the beneficiary's Social Security check. The Part B premiums amount to approximately 25 percent of the cost; the federal government or taxpayers subsidizes the other 75 percent through general revenues.

A coinsurance applies to the covered services under Part B. That is, the government pays for a portion of the services while the patient is responsible for the remaining amount. If the beneficiary's income is less than 100 percent of the federal poverty level, Medicaid will pay Part B premiums; if income is higher than the federal poverty level Medicare will pay Part B premiums.

Copayments, deductibles, and coinsurance have been increasing since 1965. These components are used as strategies to shift the cost of care from Medicare to the user of services; it is one way that the government has dealt with the rising cost of Medicare.

Psychiatric Hospital Coverage

Inpatient hospital coverage is limited to a maximum of 190 days. Psychiatric care provided in a general hospital is not subject to the 190-day limit.

Medicare added skilled nursing facility (SNF), home health, and hospice coverage because they are less expensive than inpatient hospitalization.

Skilled Nursing Facility (SNF)

Medicare insurance covers up to 100 days for care provided in a skilled nursing facility (SNF). Medicare pays the full cost for first 20 days; during the 21st through the 100th day, the patient pays $99 per day copayment; after the 101st day, the patient is responsible for all charges.

Home Health

Medicare pays the entire bill for covered home health services as long as the services are medically reasonable and necessary. Medicare also covers the full cost of some health care supplies and 80 percent of the approved amount for durable medical equipment such as hospital beds, wheelchairs, oxygen, and walkers.

Hospice Care Services

Patients can elect to receive hospice care rather than regular Medicare benefits if they are terminally ill. If patients elect to receive hospice care, Medicare pays up to 210 days and sometimes longer. There may be a $5 copayment for each drug prescription and usually a $5 per day copayment for inpatient respite care. Respite care provides temporary relief to persons, often a family member or other informal caregiver, who regularly care for the patient.

Medicare Certified Facilities

The certification of provider facilities ensures that institutional health care providers serving Medicare beneficiaries meet the minimum health and safety requirements. State survey agencies or private accrediting organizations conduct the certification. The **Joint Commission** is one such private accrediting organization.

■ Gaps in Medicare Coverage

Medicare is less generous than most employer health plans. Medicare has no stop loss coverage; it covers less than half of all beneficiaries' total health spending. On average, more than 20 percent of household income goes toward direct payment of health services, Part B premiums, and supplemental insurance premiums. The 20 percent figure does not include additional long-term care expenses.

Beneficiaries fill gaps in their health insurance coverage by enrolling in health maintenance organizations (HMOs) and purchasing private insurance. Nearly two-thirds of enrollees purchase some form of supplemental insurance, such as **Medigap** insurance, or are covered under employer-sponsored retiree health benefits. Another method of filling gaps in Medicare is through coverage from Medicaid. The members of the lowest income Medicare population are eligible for Medicaid.

Voluntary supplemental insurance coverage is offered by Blue Cross/Blue Shield and commercial insurers to help enrollees pay for the gaps in Medicare coverage—particularly coinsurance requirements for hospital care.

Medigap policies pay most, if not all, of Medicare coinsurance amounts and may provide coverage for Medicare's deductibles. Some pay for services not covered by Medicare such as outpatient prescription drugs, preventive screenings, and emergency health care while traveling outside of the United States. Some benefits have dollar limits.

Medigap policies are not comprehensive; they may not succeed in filling all "the gaps" that the elderly need covered. The elderly poor have the greatest need for Medigap insurance but are less likely to have it because they cannot afford it.

The elderly choose from 10 standard Medigap policies (A–J), each offering a different combination of benefits. The very comprehensive plans are very expensive, and only three plans offer prescription drug coverage.

■ Medicare Health Maintenance Organizations

For Medicare beneficiaries to be eligible to enroll in a managed care plan, they must have Medicare Part B and continue paying Part B premiums. They must live in the plan's area, cannot receive care in a Medicare-certified hospice, and cannot have permanent kidney failure at the time of enrollment.

The Medicare HMO is a voluntary option for the patient. Medicare HMOs are risk plans because they are paid a per-capita premium set at approximately 95 percent of the projected expenses for FFS beneficiaries.

Most Medicare HMOs provide all Medicare-covered services, and most plans offer additional services such as prescription drugs and glasses; members must obtain all their care through the plan with the exception of out-of-the area urgent care; about 90 percent of Medicare-managed care beneficiaries are in risk plans. Most Medicare beneficiaries have a choice of at least one managed care plan; half have the choice of two or more. Medicare-managed care enrollment varies greatly depending on geographic location; the majority of people enrolled under this plan live in California, Florida, Oregon, New York, Arizona, and Hawaii.

Medicare HMO enrollees enjoy several benefits. HMOs cover more comprehensive services than traditional Medicare, like case management, and cover total amounts (no copayments). However, there are drawbacks to selecting an HMO, because patients have reduced choice among providers, and some studies have demonstrated that there are poorer outcomes for chronically ill patients. In addition, the government reimburses HMOs only 95 percent of the full cost of the average patient under traditional Medicare coverage.

Medicare+Choice enrollees can contract with other types of private health plans such as **preferred provider plans (PPOs)**, **point-of-service organizations (POSs)**, and **medical savings accounts (MSAs)**.

Beneficiaries continue to pay monthly premiums but must obtain all Medicare-covered benefits through a private plan.

Enrollees in Medicare+Choice plans have several choices among products. They can enroll in an HMO where beneficiaries obtain services from a designated network of doctors, hospitals, and other health care providers, usually with little or no out-of-pocket payments. Another option for beneficiaries is the PPO, where enrollees obtain services from a network of health care providers established by a plan. Unlike an HMO, beneficiaries can see providers not in the network, and the plan will cover a portion of the services.

Beneficiaries may also enroll in a POS, which is similar to an HMO except that a group of doctors establishes them and hospitals assume the financial risk of providing comprehensive services to Medicare enrollees.

If a beneficiary decides to enroll in a medical savings account (MSA) they must select a high deductible catastrophic plan. Medicare pays the monthly premium for this plan and makes a deposit into a tax-free MSA on behalf of the beneficiary.

Finally, beneficiaries may enroll in a private fee-for-service plan. This type of coverage is a private indemnity policy where the beneficiary is not limited to a network of providers. There are no limits on monthly premiums that the beneficiary may be charged for basic Medicare benefits.

Beneficiaries may enjoy many options among plans. However, many experts have labeled the Medicare+Choice program a failure. Initially many managed care companies entered the market and enrolled patients. From 1991–1998, the number of Medicare HMOs grew from 93 to 347. Then in 1998, managed care plans found it financially unprofitable to continue to offer Medicare-managed care plans, and 100 plans withdrew. In 1999, an additional 99 plans withdrew from the Medicare+Choice program. Medicare continues to underestimate the annual cost of coverage on which Medicare HMOs are paid. This miscalculation is not by accident and is part of the ongoing strategy to shift the cost of the program back to the user and providers.

▪ Hospital Reimbursement

Before 1983, fee-for-service hospital reimbursement afforded limited incentive for efficiency, which resulted in increased costs, volume of services, admissions, and length of stay. This reimbursement mechanism fueled the utilization of high-tech, expensive treatments.

Beginning in 1983, Medicare now reimburses hospitals based on a prospective payment system. This new form of reimbursement radically changed hospital revenues under Medicare by providing preset payments for services rendered to patients rather than on costs incurred. This reimbursement scheme bases its payments on diagnosis-related groups (DRGs) and establishes fees for services that are considered by experts as required to treat specific diagnoses rather than reimbursing for discreet units of services consumed.

▪ Physician Reimbursement

Physician reimbursement under Medicare is fee-for-service based on prevailing fees for specific services within a specified geographic area. The **Omnibus Budget Reconciliation Act (OBRA) of 1989** established a new method of Medicare physician reimbursement effective in 1992, using a **resource-based relative value scale (RBRVS)**. This scheme attempts to contain costs by instituting the same pay for the same services. A national fee schedule assigns relative values to services based on the time, skill, and intensity inherent in providing them. Containing Medicare's escalating costs has been a budgetary conundrum for years. There are several possible strategies to employ to address Medicare's financial issues, such as decreasing the number of participants, increasing taxes to pay for Medicare, decreasing benefits to recipients, increasing the efficiency of the delivery of services, lowering reimbursement levels to providers, increasing copayments, coinsurance, deductibles for recipients, and requiring high-income elderly to contribute more toward the cost of their care than low income elderly. Instituting any of these interventions penalizes the provider, beneficiary, or the taxpayer, and thus will be opposed by the parties who are affected.

Vignette

MEGYN KELLY: THE CASE OF BENEFITS DENIED

Medicare beneficiary Megyn Kelly, a retired television reporter who had just turned 70, received a disturbing letter. Her gynecologist, who had been managing her ovarian cysts, informed her that she was opting out of Medicare and that Megyn was still welcome as a patient but that she would not be accepting her Medicare reimbursement any longer as payment. When Ms. Kelly asked her long time primary care doctor to recommend another gynecologist who did accept Medicare, the doctor said that she did not know of any. Further, the primary care doctor asked Ms. Kelly to please give her the name of any gynecologist that she was able to locate who was accepting new Medicare patients.

Expecting to quickly find another gynecologist near where she lived, Ms. Kelly inquired of her friends and family. Her friends said that they too were experiencing the same problem finding physicians who accepted new Medicare beneficiaries. One of her friends remarked that her regular internal medicine physician had stopped accepting Medicaid patients because of an inability to cover the costs of providing care to indigent patients. This physician had been consistently losing money over the last several years as the state had decreased its reimbursement for services delivered to Medicaid patients. The physician then decided also to stop taking new Medicare patients because of Medicare's low reimbursement rates. Fortunately, for that internist, she had a large group of patients who were insured by private commercial insurance plans.

Ms. Kelly did learn of several qualified physicians in the suburbs who were still participating in the Medicare program and were accepting new patients, but they were located a good distance away. Over the next year, Ms. Kelly was unable to find a gynecologist who was accepting new Medicare patients, and so she missed her annual gynecological exam and the various tests that were performed to determine whether any ovarian cysts had returned. This uncertainty weighed heavily on her mind as she always monitored her health closely and had never missed an annual gynecological appointment for 30 years. Her gynecologist had recommended this regular monitoring of her condition as she had a family history of ovarian cancer.

Stimulated by her journalist instinct, Ms. Kelly decided to investigate why physicians were dropping out of the Medicare program. She found that, on average, physicians are reimbursed at roughly 78 percent of costs under Medicare, and just 70 percent of costs under Medicaid (Zuckerman, Williams, & Stockley, 2009). She found that physicians make up for this shortfall by shifting costs to insured patients in the form of higher prices, or treating Medicare patients at a loss (Chou et al., 2007). In markets where there are not enough privately insured patients to support the physician's practice, there is an economic incentive to refuse new Medicare patients like herself. She found that roughly 13 percent of physicians do not accept Medicare patients, and 17 percent limit the number of Medicare patients they will see. Among primary care physicians, such as gynecologists, 31 percent of physicians limit the number of new Medicare patients that they see (Chou et al., 2007). The figures were even worse for Medicaid patients, where as many as 20 percent of doctors chose not to participate in the program (Cunningham & O'Malley, 2009). Further, about 40 percent of doctors are age 55 or over, and many may choose retirement over practice delays from hassles of government red tape and less money (Landon et al., 2006).

Finally, Ms. Kelly decided to pay out of pocket for her gynecological services and returned to her original provider for service. Although on a fixed income, during the year when she postponed care she revisited her monthly expenses, made some sacrifices, and had saved enough to be able to cover the higher costs of care. She even negotiated a payment plan with her provider that allowed her to continue receiving care. However, she continues to search for a gynecologist who is accepting new patients and participates in the Medicare program.

1. What is an affordable solution for patients who have contributed to Medicare all of their working lives but who now face obstacles in obtaining care because providers leaving the program?

2. Are you willing to pay higher payroll taxes in order to keep the Medicare program solvent and for beneficiaries to receive care?

3. Do you believe the Medicare program will be available to you when you turn 65?

4. Should wealthy Medicare beneficiaries pay a premium for the benefits they receive from the program?

▪ Medicaid

▪ Introduction and Organization of Medicaid

CMS administers Medicaid, or Title XIX of the Social Security Act; however, Medicaid is a welfare program, not an entitlement program. Medicaid is funded by personal income and corporate and excise taxes, funds transferred from more economically affluent individuals. In other words, it is a wealth transfer, or income redistribution, program.

Medicaid is a voluntary joint federal and state program, with federal funding for each state based on the per capita income of the citizens of that state. The federal government matches the funds allotted by the states by providing 50–80 percent of the overall Medicaid funds. Richer states contribute more to the Medicaid program, whereas poorer states contribute less.

Within broad national guidelines, each of the states establishes its own eligibility standards; it determines type, amount, duration, and scope of services; sets rates of payment for services; and administers its program. This method of management creates significant variation among the state Medicaid programs. Medicaid is actually 50 different programs, as each state has a unique name and method for administrating the program (KFF, 2011b).

▪ Medicaid's Role in the Health Care System

Medicaid is an essential part of the health care system. Medicaid funds substantial portions of the nation's spending on hospital care, physician services, nursing home care, and prescription drugs (KFF, 2011c). The program provides health insurance coverage to a broad spectrum of patients, such as children, adults, low-income families, elderly, and persons with disabilities. It is one of the primary sources of reimbursement for nursing home care residents and other long-term care services. Specifically, 70 percent of nursing home residents, 56 percent of low-income children, and 42 percent of poor individuals have some form of Medicaid coverage (KFF, 2011c). Medicaid is the primary payer for long-term care (LTC) services, with Medicare the second highest source of reimbursement.

Most Medicaid beneciaries, such as children and families, enroll in a private managed care plan which in turn is reimbursed by Medicaid. The managed care plans use provider networks to deliver services (KFF, 2011b).

Enrollment in Medicaid typically increases during times of economic downturn, as workers lose their jobs and their employer-sponsored health insurance. However, workers do not stop becoming ill when they lose their health insurance. People typically do not save money in preparation for losing their job and their health insurance, so they have very few resources to pay for health services if they are unemployed and are not eligible for Medicare.

Medicaid is jointly funded by the state and federal governments. Medicaid funding is typically the largest source of federal revenue for the states and due to an economic multiplier effect, enables job creation in the state. For example, a hospital may be reimbursed for caring for Medicaid patients, which enables it to pay its employees who then purchase local goods and services in the community.

▪ Coverage of Health Services

All states are required to cover a minimum set of services for Medicaid beneficiaries, such as inpatient and outpatient hospital services, physician services, nursing home services, nurse midwife and nurse practitioner services, family planning services, laboratory and X-ray services, immunizations, and early and periodic screening diagnosis and treatment (EPSDT). States have the option to cover an additional 31 services, such as prescription drugs, hospice, care for the mentally disabled, and dental and vision services (KFF, 2011b).

▪ Beneficiaries of Medicaid Coverage

The three primary groups receiving Medicaid are poor parents with children, the disabled, and the elderly who are eligible for **Supplemental Security Income (SSI)** or who are qualified Medicare beneficiaries. Specifically, Medicaid covers one in three children, one in three births, and one in four nonelderly adults (KFF, 2011b). Medicaid covers 8 million people with disabilities who require personal care assistance, transportation, and devices that allow them to remain mobile and maintain independence (KFF, 2011b).

Medicaid covers nearly 9 million low-income Medicare beneficiaries. Persons who qualify for both Medicare and Medicaid are referred to as **dual eligibles**. Dual eligibles are elderly with a low income and younger people with disabilities. Dual eligibles are typically the poorest and sickest patients who have very limited resources. More than half have income below $10,000 and most have substantial health needs. Medicaid covers Medicare premiums and out-of-pocket costs, as well as critical services. Medicaid covers nursing home and other LTC services not covered by Medicare. They represent only 15 percent of enrollees but approximately 40 percent of Medicaid spending (KFF, 2011b).

▪ Long-Term Care

Medicaid is the largest single purchaser of long-term care (LTC) in the country, at 42 percent of all national spending and almost 50 percent of spending on nursing home care (KFF, 2011c). Medicaid eligibility requires the recipient of long-term care services to be impoverished before benefits begin; in other words, recipients must spend down their income and assets until they meet state income eligibility requirements.

▪ Mental Health and Medicaid

Medicaid for mental health typically covers inpatient services for 30 days or less per year. Medicaid reimburses for inpatient physician visits, but reimbursement is unrealistically low. Medicaid also reimburses for outpatient physician visits but is limited to 20–30 visits per year, with fees set well below prevailing charges.

▪ Medicaid and Minors

Of the 11.3 million uninsured children, an estimated 5.1 million are eligible for Medicaid or the **State Children's Health Insurance Program (SCHIP)**. Many states have initiated administrative strategies designed to reduce barriers for parents to enroll their eligible children.

Medicaid was expanded to cover additional children through the Omnibus Reconciliation Act of 1989–1990 and the **Balanced Budget Act of 1997**. The limitation of these bills is that they focused solely on the children and not the whole families of eligible children. In 1997, the Balanced Budget Act provided funds to expand health insurance coverage for children by creating the State Children's Health Insurance Program as part of title XXI of the Social Security Act. The **Children's Health Insurance Reauthorization Act of 2009 (CHIPRA)** extended and expanded the SCHIP. The passage of the bill was based on the belief that children are a vulnerable population to insure and providing preventive services to children saves future health care spending. In general, the types of care that children generally lack tend to be low cost, such as filling dental cavities and providing eyeglasses (KFF, 2011a). CHIPRA added money for children's coverage and included provisions designed to increase and strengthen children's coverage in both Medicaid and SCHIP (KFF, 2011a).

SCHIP is a state/federal partnership that permits states either to expand Medicaid coverage or develop a proposal for a new program to be reviewed by CMS. In general, states are permitted to insure kids living in families whose income is up to 200 percent of the federal poverty level. Through Medicaid and SCHIP, as of January 2011, most states cover children to at least 200 percent of poverty ($36,620 for a family of three in 2010), with 25 states covering children at or above 250 percent of the federal poverty level (KFF, 2011a). The prevailing emphasis has been on enrolling children in the programs for which they are eligible; however, millions of children may remain uninsured despite eligibility for existing programs.

Eligibility requirements are set so that uninsured children who are ineligible for Medicaid can still be covered under SCHIP. A common application for coverage under Medicaid and SCHIP does facilitate enrollment. States annually assess whether enrollment barriers exist in their state, with health insurance companies participating in SCHIP providing a range of outreach activities to educate potential enrollee families.

There are many benefits to enrolling in SCHIP, including a full range of inpatient, outpatient, and physician services. Coverage is provided for services such as laboratory, mental health, use of durable medical equipment and remedial devices, home and community-based health care, nursing care, dental care, abortion to save the life of the mother or if the pregnancy is the result of rape or incest, and case management. In addition, physical, occupational, and speech therapy; hospice; and ambulance services are covered when medically necessary.

Medicaid Costs and Managed Care

Medicaid costs are the fastest growing component of states' budgets. Many states are seeking waivers from the federal government to mandate Medicaid patient enrollment in managed care plans, to contain costs. Some states are also experimenting with voluntary Medicaid managed care enrollment.

In theory, the economic incentives inherent in managed care promote timely, appropriate access to preventive care. This motivation should increase access for Medicaid patients. However, low Medicaid fee-for-service reimbursement has made clinicians reluctant to accept them as new patients.

▪ Welfare Reform and Medicaid

The Welfare Reform Act of 1996 changed Aid to Families with Dependent Children (AFDC) to **Temporary Aid for Needy Families (TANF)**. This change ended the welfare system where mostly single women with children were provided with cash assistance, housing, and health insurance. Before its passage, individuals qualifying for welfare automatically qualified for Medicaid coverage. This Act separated the provision of cash assistance from the provision of Medicaid coverage. After the Welfare Reform Act, cash assistance was provided for up to 6 months and qualifying for cash assistance no longer equated with qualifying for Medicaid coverage.

▪ Distribution of Medicaid Coverage and Expenditures

Although Medicaid has many advantages, it does have shortcomings. For instance, it covers only 45 percent of the poor, and many working poor do not qualify for the program (Galewitz, 2011). The eligibility for the program varies significantly from state to state, and poorer states typically have less comprehensive coverage, but sicker populations. Medicaid also provides lower reimbursement levels to clinicians who refuse to take new patients who need services. This policy has reduced provider participation in the program. Because of these reimbursement and access barriers, the poor have had unequal access to care.

Medicaid, however, has been responsible for many improvements in health care. Medicaid covers large numbers of children and is the largest payer for maternity and long-term care services. It is the largest insurer of persons living with AIDS and provides a safety net for nearly 6 million low-income Medicare beneficiaries.

As with Medicare, cost containment under Medicaid has been a contentious issue. Several factors drive Medicaid spending in a state, such as the number of enrollees, the price of medical and LTC services, enrollees' use of services, and the effectiveness of managed care plans.

Medicaid expenditures can be reduced through increasing the requirements for eligibility and therefore removing people from the program, lowering the rate of reimbursement to providers, reducing the benefit package or the number of covered services, and shifting recipients into managed care. Similarly, all of these measures have an impact on the recipients of care.

▪ Summary

This chapter addressed the federal programs of Medicare and Medicaid, their administration, who is covered, and their funding. The government is a major purchaser of health care services on behalf of the beneficiaries of the two programs. Spending by the two programs is slightly more than one-third of the country's total health care expenditures and almost three-fourths of all public spending on health care.

The federal government created Medicare as a health insurance program for the elderly and disabled in 1965 when President Johnson signed into law the 18th

Amendment to the Social Security Act of 1935. The Social Security Act was part of Roosevelt's New Deal social program. CMS administers Medicare and is one of the largest purchasers of health care services.

Medicare will face increasing pressure to remain financially solvent as more baby boomers reach age 65 and fewer active workers remain to contribute through payroll taxes. The focus on the financial solvency of the program increases as the U.S. economy goes through periods of recession with less tax revenue and fewer workers paying for the program. Estimates vary, but some experts predict that Medicare outlays will exceed revenues by 2019, and they are projected to consume an increasing percentage of the federal budget.

Medicare was passed in a critical time of the Great Society program, and since its passage it has contributed to significant increases in access to care for America's elderly and most disabled citizens. It is also one of the fastest growing entitlements in the federal budget. As a result, experts have suggested that the only way to ensure the sustainability of these programs is to increase immigration rates, accelerate productivity growth well beyond historical experience, increase the age of eligibility for benefits, decrease benefits, or use general revenues to fund benefits. Thus, there are quick solutions, and most of these alternatives will face significant opposition from stakeholders.

Medicaid is a voluntary joint federal and state program, with federal funding for each state based on the per capita income of the citizens of that state. The federal government matches the funds allotted by the states by providing 50–80 percent of the overall Medicaid funds. The three main groups receiving Medicaid are poor parents with children, the disabled, and the elderly who are eligible for Supplemental Security Income (SSI) or who are qualified Medicare beneficiaries.

In general, states are permitted to insure children living in families whose income is up to 200 percent of the federal poverty level. The dominant emphasis has been enrolling children in the programs for which they are eligible. However, millions of children may remain uninsured despite eligibility for existing programs.

While Medicaid has many advantages, it does have shortcomings. The program covers only 45 percent of the poor and many working poor do not qualify for the program. The eligibility for the program varies significantly across states, and poorer states typically have less comprehensive coverage, but sicker populations. Medicaid also provides lower reimbursement levels to clinicians who refuse patients who need services. This policy has reduced provider participation in the program.

Medicaid coverage has a strong positive impact in health care. Medicaid covers large numbers of children and is the largest payer for maternity and long-term care services. It is the largest insurer of persons living with AIDS, and provides a safety net for nearly 6 million low-income Medicare beneficiaries.

■ Review Questions

1. What is the chief funding source for Medicare?

2. What is the chief funding source for Medicaid?

3. What does Medicare Part A cover for beneficiaries?

4. What does Medicare Part B cover for beneficiaries?

5. What does Medicare Part C cover for beneficiaries?

6. What does Medicare Part D cover for beneficiaries?

7. How does the funding of Medicaid differ from the funding for Medicare?

8. Does Medicare provide comprehensive coverage for the elderly?

9. Does Medicaid provide sufficient health care coverage for pediatric patients?

10. When is Medicare expected to run out of funding, and why?

▪ Additional Resources

Centers for Medicare and Medicaid Services (CMS) www.cms.gov/

Children's Health Insurance Program (CHIP) www.cms.gov/home/chip.asp

Children's Health Insurance Program Dental Coverage www.cms.gov/CHIPDentalCoverage/

Kaiser Family Foundation Medicaid www.kff.org/medicaid/index.cfm

Kaiser Family Foundation Medicare www.kff.org/medicare/index.cfm

Kaiser Family Foundation—Medicaid Children's Health Insurance Program www.kff.org/medicaid/children.cfm

Medicaid Eligibility Are Your Eligible? www.cms.gov/MedicaidEligibility/02_AreYouEligible_.asp#TopOfPage

Medicaid Eligibility General Information www.cms.gov/MedicaidEligibility/

Medicare Coverage General Information www.cms.gov/CoverageGenInfo/

Medicaid Program General Information www.cms.gov/MedicaidGenInfo/

Medicare General Information www.cms.gov/MedicareGenInfo/

Medicare Part A General Information www.cms.gov/MedicareGenInfo/02_Part%20A.asp#TopOfPage

Medicare Part B General Information www.cms.gov/MedicareGenInfo/03_Part%20B.asp#TopOfPage

Medicare Prescription Drug Coverage General Information www.cms.gov/PrescriptionDrugCovGenIn/

Prescription Drug Coverage—General Information www.cms.gov/PrescriptionDrugCovGenIn/01a_bridgingthegap.asp#TopOfPage

Prescription Drug Plan Resources www.cms.gov/PrescriptionDrugCovGenIn/03_Resources.asp#TopOfPage

■ References

Chou, W., Cooney, L., Van Ness, P., Allore, H., & Gill, T. (2007). Access to primary care for Medicare beneficiaries. *Journal of the American Geriatrics Society, 55*(5), 763–768.

Centers for Medicare and Medicaid Services (CMS). (2010). Data Compendium 2010 Edition. Baltimore MD. Retrieved October 1, 2011, from https://www.cms.gov/DataCompendium/14_2010_Data_Compendium.asp#TopOfPage.

Cunningham, P., & O'Malley, A. (2009). Do reimbursement delays discourage Medicaid participation by physicians? *Health Affairs, 28*(1), w17–w28.

Galewitz, P. (2011 July). Medicaid: True or false? Kaiser Health News. Low Cost Health Insurance for Families and Children. Retrieved October 1, 2011, from http://www.cms.gov/LowCostHealthInsFamChild/

Johnson, A (2010), Private medicare plans are retrenching, *The Wall Street Journal*, November 19. Retrieved October 1, 2011, from http://online.wsj.com/article/SB10001424052748703374304575622480028578008.html.

Kaiser Family Foundation (KFF). (2011a). Kaiser Commission on Medicaid and the Uninsured. CHIP Enrollment. Washington, DC: Author. Retrieved October 1, 2011, from http://www.kff.org/medicaid/upload/7642-05.pdf.

Kaiser Family Foundation (KFF). (2011b). Kaiser Commission on Medicaid and the Uninsured. Medicaid facts. Washington, DC: Author. Retrieved October 1, 2011, from http://www.kff.org/medicaid/upload/8050-04.pdf.

Kaiser Family Foundation (KFF). (2011c). Kaiser Commission on Medicaid and the Uninsured. Medicaid and long term care services and supports. Washington, DC: Author. Retrieved October 1, 2011, from http://www.kff.org/medicaid/upload/2186-08.pdf.

Landon, B., Reschovsky, J., Pham, H., & Blumenthal, D. (2006). Leaving medicine: The consequences of physician dissatisfaction. *Medical Care*, 44(3), 234–242.

U.S. General Accountability Office (GAO) (2009 August). Medicare Physician Services. Utilization Trends Indicate Sustained Beneficiary Access with High and Growing Levels of Services in Some Areas of the Nation. Report to the Committee on Finance, U.S. Senate. Washington DC, GAO 09-559.

Zuckerman, S., Williams, A., & Stockley, K. (2009, May/June). Trends in Medicaid physician fees, 2003–2008. *Health Affairs, 28*(3), w510–w519.

Key Terms

ambulatory surgical center

bad debt

charity care

critical access hospital (CAH)

diversification strategies

Hill-Burton Act

horizontal integration

hospital

independent living facility

joint ventures

long-term care hospitals (LTCHs)

medical home

Rural Hospital Flexibility Program (Flex Program)

specialty hospital

underpayment

vertical integration

Learning Objectives

- Differentiate among various types of hospitals.

- Describe basic concepts of hospital governance.

- Discuss the likely future role of inpatient care in the U.S. health care system.

- Describe and differentiate the types of health services provided in outpatient settings from those provided in inpatient and long-term care settings.

- Understand the difference between for-profit and not-for-profit facilities and the issues surrounding this tax status.

- Discuss the political, economic, social, and regulatory factors that led to dramatic growth in outpatient services.

- Understand critical techniques for measuring hospital clinical and financial performance.

- Identify the main financial drivers in hospitals.

- Describe the main differences between horizontal and vertical integration among health care facilities.

- Identify ethical issues related to hospitals and their delivery of care.

▪ Introduction

Hospital care is the largest component of the health services sector. Hospitals have a significant impact on employment in the United States, supporting nearly 1 out of every 10 jobs. The number of hospital employees has grown significantly, as hospitals have expanded their capacity and the population has demanded more care. Hospitals also are typically one of the main drivers in the local economy, offering stable employment throughout economic cycles. In 2008, hospitals employed more than 5.3 million people (Health Forum LLC, 2010).

Despite recent economic turmoil, in 2008 hospitals spent approximately $322 billion on staff salaries and $268 billion on other goods and services (Health Forum LLC, 2010). Hospital employees purchase goods and services that support other businesses and create new jobs in the local economy. According to the American Hospital Association (AHA) (2006), each hospital job supports about 1.6 additional jobs, and every dollar spent by a hospital supports more than $2 of additional business. Economists call this phenomenon the multiplier effect; thus, shifts in health policy that affect the financial health of the hospital also affect the local economy.

▪ Hospital Origins

▪ Historical Development of Hospitals

The Latin root for **hospital** is *hospes*, meaning "a stranger" or "a guest: it is also the root for *hostel* and *hotel*. In ancient times, Egyptians, Chinese, and the Greeks had military field hospitals to care for injured soldiers after battle. During the Middle Ages, monasteries and almshouses often served as a refuge for the sick, poor, old and orphaned, and as shelters for sick travelers. A personal physician cared for the wealthy in their homes.

The Pennsylvania Hospital was founded in 1751 by Benjamin Franklin (1706–1790) and Dr. Thomas Bond (1712–1784) to care for the sick, poor, and insane of Philadelphia and was the first hospital in the United States. Almost from its beginning, Pennsylvania Hospital was the teaching hospital for the University of Pennsylvania Medical School.

Hospitals as a refuge for the sick and poor persisted until the later part of the 1800s, when hospitals began focusing primarily on providing health care. Before the late 1800s, wealthy persons received care at home, because hospitals were often places of rampant infection.

▪ Medical Breakthroughs Impact Hospitals

Two major medical breakthroughs in the late 1800s led to the dramatic growth in the number of hospitals. The first was the development of the germ theory of disease by Louis Pasteur (1822–1895) and Robert Koch (1843–1910). Before this discovery, the majority of invasive surgeries were lethal because infection set in after the surgery. The need for cleanliness and sterility in the hospital was not recognized. Prior to germ theory, the more a surgeon's apron was covered with blood and pus, the more he was viewed as experienced.

With the introduction of antiseptic strategies such as carbolic acid sprayers, surgeries could be performed far more successfully because infection could be better controlled. This process was later replaced by antisepsis methods such as sterilizing surgical equipment and the physician "scrubbing" before surgery. Before Robert Koch and Louis Pasteur, Ignaz Semmelweis (1818–1865) in 1847 discovered the connection between hand washing and the prevention of the spread of puerperal fever, known also as childbed fever, which was caused most commonly by staphylococcus and streptococcus in maternity wards. Because his peers rejected his work for decades, the work of Ignaz Semmelweis was largely unrecognized and unappreciated. However, Ignaz Semmelweis's hunch proved to be correct, demonstrated by Louis Pasteur's now famous research.

The second major development that affected hospitals was the discovery of safe anesthesia. Before the use of safe anesthesia by physicians, surgeons relied on the speed with which they could perform an amputation or other surgery and employed opium and alcohol to dull the patient's sense of pain. These primitive anesthetics were often ineffective or, when given in sufficient dose to kill pain, resulted in dangerous side effects such as nausea or vomiting, or even death. However, with the development of safe anesthia in 1846, hospitals began to use it for surgical procedures. In the twentieth century, scientific medicine became increasingly effective and complex, and physicians became more dependent on hospitals as their primary place to deliver care.

With these and other medical breakthroughs, the functions of hospitals changed as they began to provide patient care and medical educational opportunities for physicians, nurses, dentists, and pharmacists, and to conduct research activities. The hospital evolved into a multiservice institution and became the center of the health care system.

■ Hospital Types

There are many types of hospitals in the health care industry. They can be separated based on ownership, such as for-profit, not-for-profit, government, or physician-owned. Bed size categories, such as 1–50, 51–100, and 100–500, can be used to differentiate based on the scale of operation. Hospitals are defined based on the type of care provided, such as general acute care or specialty. Urban hospitals are different from their rural community hospital counterparts. We assess hospitals by identifying their main characteristics and roles in health care delivery. A hospital can be more than one type and no category is exclusive.

■ General Acute Care General Hospitals

General hospitals provide emergency care, general surgery, and admit patients for a wide range of general conditions and procedures. This type of hospital provides services for short-term illnesses or conditions (DHHS, 2010a). The majority of short-term general hospitals are nongovernmental and not-for-profit.

Teaching Hospitals

The Role of Teaching Hospitals

Teaching hospitals train future physicians and conduct research through clinical trials. Compared to the average hospital, they tend to have more sophisticated diagnostic and treatment technologies and treat the sickest patients. Most are nonprofit, and they are located in each state. In 2007, there were more than 1,000 teaching hospitals throughout the United States (AHA, 2009a). Teaching hospitals typically have additional training programs for nurses, nurse practitioners, and physician's assistants.

Reimbursement for Teaching Hospitals

Teaching hospitals receive substantial support from the National Institutes of Health (NIH) to fund clinical research and develop innovative applications of clinical science. They typically deliver specialized services that are not available at general community hospitals. Adult intensive care, neonatal intensive care, burn treatment, and organ transplant services are delivered at teaching hospitals.

Teaching hospitals receive extra reimbursement through Medicare and Medicaid to fund training and support of medical residents. Like all hospitals, teaching hospitals are affected by changing economic environments, and the recent economic recession has depleted their profit margins. Such changes strain the teaching hospital's resources to support their teaching and training and their role as a safety net hospital.

Historically, teaching hospitals have served as a critical safety net system for vulnerable patient populations. Many uninsured or underinsured patients receive care at teaching hospitals. Teaching hospitals provide a majority of all uncompensated care in the United States (AHA, 2009a).

Specialty Hospitals

Specialty hospitals provide inpatient care with highly technical tertiary or specialized services for specific conditions, such as cancer or pediatrics. The primary distinction between a general acute care hospital and specialty hospital is the breadth of services that are offered. Specialty hospitals typically focus on providing a select core of services. Examples of specialty hospitals include facilities for orthopedics, cardiology, surgery, rehabilitation, eye and ear care, arthritis, and mental health. Specialty hospitals may also be dedicated to a specific category of patients, such as children or women.

Rehabilitative Hospitals

Rehabilitative hospitals specialize in providing services to stabilized patients who are diagnosed with trauma or disease and need to learn how to function again in an inpatient setting. The patient may require speech, physical, or occupational therapy. Patients in a rehabilitation hospital are stable, but 24-hour nursing care is provided. This type is called a post-acute hospital (DHHS, 2010a).

▪ Critical Access Hospitals (CAH)

Critical Access Hospital Eligibility Requirements

Critical access hospitals (CAHs) must be located in a rural area and be more than 35 miles from any other hospital or 15 miles from another hospital in mountainous terrain or areas with only secondary roads (Rural Assistance Center, 2010). A CAH must be certified by the state as a necessary provider of health care to area residents and must provide emergency services 24 hours a day. They must maintain an annual average length of stay of 96 hours or less for their acute care patients and have a maximum of 25 acute care inpatient beds (Rural Assistance Center, 2010). CAHs are predominately not-for-profit institutions and operate with very limited resources. CAHs are located throughout the United States, with a concentration in the Midwest and Northeast.

Critical Access Hospital Reimbursement

CAHs receive cost-based reimbursement from Medicare, typically the largest payer. Medicare reimburses CAHs on the basis of the necessary cost of care for a patient plus 1 percent. The reimbursement is intended to improve their financial performance and reduce risk of closure. As of July 2009, there were 1,305 certified CAHs (Rural Assistance Center, 2010). Cost-based reimbursement differs from other rural and urban hospitals that are paid under the Medicare Prospective Payment System.

Critical Access Hospital Benefits

There are many benefits to being classified as a CAH: one such advantage is reimbursement based on cost of care plus 1 percent that allows additional focus on providing critical care for the community. CAHs typically network with acute care hospitals for support for services they are unable to provide. They are able to account for needed capital improvements to the hospital when determining the costs on which Medicare reimbursement is based. CAHs have access to state grant monies through the **Rural Hospital Flexibility Program (Flex Program)**, which provides assistance to CAHs, encourages the development of rural health networks, assists with quality improvement efforts, and improves rural emergency medical services (Rural Assistance Center, 2010).

CAHs typically have an agreement with a general acute care hospital for the transfer and referral of patients who require more intensive acute care. These transfers may be on an emergency or nonemergency basis. CAHs are required to have at least one physician with oversight responsibility on call. Mid-level providers such as a nurse practitioner or physician assistant typically direct patient care. This flexibility allows CAHs to provide care in rural underserved areas where recruitment and retention of full-time physicians and specialists is difficult (Rural Assistance Center, 2010).

CAHs are critical to providing primary care to rural underserved areas. They typically are the only provider within a 1- to 2-hour drive for patients. The distance from acute care and trauma care is critical during medical emergencies or accidents. Lack of access to primary and specialty care in rural areas affects the mortality rate and life expectancy of patients. They provide care in medically underserved areas with few physicians and where specialists may only visit several times a month. They represent a vital link in the continuum of care and a critical source of primary care for patients, many of whom may lack insurance in rural areas.

CAHs have addressed the importance of primary care by providing additional primary care services, public health screenings and health fairs, recruitment and retention of physicians, chronic illness prevention and education, and capital improvements to enhance their ability to provide care (Coburn & Gale, 2008).

■ Behavioral Hospitals

Behavioral hospitals specialize in treating individuals with a mental health diagnosis. Originally called psychiatric hospitals, these facilities have expanded their mission to treat a broader array of mental health disorders other than the most serious. Behavioral hospitals provide effective intervention to treat addictions and behaviors, and offer a safe therapeutic environment that helps to stabilize and motivate individuals to live their lives to the fullest.

■ Physician-Owned Specialty Hospitals

Most physician-owned specialty hospitals are for-profit and fall into four categories of specialized care: cardiac, orthopedic, general surgical, and women's health. Often referred to as boutique hospitals, these facilities are typically located in urban areas and owned by physicians who have admitting privileges. They are concentrated in states favorable to their growth, with most located in the western and southern regions of the United States. Texas leads all states, with 39 physician-owned specialty hospitals (AHA, 2008). General acute care hospitals face competition from specialty hospitals whose owners or investors include physicians who admit patients to the facility (GAO, 2006).

Physician-owned specialty hospitals raise concerns in the hospital industry. Federal law, or the Stark law, generally prohibits physicians from referring Medicare patients for specific services to hospitals or other facilities in which they have a financial stake (GAO, 2006). However, the Stark Law has an exception that allows physicians to refer patients to a hospital in which they have an ownership stake in the entire hospital and where they have staff privileges (GAO, 2006).

Specialty hospitals compete with general acute care hospitals, and several issues have been raised about their impact on community hospitals. First, there are concerns regarding how physician-owners make decisions when treating patients. Physicians-owners may have incentives to refer patients to hospitals in which they have a financial stake rather than another hospital, perhaps one that is more appropriate for the patient's condition. Physicians are permitted to refer patients to hospitals in which they have an ownership interest if they have a stake in the whole hospital (Guterman, 2006). Opponents argue that physicians should not be allowed to refer to such hospitals because they are providing only a limited service.

Second, specialty hospitals may attract only the least complex and most profitable cases. This phenomenon is driven by reimbursement that provides payment to hospitals upon discharge based on the diagnosis rather than the costliness of each case. Specialty hospitals that focus on cases that are less complex, easy, and more profitable, benefit financially, often called "skimming the cream."

Third, specialty hospitals have an incentive to avoid patients that are unable to pay because of a lack of financial resources. These patients may be uninsured or on governmental assistance, and they represent potential financial losses for the hospital. Community hospitals may be left with the responsibility of providing care for these patients while also contending with a diminishing patient population that is covered by commercial insurance plans (Guterman, 2006).

Fourth, specialty hospitals may harm the financial health of community hospitals that are specifically directed at providing affordable health care for their communities. Physicians who have a financial stake in their hospital have incentive to realize a financial reward from their investment. When physicians act on those incentives and direct patients who generate the most revenue away from community hospitals and toward specialty hospitals, then community hospitals will suffer. Such harm results because privately insured patients typically cross-subsidize the care that is provided to patients who cannot pay or to patients whose conditions cause the hospital to absorb financial loss (Guterman, 2006).

Although specialty hospitals may threaten the financial viability of community hospitals, they do have some advantages. Like specialists, specialty hospitals perform many procedures with a higher level of frequency than elsewhere, which results in better clinical outcomes. Specialty hospitals become very adept at their narrow realm of services, and physicians hone their skills and expertise, which results in benefits for patients.

The evidence regarding the response by community hospitals to the entrance of physician-owned specialty hospitals has been mixed. According to the Medicare Payment Advisory Commission (MedPAC), hospitals have responded by engaging in aggressive cost-cutting and pricing strategies (MedPAC, 2006). MedPAC is an independent Congressional agency established to advise Congress on issues related to Medicare reimbursement for health care services. Competitor community hospitals have responded by cutting expenses by cutting staff, raising revenue from private payers, and expanding profitable business lines such as imaging, rehabilitation, pain management, cardiology, and neurosurgery (MedPAC, 2006). These responses to competition from specialty hospitals, along with the growth in the patient population, have allowed community hospitals to maintain their financial health in line with national averages (MedPAC, 2006).

Operational challenges have emerged for community hospitals because of more competition from many types of facilities such as other general hospitals, ASCs, and imaging centers that far outnumber the relatively few specialty hospitals (GAO, 2006). The GAO found relatively few differences operational and clinical service changes between general hospitals with and without specialty hospitals in their market (GAO, 2006).

It is unclear whether community hospitals will be able to maintain their financial performance in the face of competition from specialty hospitals. As specialty hospitals continue to capture more profitable service lines and treat less complex and more profitable cases, the impact on community hospitals may be significant (Greenwald et al., 2006; MedPAC, 2006). The financial health of community hospitals has remained stable through 2004, even in those markets where physician-owned specialty hospitals have captured a significant share (10%) of the market (MedPAC, 2006).

The long-term impact of multiple providers expanding their delivery of profitable service lines may lead to overall higher health care costs. Providers have been expanding their profitable service lines, are providing a large number of services per Medicare beneficiary, and may threaten the viability of the Medicare system (MedPAC, 2006).

In summary, studies of the impact of specialty hospitals show that physician-owners do respond to the financial incentives to generate maximum revenue from hospitals in which they have a stake. On average, specialty hospitals treat less complex cases that generate more revenue for the hospital (MedPAC, 2006). This trend has led to calls for payments and the current diagnosis-related groups (DRGs) to be adjusted to reflect the complexity of cases. That is, more complex cases that are treated at community hospitals would receive higher reimbursement than the less complex cases treated at physician-owned specialty hospitals (Guterman, 2006). Specialty hospitals treat fewer patients who are uninsured or underinsured when compared with community hospitals (MedPAC, 2006). Perhaps most importantly, there is no concrete evidence that physician-specialty hospitals harm the financial health of community hospitals (MedPAC, 2006). This conclusion is based on a few studies at a relatively early point in the development of specialty hospitals.

■ Long-Term Care Hospitals

Long-term care hospitals (LTCHs) provide care to patients with clinically complex problems (e.g., multiple acute or chronic conditions), who need acute care for long time periods. To receive Medicare payment, an LTCH must meet Medicare's conditions of participation for acute care hospitals and have an average length of stay greater than 25 days for its Medicare patients. There are approximately 386 long-term care hospitals that receive Medicare reimbursement (MedPAC, 2010).

LTCHs may be a freestanding facility or be located within a short-term hospital as a hospital within a hospital. Patients that receive care in long-term care hospitals require concentrated care as they suffer from comorbidities and chronic conditions that are expensive to manage and control (MedPAC, 2010). Examples may include chronic obstructive pulmonary disease (COPD), respiratory conditions that may require respiratory support, complications due to diabetes or obesity, or renal failure (MedPAC, 2010). Most patients who receive care in a LTCH are female, white, and over 75 years of age (MedPAC, 2010).

State or federal government owns the majority of long-term general hospitals. The majority of long-term psychiatric hospitals are state-owned hospitals. An LTCH may also be owned by for-profit organizations and operated as a national chain. Examples include the top three for-profit LTCH chains: Kindred, Select Medical Corporation, and RehabCare Group (MedPAC, 2010).

Long-Term Care Hospital Reimbursement

Medicare is the predominant payer for LTCH services, accounting for about two-thirds of LTCH discharges. In 2008, Medicare spent $4.6 billion on care furnished in LTCHs (MedPAC, 2010).

■ Hospital Organization

The final authority for hospital operations rests with the board of directors or trustees. In the Darling Case (1968), the Board of Directors was held liable because it failed to put a quality-control mechanism in place to oversee the granting of admitting privileges for physicians. Most hospital boards are comprised of prominent community members or business or political leaders who have special administrative or political skills.

The board of directors in a hospital typically has several important functions in the hospital. It selects the CEO of the hospital, exercises control during a major crisis, reviews major managerial decisions and performance, establishes political and social contacts, raises funds, enhances the reputation of the organization, provides advice and technical assistance to the administrators, and develops political and community influence.

A unique organizational characteristic of hospitals is that they have physicians who are not employees, but who are staff with admitting privileges. These medical staff members, although not employees, have the main legal responsibility for patient care. They possess the power to admit patients and have the immediate primary responsibility for patient care. The hospital does not have the same power over the physician staff that it does over its traditional employees.

Historically, physicians have been a powerful influence in determining how hospitals operate because they could admit their patients at competing hospitals, and the hospital would lose patients. This behavior is problematic for the hospital in an area with a shortage of physicians. However, in an area with a surplus of physicians or a strong managed care presence, the physician advantage is much less or even reversed.

▪ Hospital Closure

Small nonprofit hospitals and publicly owned hospitals have the highest risk of closing and having poor financial as well as clinical performance. Small hospitals, with fewer than 100 beds are predominantly located in rural areas and are at high risk of closure. They are at risk because larger hospitals offer a larger mix of equipment, personnel, and services, and are usually located in more densely populated areas.

Rural areas are less densely populated, leading to lower hospital occupancy rates. Small hospitals lack high-tech equipment because there is not enough patient demand for it to be efficiently used. There are also fewer specialists in rural hospitals due to fewer patients and the lack of the latest technology in the hospitals. Furthermore, mortality rates, infection rates, and other complication rates have been higher in small hospitals. Given the extensive interstate highway system, many people who reside in rural areas are within a 3-hour or less drive from a large hospital.

Public hospitals are also at risk of closure because they deal with a disproportionately poor patient population; therefore, they are more likely to provide care that is not reimbursed. Studies have shown that publicly owned hospitals provide most of the uncompensated care in the health industry. The demand for such care is related to the fact that more than 45 million persons in America lack health insurance. Medicaid only covers about 40 percent of the poor, and both Medicare and Medicaid reimburse hospitals at a rate that is lower than the cost the hospital incurs for providing care.

Hospitals must charge a higher rate to patients who are privately insured to cover the costs of care for those that lack health insurance. This process is called "cost-shifting" to paying customers. However, patients that have employer-sponsored health insurance typically do not go to public hospitals, so there is no one to whom the costs can be shifted. As a result, these community hospitals are at far greater risk of closing their doors.

■ Hospital Economics

■ The Cost of Empty Beds

Empty beds are a cost to hospitals because they are associated with fixed costs, which include heat, electric, and staffing, as well as some ancillary services such as lab and X-ray. These costs do not change in the short term when the occupancy of the hospital changes. The fixed costs associated with those empty beds exist regardless of whether they are filled or empty. When hospital beds are empty, they cost approximately 70 percent of what the full cost is when beds are filled. The cost of empty beds as well as that of uncompensated care is covered through cost shifting when other patients in the hospital pay more for their care (e.g., private pay or private insurance pay). This move in turn drives up the cost of private health insurance and leads to increased taxes to support Medicare and Medicaid.

For example, consider when one hospital has a 90 percent occupancy rate and another has a 40 percent occupancy rate. If both hospitals were reimbursed for $5,000, the 40 percent occupancy rate hospital would be at a disadvantage because it would have to use the funds to pay for the empty beds, whereas the 90 percent occupancy rate hospital has revenues from its filled beds. The lesson is that it is always better, on average, to have higher occupancy when those patients occupying the beds generate revenue for the hospital.

Since 1980, hospital occupancy rates or average length of stay has decreased because of the introduction of a prospective payment system (PPS). This method of payment uses diagnosis-related groups (DRGs) to reimburse hospitals based on the primary diagnosis of the patient they treat. The primary diagnosis is part of a diagnostic-related group for which there is a set amount of money paid to the hospital. The hospital is reimbursed for delivering care to the patient, and the extent to which the hospital keeps its costs below the amount it is reimbursed, it makes a profit. This method of payment provides incentives for hospitals to discharge patients quickly to save money.

■ Impact of the Changing Economy on Hospitals

A hospital is in the business of producing health care services for patients. Like all other businesses, it is affected by cyclical changes in the economy. Starting in 2008, the economy of the United States experienced a recession and downturn, and hospitals were affected. In 2009, the median total margin of all hospitals, the difference between expenditures and revenues, had fallen to zero (AHA, 2009a). High unemployment means that fewer patients can afford care because they have lost their health insurance or are unable to pay. Business closings mean fewer patients covered with employer-sponsored health insurance.

Access to capital, dollars used for physical expansions and improvements, through capital markets was reduced because of the collapse in the housing and capital markets (Health Forum LLC, 2010). Hospitals are affected when access to capital is reduced during economic downturns (Health Forum LLC, 2010). Capital is required for hospitals to fund expansion and meet daily financial obligations. Hospitals reacted by delaying or stopping expansion projects, improvements in clinical technology, and information technology (Health Forum LLC, 2010). Deteriorating economic conditions impact the value of hospital investments, as do decreased charitable donations (Health Forum LLC, 2010).

Hospitals respond to changes in economic conditions by cutting expenses, reducing staff, and reducing services that are poorly reimbursed. Such services may include behavioral health, clinics, patient education, and post-acute care (Health Forum LLC, 2010).

▪ Uncompensated Care and Bad Debt

Under federal law, hospitals must provide care for patients with life-threatening conditions that present in their emergency department. Hospitals must provide care to stabilize the patient and then either admit the patient or transfer him or her to another hospital for ongoing care. Hospitals also provide care to many patients who are uninsured or underinsured and are not able to pay their hospital bill. Millions of dollars are written off by hospitals each year when providing such care to patients. Economic conditions such as recessions, layoffs, and changes in reimbursement from payers adversely impact how much uncompensated care hospitals are able to deliver.

The monies that hospitals write off each year fall into several categories. Uncompensated care is a large category that includes all care for which there was no payment received from a patient or a payer. **Charity care** is patient care for which a hospital does not expect to be reimbursed (AHA, 2009b). Charity care is typically provided to patients who are uninsured and have no means to pay the hospital.

Bad debt is incurred from services not reimbursed that are provided with the expectation of being reimbursed. For instance, an insured patient may be unable to afford the copayments or coinsurance portions of their payment. Hospitals have faced increases in uncompensated care costs for the last two decades, starting in 1980 (AHA, 2009b).

▪ Reimbursement by Medicare and Medicaid

Hospitals are not required to provide services for patients covered by Medicare and Medicaid unless they present with a life-threatening condition. However, for many hospitals the revenue from Medicare and Medicaid is a substantial portion of their revenue. For most hospitals the amount that is paid to hospitals for providing services to such patients does not cover their cost. The difference between the hospital cost of care and the amount paid to the hospital for providing care is called an **underpayment** (AHA, 2009c).

Hospitals have been experiencing growing underpayments from Medicare and Medicaid. From 2000 through 2008, underpayments to hospitals from Medicare and Medicaid have grown from $3.8 billion in 2000 to $32 billion in 2008 (AHA, 2009c). In 2008, the average hospital was reimbursed approximately 90 cents for every dollar spent caring for Medicare and Medicaid patients (AHA, 2009c).

▪ Community Hospitals

Community-hospital inpatient days have decreased, while their outpatient visits have increased. Occupancy rates in community hospitals have decreased since the 1970s for several reasons, primarily because of a shift to outpatient care and advances in health care technology.

Hospital revenue sources for community hospitals have shifted toward outpatient services due to technological advances, more outpatient services, and government and industry curtailing costs. There has been a significant decrease in the number of community hospitals in rural areas compared to urban areas. In the 1980s, nearly 10 percent of rural hospitals closed, and although that rate decreased in the 1990s, rural hospitals continued to close (Cecil G. Sheps Center, 1998). These closures had a marked effect on rural residents' access to care such that one-third of rural residents' hospitalizations in 2003 were in urban hospitals (Hall et al., 2010).

Community hospital closures affect access to care, as patients must find somewhere else to receive care. Closure also influences the local economy and employment, as the community hospital may be the largest employer in a community, especially in rural communities. Patients who need care, as well as persons who are seeking employment, are adversely affected when they close.

Hospitals and Their Feeder System

Hospitals obtain patients from a feeder system composed of office-based physicians who typically refer patients needing further care to hospitals. During the 1980s, multi-hospital systems formed, and they purchased physician offices, stimulating a trend in the growth of multi-specialty physician group practices. Affiliated hospitals, hospital-owned urgi-care centers, hospital-owned physician practices, and hospital-owned nursing homes continue to provide patient referrals to hospitals.

Trends in Health Care Facilities

Formation of Integrated Delivery Systems

The major trend in the nation's hospital system is the development of multi-hospital chains and hospital mergers. A multi-hospital chain is an example of **horizontal integration** of corporate structure. Horizontal integration is the merger of similar organizations, such as hospitals with hospitals, and nursing homes with nursing homes. Horizontal integration reduces the costs associated with market competition. By merging with the competition, a hospital no longer needs to expend extra effort to compete.

There are several advantages to hospitals forming multi-hospital systems. Multi-hospital systems improve access capital. A multi-hospital system will have a higher bond rating and therefore pay lower interest rates because it is spreading the risk over multiple hospitals and, thus can "buy money" more cheaply. With horizontal integration, other operational advantages are expected. Separate providers may realize economies of scale through merging together as they expand the scope of their operation. That is, as the breadth of the operation increases, the overall cost may decrease for the provider. A hospital system may be able to operate more efficiently by purchasing supplies at a higher volume and a higher discount. This formation is similar to the advantages the discount retail gaint Walmart has over smaller specialty stores. Brand recognition may increase when the hospital system expands its marketing to a wider patient audience. Patient referral patterns may be more predictable within the system as physicians refer to specialists who are within its network. Physician recruitment and retention is enhanced as the resources and technology of a larger system improves patient care and outcomes.

Second, a health system has the advantage of both recruitment and retention of high-quality employees because it can often offer more competitive benefit packages to employees than freestanding institutions. Third, a multi-hospital chain can have a regional focus and thus maximize its political influence. The larger the organization, the more likely it will be able to affect state, local, and even national law, regulation, and policy. If the hospitals and other component facilities are concentrated over several bordering state areas, they can have a regional political influence as well as develop a large health care referral network.

▪ Vertical Integration

Another trend among hospitals is integration among health care organizations, or **vertical integration**. Vertical integration improves the ability of providers to capture patients by controlling the continuum of care that is delivered to patients. This purview provides the organization with a market advantage over competitors and potentially higher profits.

A vertical merger exists when a hospital joins with one or more health maintenance organizations (HMOs), outpatient clinics, home health agencies, rehabilitation centers, long-term care facilities, urgi-centers, and technical laboratories, or wellness clinics.

Vertical integration can include *forward* vertical integration, where hospitals purchase health maintenance organizations (HMOs), wellness clinics, surgi-centers, or rehab centers. This form of integration brings the hospital providers closer to the patient. Vertical integration can also encompass *backward* vertical integration, where hospitals purchase a manufacturer of health care supplies or technology, a biotech company, or a producer of biotech products used in hospitals. This form of integration brings the provider closer to their suppliers.

▪ Competitive Strategies of Hospitals

The ultimate purchasers of hospital services are physicians on behalf of patients (Devers, Brewster, & Casalino, 2003). Physicians also have incentives to use the most technological advanced hospital services, and they may benefit financially by performing more tests and procedures. In addition, hospitals compete with one another by marketing and providing highly specialized services that generate significant revenue through higher prices.

Inpatient Specialty Services

Hospitals compete by developing specialty care in areas such as cancer treatment, invasive cardiology, orthopedic surgical centers, hospital–physician **joint ventures**, and heart hospitals (Devers et al., 2003). In many instances, these services are developed despite the fact that a competitor may already offer the service. Duplication of service occurs when two or more competitors offer the same type of service in a patient market. Thus, when two hospitals compete with one another, each may offer sophisticated imaging services, both of which are used at perhaps 60 percent capacity. Hospitals rationalize this apparent inefficiency by arguing that such services maintain or enhance the reputation of the facility in the eyes of the community, and such services are necessary to maintain the support and loyalty of their medical staff. Nevertheless, this inefficiency is detrimental to the health care system because valuable resources could otherwise be used to develop forms of care that would benefit patients.

Outpatient Facilities

Hospitals also compete by adding outpatient centers, ambulatory surgery, diagnosis, testing, and treatment (Devers et al., 2003). Hospitals face pressure to reduce costs, and patients prefer outpatient settings that offer fewer risks of adverse events than inpatient hospitals. Outpatient testing and diagnosis facilities also lead to a predictable stream of patients to the main hospital facility. For instance, mammograms and colonoscopies may lead to further cancer treatment and surgery. Hospitals are increasingly losing market share to other providers of outpatient services.

Hospital–Physician Joint Ventures

Hospitals compete by forming joint ventures with physicians. For example, in some states physicians are not reimbursed for imaging services unless they are part of a multimodality-imaging center with full-time radiologists. Physicians would form a joint venture with a hospital meeting those requirements. In addition, hospitals and physicians may joint venture to form a new company that might provide cardiac catheterization services. For hospitals, a joint venture with physicians provides them with a smaller percentage of the market share, but a reduced share is better than none (Berenson et al., 2006). It is a win–win proposition for the hospital and physicians. Hospital quality is enhanced, service lines generate revenue, and physicians are retained in the market through joint venture activities (Berenson et al., 2006).

Hospitals also benefit from joint venture activity by preempting possible competition from specialists in ambulatory care and referring patients to other hospitals (Lake, Devers et al., 2003). As specialty groups have consolidated, hospitals face stiffer competition for outpatient services because the specialty groups have more market power and access to capital (Lake et al., 2003).

Joint ventures with specialists can be critical for hospitals that depend on them for referrals. Specialists can attract patients needing profitable services to hospitals, bringing in added revenue under fee-for-service arrangements. They can also harm a hospital through directing patients to other hospitals if they are not satisfied with the hospital or hospital system (Lake et al., 2003).

Physicians also benefit from forming a joint venture with a hospital. They gain access to capital, management expertise, a larger pool of potential patients, and preemption of head-on competition with the hospital (Berenson et al., 2006).

One of the concerns of joint integration between hospital and physicians is the impact it can have on the prices charged for services. A joint venture is able to capture more of the local market for certain services, thereby potentially lessening competition among providers and increasing prices (Ciliberto & Dranove, 2006).

A national study of hospital joint ventures identified positive outcomes for financial performance for hospitals with joint ventures with physicians (Harrison, 2006). Hospitals that operate joint ventures were also found to be operating at higher clinical and financial complexity than their counterparts. They had a higher occupancy rate and a longer average length of stay, more **diversification strategies**, lower long-term debt, and more managed care contracts (Harrison, 2006).

Hospital Specialized Services and Centers of Excellence

Teaching hospitals frequently develop unique services to attract patients with specific diagnoses who require specialized care by highly trained specialists. Services such as eye surgery or ophthalmology, brain surgery, pain management, hernia repair, gamma-knife brain surgery, rehabilitation, and prostate treatment are specialized services that hospitals use to capture unique patient groups.

Hospitals can declare that they offer center of excellence care in areas such as cardiology, transplantation, surgery, cancer treatment, patient safety, minimally invasive surgery, surgical weight loss, and robotic surgery. Hospitals typically invest in specialists, marketing, and the technology, and announce they operate a center of excellence. Hospitals may determine that they operate a center of excellence without a formal accreditation (Devers et al., 2003).

Hospital Diversification Strategies

Hospital diversification strategies include freestanding outpatient diagnostic services, inpatient rehabilitation, freestanding outpatient surgery services, industrial medicine, and women's medicine. These strategies are implemented to increase both profits and patient volume.

Other diversification strategies for hospitals include developing emergency departments, outpatient alcohol or chemical treatment centers, hospices, outpatient departments, outpatient rehabilitation, home health care, and occupational therapy. Hospitals may also develop other special services such as organ transplants, cardiac catheterization, advanced cancer treatments, and other advanced treatments.

Competition between hospitals has led to an increase in the diversity of services that are offered. Services that are more complex enhance the prestige of a facility. Hospitals are offering more technological services because health care is increasing in complexity and hospitals must maintain their market share of patients. They may lose customers to competitors if they are not offering the latest advances in health care such as cardiac catheterizations. Physicians also want to admit patients to hospitals that are offering the best health care with the best technology.

Hospitals have increased their focus on delivering ambulatory services due to their lower cost. The reimbursement method for inpatient care is a prospective payment system (PPS) where the provider is reimbursed a specific amount for the primary diagnosis. This method of payment has forced the hospital to cut costs and consequently the profits for some diagnoses have been lowered. Thus, by shifting the patient away from inpatient care to less stringently controlled outpatient care, there is the potential to increase profits.

▪ Hospital Personnel

More than half of hospital expenses go to pay salaries, wages, and benefits for its employees. Hospitals typically are one of the largest employers in their market and consistently rank among the top 10 employers in the large urban areas such as Boston, New York, Pittsburgh, and Cleveland. In Cleveland, the two largest hospital systems, the Cleveland Clinic Health System and the University Hospitals Health System, are the top two employers and together employ more than 43,000 workers (AHA, 2006). From a regional perspective, hospital positions can account for more than 4 percent of employment (AHA, 2006).

Between 1993 and 2009, the number of employees in community hospitals had experienced a steady growth. Hospitals are the second largest source of private sector jobs and spend billions of dollars on goods and services provided by other businesses (AHA, 2011a).

The impact of hospitals in rural areas is significant because they are usually the largest or the second-largest employer (AHA, 2011b). The hospital provides a source of positions for high-level technicians, physicians, and pharmacists. The impact of a rural hospital on its local economy is usually higher than in urban areas because it is likely to be the main employer. Total direct and indirect employment generated by health care is often 10–15 percent of a rural community's employment (AHA, 2011b).

Although hospitals are typically the primary employer in their market, they do face serious workforce shortages in key caregiver positions. An America Hospital Association survey of hospital leaders found that hospitals face workforce shortages that affect patient care (AHA, 2006).

Hospitals are combating the current difficulties in recruiting nurses through an array of strategies. Some hospitals offer tuition-reimbursement programs, partner with local colleges to offer training, or recruit nurses from overseas locations such as India, the Philippines, or Africa. Overseas recruitment has been criticized for causing a "brain-drain" of skilled clinicians from third-world countries. Nursing recruiters insist, however, that providing well-paying jobs in the United States offers nurses a secure high-paying job and a significantly improved lifestyle.

Hospitals offer a wide array of high-tech services and therefore require a wide range of skill levels. They employ caring physicians, nurses, and therapists, as well as offer blue-collar positions in environmental and food services.

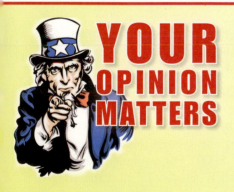

YOUR OPINION MATTERS

Should Robots Be Allowed to Provide Care and Support for Patients in Hospitals?

Background: Using Robots in Hospitals

Robots are the newest development in providing care and support for patients in hospitals. They are able to dispense medication, make deliveries, visit patients, and perhaps improve the way hospitals function. Robots are helping doctors reach patients across distances.

Yes

Advantages of Robots in the Hospital

Robots perform tasks for nurses, support staff shortages, and streamline many tedious administrative tasks (Andrews, 2009). They transport materials

(Continued)

like food, X-rays, and linens throughout the hospital. They are able to travel a set path and avoid collisions by using sonar. Robots do not have many of the disadvantages of humans in carrying out menial tasks. For instance, robots do not require bathroom breaks or vacation and benefits, nor do they waste time when working (Grey, 2007). Robots also follow commands without complaint.

Robots use a wireless system, Wi-Fi, or an active radio frequency identification (RFID) network to navigate throughout the hospital and perform its tasks (Grey, 2007). The manufacturer maps a wireless route and programs it for the robot before the robot is expected to navigate throughout the hospital. Robots rarely have any technical glitches and can haul up to 500 pounds. Whenever a technical problem does arise in a robot, it can automatically call a technical support desk, and the problem can be addressed remotely by the manufacturer (Grey, 2007). Studies have shown that a fully functioning robot performing routine hospital tasks can do the job of 4.2 people, and hospitals can realize a return on their investment in the range of 30–50 percent (Grey, 2007).

Robots enable virtual physician visits (Andrews, 2009). Physicians can remotely examine patients from afar with hi-tech visuals, provide faster service to patients, and increase doctor–patient contact, although remotely. Medical robots are fully mobile, with computer screens for heads and real-time video cameras for eyes and ears. Doctors or nurses can operate them using a joystick and wireless technology, while saving staff from cross-infection (Andrews, 2009). For example, when a nurse measures a patient's pulse or heart rate every 15 minutes, it disturbs the patient and infection can occur with diseases like MRSA. But these robot systems allow for a no-touch situation that can still read vital signs (CNN, 2006).

Future robots may be able to directly assist nurses in performing menial tasks such as cleaning bed pans, giving injections, and lifting patients (CNN, 2006). However, they will never be able to replace the caring nurse.

Robotic Surgery

Robots, as with all investments in expensive health care technology, are used in hospitals to improve clinical care and slash error rates, reduce patient stress, and encourage healing (Andrews, 2009). For example, robots are increasingly used to perform operations such as general abdominal procedures like gallbladder removal, heart surgery, prostate cancer surgery, gynecologic procedures, and bariatric surgery, among others (Andrews, 2009). The robotic procedure is performed as a surgeon manipulates computer controls rather than a scalpel (Andrews, 2009). During surgery, the surgeon views the surgical field on a screen while in the operating room. Instruments are guided through ports to the surgical site and then controlled by the physician via a joystick and buttons (Andrews, 2009). The operator has three-dimensional (3-D) stereo imagery available and a motion-scaling concept, which can be scaled down to five-to-one, to be more precise than a human hand (CNN, 2006). In addition, the surgeon feels very similar sensations to those he or she would feel working with their hands (CNN, 2006). Robots help surgeons cope with the exhaustion of long procedures, and some have been programmed to compensate for the hand tremors tired surgeons experience (CNN, 2006).

Robotic surgery has grown in the field of laparoscopic surgery (Corcione et al., 2005). In laparoscopic surgery, a surgeon operates on patients with the aid of a small camera or laparoscope, and instruments inserted through small incisions. Applications of laparoscopic surgery include operations on the colon and hernia repair, among others. Robotic surgery offers the following advantages over laparoscopic surgery techniques: a stable camera platform, replacing two-dimensional (2-D) with three-dimensional (3-D), imaging, improved mobility when compared with the straight laparoscopic instruments, and offers the surgeon a comfortable and ergonomically optimal operating position (Corcione et al., 2005).

Potential future applications call for the surgeon to be located in even more remote locations, such as across a city or the world. This use raises the potential of increased access to care in remote locations or battlefields (Andrews, 2009). Advantages of robotic surgery are less pain and blood loss, and potentially better clinical outcomes. Experts say this benefit is due to the robot's steadier "hands" and wider range of motion than human hands. In addition, the instruments are more flexible than traditional laparoscopic instruments (Andrews, 2009).

No

Limitations of Robots in the Hospital

There are limitations to using robots in a hospital. They do not replace the human-to-human touch that "laying on of hands" provides. Patients in the hospital are sick, vulnerable, scared, and overwhelmed. Another human being at the bedside who shows compassion, caring, and concern is not replaced with a machine-like device. Overuse of robots may alienate patients who expect a human caregiver providing bedside care, listening to their concerns, and providing verbal and nonverbal direct communication. Robots are also very expensive and require a significant investment in wireless networks required for their navigation.

With surgical robots, the instruments are also expensive and need to be replaced after a number of surgeries (Corcione et al., 2005). Larger operating rooms are required for surgical robots that make small operating theaters impractical. Each type of surgical procedure requires the surgical robot to be prepared in a unique manner that is time-consuming for staff (Corcione et al., 2005). Further, operating with a robotic instrument is not the same as a surgeon using his or her own hands and having contact with the tissue, sutures, and scalpel during the procedure. Surgeons must rely on visual cues to estimate the impact of their instruments on tissue (Corcione et al., 2005).

(Continued)

Limitations of Robots in Surgery

Robots have limitations in performing surgery. For instance, complications may arise during the procedure, and emergency measures would be required. A patient could suddenly start to bleed extensively, experience an irregular heart rate, or suffer complications in breathing. A robot would have to be replaced with a human able to manage the complications and adjust the manner in which the procedure was performed (Corcione et al., 2005).

Other limitations include the liability of the surgeon in the event of robotic equipment failure. Yet another barrier is the liability for the delay in the transmission of electronic commands if the surgeon is in a remote location. There may also be state and international licensure issues that would limit surgeries being performed remotely (Marescaux & Rubino, 2006).

You decide:

1. If you were a patient in a hospital, suffering from pain and discomfort, would you prefer a human being or a robot to monitor your vital signs and deliver your medication to your bedside?

2. What would expect of a robot before you would feel comfortable as a patient?

3. Would you allow your surgeon to use robotic instruments in your surgical procedure?

4. What would you need to know before you would agree to the use of robotics in a medical procedure?

■ Hospitalists

A hospitalist is a physician who specializes in the care of inpatients in place of the primary care physician (Wachter, 2008). The number of hospitalists has grown throughout the United States, making it the fastest growing specialty (Wachter, 2008).

■ Hospital Accreditation

Smaller hospitals are less likely to be accredited by the Joint Commission because they have greater difficulty meeting the criteria for accreditation. Costs of preparing for accreditation are significant, and smaller hospitals are less likely to have the latest health care technology, they offer fewer services because they do not have the population density to support them, and their staff is less likely to be certified in their area of care. Smaller hospitals are also at greater risk of closure. A "survival" strategy that small hospitals are utilizing is to convert their empty floors into nursing homes and engage in vertical integration with other providers to diversify care offerings.

Accreditation by the Joint Commission is voluntary, but there are strong legal and financial incentives to seek it. Many assume that accreditation by the Joint Commission is necessary for improving the quality of care delivered in a hospital, as Joint

Commission requires periodic reviews. Because a high priority is placed on delivering high-quality care in the United States, there are dozens of agencies that regulate components of the health care delivery system. Among them are the Community Health Accreditation Program, Inc. (CHAP), a subsidiary of the National League of Nursing (NLN) that certifies home care and community health organizations; the Accreditation Commission for Health Care, Inc. (ACHC), which approves home care services; the Continuing Care Accreditation Commission (CCAC), which oversees continuing care retirement communities; the Commission for Accreditation of Rehabilitation Facilities (CARF), which certifies hospital-based or freestanding medical rehabilitation centers, adult day services, and assisted living centers; American College of Surgeons Commission on Cancer (ACS-CoC), which certifies cancer treatment programs in hospitals, outpatient centers, and freestanding facilities; Council on Accreditation (COA), which covers outpatient mental health, residential treatment centers, alcohol and other substance abuse treatment centers, and therapeutic foster care; and Accreditation Association for Ambulatory Health Care (AAAHC), which certifies ambulatory surgical centers, medical and dental group practices, community and university, student health centers, and diagnostic imaging centers.

▪ History of Hospital Funding

▪ Hill-Burton Act 1948

After WWII, the United States shifted from a wartime to a peacetime economy. During the 1950s and the 1960s, there was unprecedented economic prosperity, which gave rise to concern for those who were less fortunate and not experiencing these benefits. There was a perceived shortage of hospital beds in rural areas and less access to care, followed by an increase in government financing of health care institutions in an effort to build or expand nongovernmental, not-for-profit hospitals.

The **Hill-Burton Act**, or the Hospital Survey and Construction Act of 1948, was designed to bring hospital beds to areas that were previously underserved. Two-thirds of the beds built during this time were in rural areas, and 40 percent of the money went to rural hospitals. In addition, Hill-Burton increased the quality of hospitals in that a number of physician-owned hospitals with six to seven beds were replaced by larger hospitals with 20–40 beds. The government also believed that if more hospitals were built in rural areas, they would attract physicians to these areas. Today, however, the modern interstate highway system allows a majority of patients to bypass these smaller community hospitals.

Another downside to the Hill-Burton Act was that it increased the number of small hospitals and created a surplus of short-term beds in rural areas. Small hospitals with less than 200 beds often are less efficient and have lower quality with less technical competence than larger facilities. The federal funding for the Hill-Burton Act was eventually phased out in 1979.

▪ Funding Sources for Hospital Construction

During the 1960s, the government played a large role in constructing new hospitals. As a result, the number of hospital beds per 1,000 of the population peaked in 1960.

During the late 1970s, policy makers believed that there were too many hospitals, physicians, and beds, leading to unnecessary utilization of those beds. Between the date of passage of the Hill-Burton Act and today, many hospitals closed. Overall, funding sources for hospital construction shifted from government and philanthropy to mechanisms used by other private construction ventures like obtaining debt financing from banks and other money institutions and establishing capital reserves from yearly revenues for expansion.

Trends in Hospital Financing

Uncompensated Care

Hospitals provide millions of dollars in uncompensated care every year when patients are unable to pay their bills. The amount of uncompensated care has increased as the number of uninsured and underinsured patients has grown. Because Medicaid only covers approximately 40 percent of the poor, they are disproportionately more likely to be without health insurance and less likely to have a job that offers health benefits. Furthermore, Medicaid and Medicare typically reimburse a hospital less than the actual cost of delivering care, which has exacerbated the uncompensated care problem. Private commercial insurance companies usually reimburse hospitals at 129 percent of costs.

Although the amount spent on uncompensated care continues to increase, it has remained relatively constant as a percentage of health care costs. Hospitals engage in cost-shifting and pass the cost for providing uncompensated care to patients with private commercial insurance, which results in higher premiums. Hospitals in high-poverty areas frequently do not have anyone to whom they can shift their uncompensated costs. Hospitals offer services to some needy patients through Medicaid, a federal-state program that does not fully reimburse hospitals for the cost of their care.

Advertising

Hospitals, physicians, or other health professionals did not engage in advertising before the 1980s, as it was considered unethical. Today, advertising by hospitals and other health care providers is critical to maintaining their market share and brand recognition. Many health care markets are extremely competitive, with too many beds, and in some areas, too many physicians. Many companies engage in health care advertising that is directed at consumers bypassing physicians in favor of direct marketing to patients.

Hospital Ownership Status

For-profit hospitals are not more efficient. With the implementation of diagnosis-related groups (DRGs) and the prospective payment system for hospital reimbursement, the rate of closure of for-profit hospitals increased over that of not-for-profits. The reason was that before DRGs and a prospective payment system, for-profits were reimbursed on a cost-plus basis, which established a reasonable profit margin above actual costs. Not-for-profit hospitals were reimbursed strictly on a cost basis. After the advent of the prospective payment system, both types of hospitals were reimbursed on the same basis, eliminating the profit margin. In addition, for-profits have to pay taxes and pay dividends to shareholders.

For-profit hospitals also attempt to attract the healthiest, wealthiest patients, or "skim the cream" off of the patient population. For-profit hospitals are typically located in suburbs where healthier and wealthier patients live and where they are less likely to encounter poor patients who lack health insurance. They tend to not participate in research and teaching, which often entails higher costs of care that may not be covered by private insurance companies. Overall, for-profit hospitals have lower rates of uncompensated care than not-for-profit hospitals, and shorter average lengths of stay.

◾ Hospital Performance

Many factors affect the performance of hospitals. The government and other third-party purchasers apply significant pressure to contain cost through managed care and prospective payment plans. With a prospective payment system, hospitals are paid based on the primary diagnosis that is made by their physician. Second, hospitals face competition from other delivery sites such as other hospitals in their market, physician offices, and local clinics. This competition also requires hospitals to invest in marketing campaigns that increase brand recognition.

Third, the cost of investment in health care technology has increased in accord with the increased availability of such technology. Health care technology is a significant investment for a hospital and required to provide the best clinical care for patients. The hospital then is required to utilize the technology to recoup their invested dollars. Fourth, hospitals are constrained when the economy is in a slow growth period. The economy always has periods of slow growth and faster growth. When the economy is strong and more people are employed, there are more patients who are insured by commercial insurance companies. Commercial insurance companies typically reimburse hospitals for their services at a higher rate than the government, through Medicare or Medicaid.

Finally, the changing governmental philosophy about health care is always in flux, depending on who is president and which party controls Congress. The president may place a high priority on funding for hospitals and reimbursement of health care services. The president's annual budget is submitted to Congress and reflects these priorities. Congress must approve the increases in spending and may or may not have the same priorities as the president.

Hospitals also are subject to forces that propel them to expand and grow. For instance, new demand for health services such as wellness programs, outpatient care, and outpatient surgery provide opportunities for hospitals to invest in those markets. Second, hospitals have more discretion in attracting patients and developing more markets as the power of physicians in hospitals has weakened. Third, new organizational structures influence hospitals. Whether a hospital is a member of a hospital system, affiliated with other hospitals, or is an independent not-for-profit community-owned hospital will impact its investment decisions.

Fourth, management teams of hospitals have become more focused on treating hospitals as a business organization. Hospital leaders concentrate on delivering care in an efficient manner, improving quality, and increasing the revenue of the organization.

Finally, the aging population means that there are more elderly patients and their health care needs are more acute. Hospitals are required to invest in resources that provide care to a larger population of patients who suffer from chronic conditions such as diabetes, heart disease, memory loss, dementia, pain management, and cancer treatment.

Changing customer expectations for services at hospitals could influence hospitals to expand or restrain their growth. For instance, many people view rationing of care as acceptable in the modern health care industry with escalating costs—just as long as their personal health care is not rationed.

■ Ambulatory Surgical Centers

An ambulatory surgical center (ASC) furnishes outpatient surgical procedures to patients who do not require an overnight stay following the procedure (MedPAC, 2010). The majority of surgeries in the United States are performed in the outpatient setting, and Medicare spending on outpatient services has increased significantly (Chukmaitov et al., 2008). Many ASCs are owned by physicians or have at least one physician-owner. They may also be a joint venture between a physician group and a hospital (MedPAC, 2010).

■ Growth in Ambulatory Surgical Centers

Hospitals face increasing competition from **ambulatory surgical centers (ASCs)**. They are typically located in physician offices and freestanding facilities. Since 1981, there has been a steady decline of surgeries performed in hospital outpatient settings and a steady increase in surgeries performed in freestanding ASCs. In addition, there has also been an increase in the percentage of outpatient surgeries performed in physician offices (Koenig et al., 2009). The number of ASCs has increased steadily throughout the last 10 years because of incentives provided through favorable reimbursement and increased efficiency. The number of Medicare-certified ASCs grew at an average yearly rate of 7.1 percent from 1997 through 2008 (Koenig et al., 2009). In 2008, ASCs provided care to 3.3 million Medicare beneficiaries, an increase of 2.8 percent over 2007, and the number of Medicare-certified ASCs was 5,175, an increase of 3.7 percent over 2007 (MedPAC, 2010).

In 2008, there were approximately 5,175 Medicare-certified ASCs, with the majority being proprietary (MedPAC, 2010). On the other hand, the number of hospitals has remained fairly stable at roughly 4,800 in 2008. ASCs are concentrated heavily in California, Florida, and Texas (Koenig et al., 2009). Most ASCs are multi-specialty facilities offering a variety of outpatient surgical services, with the next two largest categories comprising facilities that specialize in gastrointestinal and ophthalmology services, respectively (Koenig et al., 2009).

A number of factors account for the high growth rate, including guidelines for disease screening (e.g., colorectal cancer screening), growth in outpatient surgeries performed in ASCs versus the hospital outpatient setting, reimbursement that provides incentives to perform surgeries in the most cost-effective setting, demographic changes, consumer and physician preferences, and physicians investing in ASCs to receive more favorable professional fees (MedPAC, 2010). The federal anti-referral law, also known as the Stark law, does not apply to surgical services being performed on an outpatient basis (MedPAC, 2010).

■ Technology in Ambulatory Surgical Centers

Improvements in surgical technology have enabled ASCs to perform many different types of surgeries in an outpatient setting. Such improvements have enabled patients to recover faster, experience less pain, and enjoy overall better clinical outcomes. Such technologies include minimally invasive surgical procedures, anesthesia, and improved pain management after discharge (Koenig et al., 2009).

■ Services Provided by Ambulatory Surgical Centers

Ambulatory surgical centers provide outpatient services. The following are the most common areas: eye procedures such as cataract removal and lens insertion, gastrointestinal procedures such as colonoscopies and endoscopies, pain management, and orthopedic surgery (Koenig et al., 2009). Most of the growth in services provided in ASCs has been for cataract surgeries, colonoscopies, and upper gastrointestinal procedures. These services are critical for patients covered by Medicare as they are preventive cancer treatments and screenings (Koenig et al., 2009).

There are differences between patients that receive care at an ASC and those that receive care at a hospital outpatient surgery service (MedPAC, 2010). Physicians can choose which patients to serve and which patients to refer to the local hospital outpatient surgery department. A physician-owner may also have a motive not to treat patients who would increase the cost of care as a consequence of complications. Overall, ASCs are less likely to serve patients who may have medical complications, who are covered by Medicaid, who are members of minority groups, and who are Medicare beneficiaries due to age or a disability (MedPAC, 2010).

■ Competitive Advantages of Ambulatory Surgical Centers

The growth in ASCs has been driven by patient and physician preferences. ASCs operate more efficiently than hospitals and have lower fixed costs. Overall, patients have lower copayments, more locations that are accessible, shorter wait times, and easier scheduling procedures than they do at hospitals (Koenig et al., 2009).

Physicians prefer to operate in ASCs as they can concentrate on one type of procedure and develop expertise and efficiency by performing high volumes of the same operation. They are able to manage their work environment more effectively by making personal decisions regarding equipment use, nursing staff composition, and operating schedule. The nursing staff is also able to be more efficient because staff members are concentrating on a select number of surgical procedures that are performed at high volumes. The combination of experienced physicians and nurses enables ASCs to increase productivity and maximize their revenue (Koenig et al., 2009).

It has been suggested that ASCs may have better clinical outcomes because physicians can pick and choose which patients to operate on and which to refer to the local hospital. Perhaps sicker patients may be referred to the local hospital that has sufficient resources to care for a patient that may develop complications (Chukmaitov et al., 2008). However, if an ASC specializes in certain types of procedures, it may improve patient outcomes. There have been several empirical studies performed that have shown a correlation between hospital procedural volume and better clinical outcomes. Overall, the specialized, high volume focus of many ASCs may improve patient outcomes and lower the cost of care for patients and the health care industry (Chukmaitov et al., 2008).

Vignette

THE GEISINGER EXPERIENCE

Geisinger Health System (Geisinger), headquartered in Danville, PA, is one of the premier academic medical centers in the United States. It is an example of how a major medical center has adopted health care technology and case management strategies to reduce the cost of care for its patients and improve clinical outcomes. President Barack Obama has highlighted Geisinger in several of his speeches as an example of successful use of health care technology and efficient care of chronic conditions. It has been recognized as a leader in the specialty care of the elderly (Steele, 2009).

Founded in 1915, Geisinger provides care in 43 Pennsylvania counties and serves 2.6 million patients a year (Geisinger, 2010). The patient mix at Geisinger is rural, older, sicker, suffering from multiple chronic conditions, and covered by either Medicare or Medicaid (Geisinger, 2010). Geisinger employs approximately 800 physicians who see patients in more than 50 clinical practice sites throughout Pennsylvania. Geisinger has successfully implemented innovative programs to address the special challenges it faces in providing care to its patients (McCarthy, Mueller, & Wrenn, 2009). The system has bundled payments for acute care procedures, improved support for its primary care physicians and care teams, and better managed chronic disease and the transitions of care for patients from caregiver to caregiver. Overall, these programs have led to reduced admissions for patients with multiple chronic conditions by 25 percent and readmissions following discharges has decreased by as much as 50 percent in community sites (Steele, 2009). The following sections provide an overview of several of the successful strategies that Geisinger has implemented to improve clinical outcomes, harness technology, and reduce costs.

I. Health Care Technology

Geisinger provides care to 2.6 million patients in central and northeastern Pennsylvania. The organization has an enterprise-wide electronic health record (EHR) that was implemented 14 years ago, with more than 3 million individual patient records (Steele, 2009). With the adoption of health care technology, Geisinger has been named as "MostWired" by *Healthcare's MostWired* magazine seven times (*Healthcare's MostWired*, 2010).

Geisinger's EHR allows customers to book their own appointments, leading to 95 percent attendance, compared with 60 percent if receptionists schedule the patient. During office visits, physicians are able to determine immediately what diagnostic tests have been performed, reducing duplicative care and delays (Fifield, 2010).

Geisinger has implemented an innovative tool to connect with and monitor their patients—their own electronic medical record. Patients access their lab results, radiology results, request prescription refills, and email their doctors, nurses, and staff with questions. Appointments can also be scheduled online (Steele, 2009).

Geisinger's size allows it provide a health care insurance product, the Geisinger Health Plan, which enrolls nearly 250,000 members, 35,000 Medicare beneficiaries, 18,000 network physicians, and 90 hospitals, not including Geisinger hospitals, and it spans most of Pennsylvania (Abelson, 2010).

II. Medical Home Initiative

Geisinger's Medical Home program is called ProvenHealth Navigator and strives to improve patient care coordination throughout the system. The program covers more than 30,000 Medicare recipients and 3,000 commercial patients (Steele, 2009). It is in use in 37 physician practices, most of which are part of its own network (Abelson, 2010). The offices are targeted to have the most impact with their patients, and nurses assigned to follow their patients through the full continuum of care. The nurses become personally acquainted with their patients and their families, follow their patients' care, and help patients gain access to specialists and social services, as necessary. The nurses follow patients when they are admitted to a hospital, contact or see them when they are sent home to confirm that they are taking the appropriate medication dosages, and are available for advice 24 hours a day (Steele, 2009).

Patients can also manage their conditions through a home-based monitoring interactive voice-response surveillance (Paulus, Davis, & Steele, 2008). Patients are also provided support for end-of-life care decisions (Paulus et al., 2008).

Through its **medical home**, Geisinger provides access to an electronic health record to physicians, care managers, and patients. Patients are able to access and analyze their lab results, schedule appointments, communicate via email with providers, refill their prescriptions, and learn more about their condition through online content (Paulus et al., 2008). Through their heath record portal, patients are able to access a referral network if they are in need of medical or surgical specialists, imaging, or other ancillary services.

Geisinger physicians are given additional reimbursement to implement the medical home features. Bonus payments are based on whether the practice adds additional staff members, provides extended hours, or puts into practice other medical home initiatives, and on the reduction in cost of caring for patients (Paulus et al., 2008). Providers closely track performing reports when implementing medical home initiatives to monitor progress.

Geisinger has seen results from its investment in its medical home. In the top-performing medical practices, admissions for patients who were sickest with chronic diseases decreased by 25 percent, days in the hospital decreased by 23 percent, and readmissions following discharge decreased by 53 percent (Steele, 2009).

The success of the medical home model is dependent on nurses who work closely with the doctors to oversee the patients' care. They schedule appointments for patients at the last minute, notify physicians of early signs of trouble, keep in close contact with the patients, and monitor the patient's health through evaluating their lab results (Abelson, 2010).

III. Care Management of Chronic Conditions

Geisinger identified the most common chronic diseases, such as diabetes, coronary artery disease, congestive heart failure, and kidney disease, and applied evidence-based best practices to manage the care of their patients. The strategy is called "bundled care," and Geisinger incorporates best care practices into care pathways 100 percent of the time through its electronic medical record (EMR). Only compliance with 100 percent of the recommended bundled care practices is considered a successful implementation of the strategy. Through use of the EMR, patients' care plan needs are identified electronically and incorporated into physician care plans and automatic health maintenance alerts. A condition-specific dashboard captures relevant clinical information on a single screen (Paulus et al., 2008).

For example, care for a diabetic patient consists of nine different evidence-based best care practices. Diabetic patients are automatically identified prior to their arrival at the clinic, and a patient-specific set of orders is generated (including standing orders for routine testing such as for HbA1c and LDL) that can be accepted by the physician with a single click of a mouse (Paulus et al., 2008).

While caring for patients with chronic conditions, automatic alerts are provided to both the clinical team and the patient, and patients can schedule their own appointments through their EHR. After each visit, a patient can access his or her after-visit summary. Data show how the patient is doing in reaching goals to manage their condition. Accompanying the goals is an explanation of the risks associated with failing to achieve the goal. Patients receive their own report card through their EHR (Paulus et al., 2008).

Performance reports are presented to each physician practice, detailing both individual physician and practice-site performance compared with historical trend and other similar practices (Paulus et al., 2008). Primary care physicians are reimbursed based on how many of their patients receive best practice care services (Steele, 2009).

IV. Reimbursement for Physicians

Geisinger rewards improvements in clinical quality and reimburses its staff for better clinical outcomes financially and with recognition rewards. Physicians are benchmarked against their peers, both within Geisinger and nationally (Steele, 2009). Physician, staff, and site incentives are built into its system of reimbursement to reward quality and superior outcomes (Steele, 2009).

Salaried physicians have 20 percent of their compensation based on bonuses awarded for quality improvement rather than the number of patients they treat. This payment is different from the fee-for-service reimbursement schedule, where doctors are paid a fee for each treatment, making it worth their while to perform more tests and procedures (Fifield, 2010).

V. Acute Episodic Care Program

Geisinger has implemented a program called ProvenCare to encourage its staff to use best practices in treating patients with episodic acute procedures such as coronary artery bypass grafts (CABGs). Geisinger developed a set of best practices to provide treatment for CABG patients and programmed it into the patient's electronic medical record to prompt the physician at each step. It established one price for the bundle of services provided to CABG patients and absorbed the costs of additional treatment due to complications from the procedure (Steele, 2009).

Employers were attracted to the cost savings associated with the single-episode package price for the CABG. The package includes preoperative evaluation and workup, all hospital and professional fees, all routine post discharge care (e.g., smoking cessation counseling and cardiac rehabilitation), and care for any related complications within 90 days of elective CABG surgery (Paulus et al., 2008).

ProvenCare is an example of a new program that successfully uses evidence-based practices to cut costs and improve clinical outcomes. Three months after the program started, 86 percent of CABG patients were receiving best care, and this rate increased to 100 percent (Steele, 2009). The program has produced favorable results: complications were reduced by 21 percent, infections decreased by 25 percent, and readmissions fell by 44 percent; costs for treatment were reduced, and average length of stay decreased by half a day (Steele, 2009).

ProvenCare has been expanded to include other bundled services for the following services: hip replacement, cataract surgery, obesity surgery, prenatal care for babies and mothers from an infant's conception to birth, and heart catheterization (Paulus et al., 2008).

VI. Conclusion: Lessons Learned from the Geisinger Experience

The Geisinger experience provides insights into successful strategies for using technology, evidence-based best practices, and the medical home to deliver superior care and improve clinical outcomes. Although Geisinger is a unique provider with both a health plan and a widespread delivery network, it provides insights into proven successful strategies that cut costs while improving care for a diverse patient population.

Several factors are critical to the success of Geisinger. It is an integrated delivery system (IDS) and enjoys strong support from its physicians in implementing its initiatives (Paulus et al., 2008). It possesses substantial financial resources as an integrated delivery system (IDS) with which to invest in its electronic health record and health care technology (Paulus et al., 2008). Its physicians are committed, entrepreneurial, and willing to attempt new unproven strategies for the benefit of their patients (Paulus et al., 2008).

1. What lessons can managers learn from Geisinger to improve the operations of their hospital?

2. What lessons can patients learn from Geisinger to help them improve their hospital stay or visit with their physician?

3. Should all hospitals and physician offices use electronic medical records (EMRs) in order to reduce medical errors and improve clinical outcomes?

4. Could other health systems implement lessons learned from ProvenCare in their treatment of CABG patients?

5. Should physicians be financially rewarded and penalized based on the clinical outcomes of their patients?

6. What lessons can patients learn from the ProvenHealth Navigator?

Nursing Homes

Nursing homes have been defined by the National Center for Health Statistics (2009) as

> Facilities with three or more beds that routinely provide nursing care services. Facilities may be certified by Medicare or Medicaid (or both), or not certified but licensed by the state as a nursing home. The facilities may be freestanding or a distinct unit of a larger facility.

Nursing homes are critical to providing services along the continuum of long-term care. The most recent survey data reported that there were 1.5 million nursing home residents in approximately 16,000 facilities in the United States (NCHS, 2009).

The modern nursing home provides inpatient, outpatient, and outreach services for their patients. It may provide education for residents and staff and be engaged in research or demonstration projects to improve long-term care (Goldsmith, 1994). Nursing homes began to increase in number after the passage of Medicare and Medicaid in 1965. Demand for nursing home services is projected to double between 2000 and 2050 (NCHS, 2009).

Assisted Living Communities

Assisted living facilities (ALFs) bridge the gap between a skilled nursing facility and the patient's home. An ALF provides housing with professional support services including nursing services in a residential group setting (Evashwick, 2005). There are many different names for assisted living services, such as residential care, personal care, or adult living facility. (An in-depth discussion of long-term care facilities is in Chapter 7.)

Continuing Care Retirement Communities

A continuing care retirement community (CCRC) offers a full range of services for residents, from independent living through skilled nursing home care. The CCRC offers a wider continuum of care than other facilities. For instance, if the resident's health declines and he or she is unable to live independently, the person is able to move to the assisted living area, or receive home care in his or her unit in an **independent living facility**. If necessary, the resident can enter the onsite or affiliated nursing home (DHHS, 2010).

A CCRC may be a multi-building campus, or the facility may be housed in one building with separate floors or areas to dedicate to the respective services. A CCRC has facilities for social and recreational activities such as a cafeteria, exercise facilities, library, and computer lab, as well as areas for laundry (AAHSA, 2010). Each CCRC houses from 400 to 600 residents (Evashwick, 2005).

▪ Summary

There are many settings in which care is delivered in the health care industry. The community hospital is a major provider site but is facing increasing competitive pressure from ambulatory surgical centers, physician offices, diagnostic and imaging centers, and other specialty hospitals. Community hospitals are no longer the center of the health care system. There have been many hospital closures; for example, over 1,000 community hospital have closed in the past 20 years. Hospital admissions are down and average length of stay (ALOS) has decreased, thus reducing hospital volume and associated revenue. Competition, reimbursement changes, and advancements in health care technology have all contributed to reducing ALOS for inpatients, with a commensurate increase in the scope of services provided in ambulatory settings and in physician offices.

Many hospitals struggle to operate with lower reimbursement from Medicare and Medicaid, higher numbers of uninsured and underinsured patients, and higher costs for expensive technological equipment. Changes in economic conditions affect hospitals because patients who lose their jobs also lose their employer-based health insurance and thus their ability to pay for care. Hospitals face grim prospects as they are forced to continue to provide care to more patients who cannot pay for their care with lower reimbursement from providers.

Ambulatory surgical centers and physician-owned specialty hospitals may continue to increase their market share among patients whose care is reimbursed at higher levels than Medicaid patients. However, such facilities may offer a lower-cost alternative for select procedures than acute care hospitals. High volumes of procedures have led to improved patient outcomes, and therefore outpatient facilities may improve the efficiency and quality of care overall.

Assisted living facilities and skilled nursing homes will face a changing patient population as average life expectancy increases, more patients suffer from chronic conditions, and dementia and Alzheimer's disease become more prevalent among residents.

▪ Review Questions

1. What are the primary reasons health care facilities expand or are built?

2. What role does reimbursement for health care services, including ambulatory care, long-term care, and rehabilitative care, play in building new facilities for patients to receive care?

3. What factors should administrators consider before planning to build a new hospital or ambulatory surgical center?

4. How is the baby boomer generation going to impact the construction of new facilities for hospital care or nursing home care?

5. What is the impact of the uninsured population on hospitals and long-term care facilities and their ability to remain profitable?

6. Are wholly owned physician specialty hospitals harmful for the financial health of general community hospitals?

7. What is the impact on community hospitals from increased levels of competition from specialty hospitals, ambulatory surgical centers, imaging centers, and physician offices?

8. What is the impact on rural communities from reduction in access to hospitals and physicians due to hospital closure or reduction of services whenever physicians leave a rural community?

9. What has your experience been visiting loved ones in a nursing home? What improvements did you observe that should be made to enhance the care provided to residents in a long-term care environment?

10. What types of improvements in the layout of patient rooms can hospitals make to enhance the patient's stay at a hospital?

■ Additional Resources

Agency for Health Research and Quality (AHRQ): www.ahrq.gov/

American Hospital Association (AHA): www.aha.org

Centers for Medicare & Medicaid Services (CMS): www.cms.hhs.gov

Congressional Budget Office (CBO): www.cbo.gov

Federal Legislative Information: http://thomas.loc.gov/

Food and Drug Administration (FDA): www.fda.gov

Government Accountability Office (GAO): www.gao.gov

Health and Human Services (HHS): www.hhs.gov

Healthcare Leadership Council (HLC): www.hlc.org

HHS Assistant Secretary for Planning and Evaluation: www.aspe.hhs.gov

HHS Office of Inspector General: www.oig.hhs.gov

Hospital Care Quality Information from the Consumer Perspective: www.hcahpsonline.org/home.aspx

Hospital Compare: www.hospitalcompare.hhs.gov

Institute of Medicine: www.iom.edu

Joint Commission: www.jointcommission.org

Kaiser Family Foundation: www.kff.org

Medicare Payment Advisory Commission (MedPAC): www.medpac.gov

National Institutes of Health (NIH): www.nih.gov

National Quality Forum (NQF): www.qualityforum.org

Office of Management and Budget (OMB): www.whitehouse.gov/omb

The State-of-the-Art of Online Hospital Public Reporting: A Review of Fifty-One Websites (CMS-Funded Report, July, 2005): www.delmarvafoundation.org/newsAndPublications/reports/index.html

TRICARE: www.osd.mil

References

American Association of Homes and Services for the Aging (AAHSA). (2010, March 8). Fact sheet: What you need to know about CCRCs. Retrieved March 8, 2010, from http://www.aahsa.org/section.aspx?id=5936.

Abelson, R. (2010, June 21). *A health insurer pays more to save*. Retrieved July 24, 2010, from http://www.nytimes.com/2010/06/22/business/22geisinger.html.

American Hospital Association (AHA). (2006). *Beyond health care: The economic contribution of hospitals*. Chicago, IL: Author.

American Hospital Association (AHA). (2008). *Trendwatch chartbook*. Chicago, IL: Author.

American Hospital Association (AHA). (2009a). *Teaching hospitals: Their impact on patients and future health care workforce*. Chicago, IL: Author.

American Hospital Association (AHA). (2009b). *Uncompensated hospital care cost fact sheet*. Chicago, IL: Author.

American Hospital Association (AHA). (2009c). *Underpayment by Medicare and Medicaid*. Chicago, IL: Author.

American Hospital Association (AHA). (2011a). *Economic contribution of hospitals often overlooked*. Chicago, IL: Author.

American Hospital Association (AHA). (2011b) *Trendwatch: The opportunities and challenges of rural hospitals in an era of health reform*. Chicago, IL: Author.

Andrews, M. (2009, July 15). *The high-tech hospital of the future*. U.S. News and World Report. Retrieved July 28, 2010, from http://health.usnews.com/health-news/best-hospitals/articles/2009/07/15/the-high-tech-hospital-of-the-future.html.

Berenson, R. A., Ginsburg, P. B., & May, J. H. (2006, December 5). Hospital-physician relations: Cooperation, competition, or separation? *Health Affairs*, W31–W43.

Cecil G. Sheps Center for Health Services Research. (1998). Effects of rural hospital closure on access to care. Working Paper No. 58. Durham, NC: University of North Carolina at Chapel Hill.

Chukmaitov, A. S., Menachemi, N., Brown, L. S., Saunders, C., & Brooks, R. (2008, October). A comparative study of quality outcomes in freestanding ambulatory surgical centers and hospital-based outpatient departments: 1997–2004. *Health Services Research, 43*(5), Part I, 1485–1504.

Ciliberto, F., & Dranove, D. (2006). The effect of physician-hospital affiliations on hospital prices in California. *Journal of Health Economics*, *25*, 29–38.

CNN.com. (2006, April 26). Trust me, I'm a robot. Retrieved July 28, 2010, from http://www.cnn.com/2006/TECH/science/04/19/robmedical/index.html.

Coburn, A., & Gale, J. (2008). The flex program at 10 years: Community impact lessons and future directions. *NRHA Annual Meeting* (pp. 1–16). New Orleans, LA: Flex Monitoring Team.

Corcione, F., Esposito, C., Cuccurullo, D., Settembre, A., Miranda, N., Amato, F., et al. (2005). Advantages and limits of robot-assisted laparoscopic surgery. *Surgical Endoscopy, 19*, 117–119.

Devers, K. J., Brewster, L. R., & Casalino, L. (2003). Changes in hospital competitive strategy: A new medical arms race? *Health Services Research*, *38*,(1), Part II, 447–469.

Evashwick, C. J. (2005). *The continuum of long-term care.* Clifton Park, NJ: Thomson Delmar Learning.

Fifield, A. (2010, January 7). Innovative hospitals offer model for reforms. Retrieved July 26, 2010, from http://www.ft.com/cms/s/0/8837e026-fbbc-11de-9c29-00144feab49a.html.

Geisinger. (2010, July 23). About Geisinger. Retrieved July 23, 2010, from http://www.geisinger.org/about/index.html.

Goldsmith, S. (1994). *Essentials of long-term care administration.* Gaithersburg, MD: Aspen Publishers.

Greenwald, L., Cromwell, J., Adamache, W., Bernard, S., Drozd, E., Root, E., et al. (2006, January/February). Specialty versus community hospitals: Referrals, quality, and community benefits. *Health Affairs, 25*(1), 106–118.

Grey, M. (2007). Hospital goes robotic. *Healthcare Informatics, 24*(7), 18–21.

Guterman, S. (2006). Specialty hospitals: A problem or a symptom? *Health Affairs*, *25*(1), 95–105.

Hall, M. J., Marsteller, J., Owings, M. (2010, November 18). Factors influencing rural residents' utilization of urban hospitals. National Health Statistics Reports No. 31. Centers for Disease Control and Prevention.

Harrison, J. (2006). The impact of joint ventures on U.S. hospitals. *Journal of Health Care Finance*, *32*(3), 28–38.

Healthcare's MostWired. (2010, July 23). 2010 Most Wired results announced. *Healthcare's MostWired.* Retrieved July 23, 2010, from http://www.hhnmostwired.com/hhnmostwired_app/index.jsp.

Health Forum LLC. (2010). *Trends: Even as health reform takes center stage, economic challenges remain.* Chicago, IL: Author.

Koenig, L., Doherty, J., Dreyfus, J., & Xanthopoulos, J. (2009). *An analysis of recent growth of ambulatory surgical centers: A final report.* Washington, DC: KNG Health Consulting.

Lake, T., Devers, K., Brewster, L., & Casalino, L. (2003). Something old, something new: Recent developments in hospital–physician relationships. *Health Services Research, 38*(1), 471–488.

Marescaux, J., & Rubino, F. (2006). Transcontinental robot-assisted remote telesurgery, feasibility and potential applications. In K. Yogesan, S. Kumar, L. Goldschmidt, & J. Cuadros, *Teleophthalmology* (pp. 261–266). Berlin, Germany: Springer.

McCarthy, D., Mueller, K., & Wrenn, J. (2009). *Geisinger health system: Achieving the potential of system integration through innovation, leadership, measurement, and incentives.* Washington, DC: The Commonwealth Fund.

MedPAC. (2006). *Report to Congress: Physician-owned specialty hospitals revisited.* Washington, DC: MedPAC.

MedPAC. (2010). *Report to Congress: Medicare payment policy.* Washington, DC: MedPAC.

Metlife Mature Market Institute. (2009). *The 2009 MetLife Market Survey of Nursing Home, Assisted Living, Adult Day Services, and Home Care Costs.* Westport, CT: Metlife Mature Market Institute.

National Center for Health Statistics. (2009). *The National Nursing Home Survey: 2004 overview.* Hyattsville, MD: National Center for Health Statistics.

Paulus, R., Davis, K., & Steele, G. (2008). Continuous innovation in health care: Implications of the Geisinger experience. *Health Affairs, 7*(5), 1235–1246.

Rural Assistance Center. (2010, March 11). *CAH frequently asked questions.* Retrieved March 11, 2010, from http://www.raconline.org/info_guides/hospitals/cahfaq.php#whatis.

Steele, G. (2009, April 21). *Healthcare reform and Geisinger.* Retrieved July 23, 2010, from http://www.geisinger.org/about/healthier/index.html.

U.S. Department of Health and Human Services (DHHS). (2010a). *Glossary of terms.* Retrieved March 5, 2010, from http://www.hospitalcompare.hhs.gov/Hospital/Static/SupportingInformation_tabset.asp?activeTab=2&Language=English&version=default.

U.S. Department of Health and Human Services (DHHS). (2010b). *Understanding long-term care.* Retrieved March 8, 2010, from http://www.longtermcare.gov/LTC/Main_Site/Understanding_Long_Term_Care/Services/Services.aspx.

U.S. Government Accountability Office (GAO). (2006). *General Hospitals: Operational and clinical changes largely unaffected by presence of competing specialty hospitals.* Washington: Author.

Wachter, R. M. (2008). The State of Hospital Medicine in 2008. *The Medical clinics of North America, 92,* 265–273.

CHAPTER

10 Cost of Health Care Services

Key Terms

cost–push inflation

demand–pull inflation

diagnosis-related groups (DRGs)

Final Report of the Committee on the Costs of Medical Care

gross domestic product (GDP)

medical malpractice

national debt

national deficit

Organization for Economic Cooperation and Development (OECD)

"pain and suffering"

quality improvement (QI) initiatives

Roemer's law

Learning Objectives

- Identify the primary factors that lead to higher health care costs.

- Describe the impact of higher health care costs on insurance premiums, Medicare and Medicaid, and personal bankruptcies.

- Assess the relationships among health costs, access, and quality.

- Describe the methods used by government to control health care costs.

■ Introduction

The cost of health care has been an issue at the forefront of debate since the inception of health insurance. Few Americans can afford expensive treatments and procedures without some form of coverage. As health care costs rise faster than other commodities, and faster than personal income, individuals and the nation have to make budget adjustments to pay for this necessity. The costs of health care far exceed the capacity of individual incomes, particularly for the majority of uninsured. In addition, for those with limited coverage—the underinsured—rising costs are barriers to obtaining some types of care.

Yet only once, in the early 1990s, has health care been a number one priority among the top 10 societal problems as viewed by the public. Consequently, for most people the economy, terrorism, and education take precedence over concerns about the health care system. However, when asked about health care, the vast majority of the public are concerned about the rapidly rising costs and expenditures.

When in the middle of an episode of serious illness like a heart attack, patients and their families tend not to focus on the cost of treatment. They do not deny themselves necessary treatment because of cost—unless, of course, they cannot afford an organ

224

transplant out-of-pocket and their insurance will not cover it. Mostly, we care about cost when it affects what we pay in taxes to fund Medicare, Medicaid, or our health insurance premiums. High-income families have the heaviest tax burden, so they bear much of the costs of financing government programs. Yet, health care spending makes up the smallest proportion of income among those high-income families. Among low-income families, approximately 20–25 percent of income is allotted to health related spending.

One of the major driving forces in rising health care costs and expenditures is the presence of the third-party payer health insurance system. Health insurance increases the utilization or demand and subsequently the expenditures in health care, because at the time services are received, someone else, such as a third-party payer, is paying for it.

Consider the following example: Suppose there is a type of insurance that insures you against the cost of buying a car. Every time you buy a car, you only have to pay $1,000–$1,500 deductible, and the insurance company pays the rest. Assume that this type of insurance business is actually profitable. Obviously, with this kind of insurance, most people would buy cars without thinking twice about it, and they would want to purchase very luxurious cars. This behavior actually resembles what we are doing in health care.

Thus, one implication of a third-party-paying insurance system is that consumers of health care services do not pay the total price of services at the time care is received. When the consumer does not have to worry about the price of care, purchasing or utilization will be determined more by the need or the desire for goods and services. The true cost of those goods and services will not be considered in the purchasing decision. This system may provide a disincentive for healthy, responsible behavior. Individuals will have less of an incentive to change behavior when they know that someone else will pay for the health care consumed to treat a serious health condition such as one that resulted because of their smoking or drinking habits.

If food prices increased at the same rate as health care prices have since the 1930s, we would be paying $69.99 per pound for bacon. However, this analogy does not account for the substantially improved quality of health care because of technology, whereas the quality of bacon has essentially remained the same. Yet, can we say that increases in quality have kept pace with increases in cost?

Health care spending has been steadily increasing for decades. One indicator of health care spending is by measuring it per person, or per capita. When health care spending is measured in this manner, it clearly shows a persistent increase over the past 20 years. In 2009, the nation spent over $8,000 per capita on health care compared to $7,000 just three years earlier; under $5,000 per capita 10 years earlier in 2000; and under $3,000 per capita 20 years earlier in 1990 (CMS, 2010).

■ What Affects Health Expenditures?

As the quantity of health care services consumed increases, total expenditures also increase. Delivering health care goods and services requires several inputs, in economic terms. These inputs can be classified as either labor or nonlabor. Nonlabor inputs include the purchase of a hospital bed, an ambulance, or aspirin, or the construction of new hospital facilities. Labor inputs include the services rendered by physicians, nurses, technicians, and administrators. Total expenditures are a function of both labor and nonlabor inputs, and influenced by the size of the patient population served by the health care system. The following formula illustrates this relationship. The residual or error factor is used to approximate changes in the quality of care:

$$\text{Expenditures} = (\text{Price of nonlabor inputs}) \times (\text{Quantity of nonlabor inputs})$$
$$+ (\text{Price of labor inputs}) \times (\text{Quantity of labor inputs})$$
$$+ (\text{Residual/error} \sim \text{quality})$$

Health Care Costs as a Portion of the Gross Domestic Product

Gross domestic product (GDP) is the value of all of the goods and services produced in the United States. Spending on health care services is a significant portion of our GDP. Health care spending is expected to reach 19.6 percent of GDP by 2016, up from 17.3 percent in 2009 (Norman, 2010). Changes in the levels of health care spending have a significant impact on our national economy. If we reduce the level of health care spending, fewer persons will be employed in the health care industry and fewer facilities would be constructed. Less spending on health care will also affect both the access to and quality of care. Conversely, increased spending can cause increases in taxes and the cost of doing business.

Health Care Costs to Society

Health care costs may be direct or indirect. Indirect costs may be in the form of lost productivity or foregone income during recovery from an illness or from "premature" death. The indirect cost of illness is significant for most diseases and may be more than the direct cost of treatment. Income is foregone when a person is sick because he or she may not be able to work, may pay fewer or no taxes, and may lose health insurance and become dependent on society.

Direct cost of illness includes the cost of a physician visit, a prescription, or a day in the hospital. Proportionally, heart disease has a smaller indirect than a direct cost to society because the loss of productivity is usually from older, retired individuals. Accidents have a much higher indirect cost, because younger people are disproportionately affected and they may not be able to earn income during their peak earning years.

The bulk of direct health care spending is consumed by hospital services (California Healthcare Foundation, 2007). This portion of health care spending is driven by the high cost of technology, inpatient services, and prices that hospitals must charge to cover losses incurred in caring for the uninsured population (i.e., uncompensated care).

Global Health Care Costs

Health care as a percentage of gross domestic product (GDP) and per capita health expenditures are higher in the United States than in other economically developed countries. Intense use of health care technology, cost of physician services, and the extensive medical research conducted in the United States are several of the primary drivers of health care spending. Health care systems of all developed nations, such as

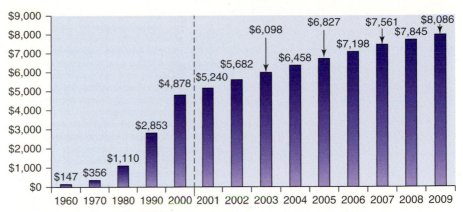

Figure 10–1 National health expenditures per capita, 1960–2009.

Source: Kaiser Family Foundation (KFF). (2010c). Kaiser Slides. Per capita total current health care expenditures, U.S. and selected countries, 2008. Menlo Park, CA: Author. Retrieved November 1, 2011, from http://facts.kff.org/results.aspx?view=slides&topic=3.

Canada and Japan, are also experiencing rapid growth in their health care costs and expenditures and the percent of the GDP they comprise. Yet health care spending per capita in the United States is more than twice that of any other developed nation. See Figure 10–1 for a graphical description of the growth in per capita health care spending from 1960 through 2009.

Figure 10–2 provides a graphical representation of the growth and the projected growth in per capita spending from 1990 through 2019.

Citizens of the United States typically do not travel to other countries to receive care. Conversely, many people from other developed countries travel to the United States to access care that is often of higher quality or not as readily available in their country.

The health care system in the United States is pluralistic, with a mix of employer-financed health care with private and government-financed health care. Our pluralistic system stands in contrast to most other developed countries that have national health

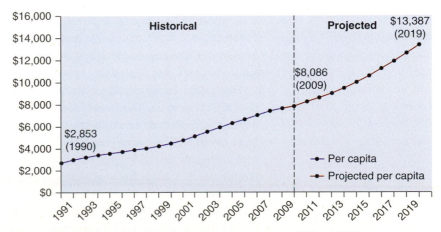

Figure 10–2 National health expenditures per capita, 1990–2019.

Source: Kaiser Family Foundation (KFF). (2010c). Kaiser Slides. Per capita total current health care expenditures, U.S. and selected countries, 2008. Menlo Park, CA: Author. Retrieved November 1, 2011, from http://facts.kff.org/results.aspx?view=slides&topic=3.

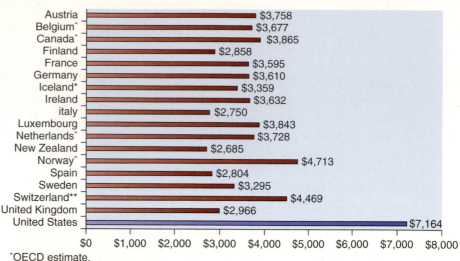

^OECD estimate.
*Differences in methodology.
**Based on 2007 data.

Figure 10–3 Per capita total current health care expenditures, United States and selected countries, 2008.

Source: Kaiser Family Foundation (KFF). (2010c). Kaiser Slides. Per capita total current health care expenditures, U.S. and selected countries, 2008. Menlo Park, CA: Author. Retrieved November 1, 2011, from http://facts.kff.org/results.aspx?view=slides&topic=3.

Notes: Amounts in U.S.$ Purchasing Power Parity, see www.oecd.org/std/ppp; includes only countries over $2,500. OECD defines Total Current Expenditures on Health as the sum of expenditures on personal health care, preventive and public health services, and health administration and health insurance; it excludes investment.

services that both provide and finance the health care of its citizens. Compared with other high-income countries that are members of the **Organization for Economic Cooperation and Development (OECD)**, the United States has a much higher annual growth in health care spending than its counterparts (White, 2007). In a study that tracked health care spending from 1970 through 2002, the United States experienced a significantly higher rate of growth than its OECD counterparts (White, 2007). See Figure 10–3 for a graphical representation of the differences in health care spending among OECD countries. Per capita spending by the United States far outpaces other similarly developed countries.

Four factors explain the disparity in growth between the United States and the rest of the OECD countries. The United States has an aging population, significant economic expansion, exploding growth in the use of technology in the provision of health care, and expansion of insurance coverage (White, 2007). Technology advancements in health care treatments have made it possible for more people to receive care at a reduced price. Health care technology has also improved clinical outcomes, reduced length of stay, and generally improved the quality of care delivered in the United States (White, 2007).

Another major driver of the higher spending on health care in the United States is the reliance on private insurance to finance health care. The United States depends on the private insurance market to finance a much higher percentage (41%) of health care than its counterparts in the OECD (12%) (White, 2007). Unlike many other OECD countries, the United States (with the exception of Medicare) does not rely on a central authority to reduce health care spending. The United States allows nongovernmental hospitals to set their own prices and provide whatever services they choose. Physicians are permitted to set their own prices and provide whatever services they are licensed to provide. Other than for Medicare, the United States government does not control what is charged or spent on health care services (White, 2007). The government does not set budgets for health care providers, and it does not determine what prices providers charge for their services (White, 2007).

■ Reasons for Concern over Rising Expenditures and Costs for Health Care

The national concern over rising health care expenditures overshadows increases in other commodities, even expensive items such as automobiles, houses, computers, health clubs, vacation travel, and music. Increases in consumption of these goods and services typically indicate a healthy economy. The following sections detail the basis of our concern over rising expenditures for health care services.

■ Cost versus Access

As the price of health care increases, it becomes more difficult for people to afford health insurance. Remaining uninsured or underinsured restricts access to health care and disproportionately affects the poor and unemployed. For instance, in 2009 the uninsured rate for children in poverty (15.1%) was greater than the rate for all children (Census Bureau, 2010).

Consistent access to a health care provider, like the necessities of food and shelter, directly affect the health of its purchasers. In 2008, 46.3 million people, or 15.4 percent of the population, lacked insurance in the United States (Census Bureau, 2010). The number of people without health insurance coverage rose to 50.7 million in 2009, and the percentage of uninsured increased from 15.4 percent to 16.7 percent over the same period (Census Bureau, 2010). In 2009, 10.0 percent (7.5 million) of children under 18 were without health insurance, a figure that remains relatively unchanged from the 2008 estimate (Census Bureau, 2010). Each year, providers render a substantial amount of uncompensated care to those who cannot afford it. Nevertheless, the fear that one cannot pay for needed health care is real.

The concern that arises from limited access to health care is the impact that it has on the health status of the persons without insurance coverage. Patients that skip having their prescription filled, their annual physical, their annual mammogram, or their dental checkup are at risk for experiencing lower levels of health than patients who have insurance and access to a customary source of care. See Figure 10–4 for a breakdown of the types of health care services that are skipped or delayed due to the lack of insurance.

■ Cost versus Quality

Quality of health care is critical to producing good health outcomes, and it requires significant investment of resources to maintain and improve. Strategies to reduce costs and expenditures, such as the rationing of care, very likely will have an adverse effect on quality. Quality may also be affected by reimbursement changes initiated by

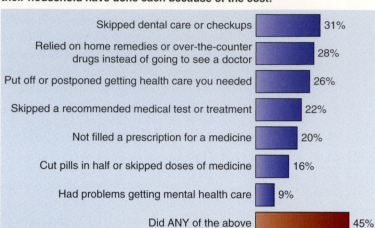

Percent who say in the past 12 months, they or another family member in their household have done each because of the cost:

Skipped dental care or checkups	31%
Relied on home remedies or over-the-counter drugs instead of going to see a doctor	28%
Put off or postponed getting health care you needed	26%
Skipped a recommended medical test or treatment	22%
Not filled a prescription for a medicine	20%
Cut pills in half or skipped doses of medicine	16%
Had problems getting mental health care	9%
Did ANY of the above	45%

Figure 10–4 Putting off care because of cost.
Source: Kaiser Family Foundation (KFF). (2010b). Health tracking poll. Conducted June 17–22, 2010. September 21. Menlo Park, CA: Kaiser Family Foundation Author. Retrieved November 1, 2011, http://facts.kff.org/chart.aspx?ch=840

containment strategies such as prospective payment systems and **diagnosis-related groups (DRGs)**.

According to one physician survey, DRGs have affected physician practices. About 31 percent of physicians reported that they were more selective in ordering diagnostic tests; 29 percent limit hospital stays; 13 percent were cost-conscious in their practice; 8 percent lowered fees; and 6 percent prescribed generic medications. Quality levels are affected in nursing homes that, to contain costs, employ untrained and inadequate staff, take inadequate safety precautions, and over- and undermedicate elders. Many of the reported poor conditions in nursing homes are a consequence of cost-cutting efforts.

▪ Growth of the National Debt and Deficits

The federal government is a major consumer and financer of health care. Approximately 47 percent of our health care expenditures comes from federal and state governments. Growth in health care expenditures have increased at a greater rate than any other commodity. The current United States debt is over $15.6 trillion, with interest on the debt exceeding $400 billion a year. The amount spent on interest on the debt is almost equal to the amount spent on Social Security or Defense (Office of Management and Budget [OMB], 2010). Thus, as health care spending consumes an increasing percentage of our federal budget, it adds disproportionately to the growth of the deficit and national debt. There are several consequences of the growing **national debt** and federal deficits. Debt and deficits reduce the government's ability to provide new and needed government services. Fewer resources are available to increase the range of services provided by government, including national defense and education.

Higher deficits may lead to higher taxes as more of the federal or state budgets are allocated to paying off government debt. It will be necessary to increase taxes if the same amounts of government services are to be provided. Increased taxes may also slow economic growth.

■ Significant Resources Spent on Delaying Death

Studies have demonstrated that much of the increase in health care spending occurs during the last months of life in an attempt to delay inevitable death. Significant resources are devoted to delaying death because of our compassion, guilt, and clinicians' limited ability to predict impending death. Even if we could be reasonably sure that someone was going to die in the near future, some family members and even some health professionals, still feel the need to "fight" for that person's life. As a society, we have alternatives to postponing imminent death by decreasing heroic interventions and maintaining a comfortable and pain-free existence through hospice care.

The priority we place on delaying death is reflected in the fact that we spend more during the last two months of a person's life than the rest of that year. We attempt heroic measures that are not likely to produce any better outcome such as operating on extremely premature babies and very sick elderly. Clinicians often employ heroic measures for some conditions because they are unable to predict with any real certainty when a patient is going to die.

■ The Effect of Health Care Expenditures on Business

During World War II, the United States began to subsidize the purchase of private health insurance when employer-sponsored health insurance became a nontaxable fringe benefit of employment. Employers can deduct the cost of providing health care insurance as a business expense, and employees are not federally taxed on insurance benefits. The vast majority of people with private health insurance receive it through their employer.

Over the past 50 years, health insurance as an employment fringe benefit has become a significant cost of production, or a cost of doing business. To manage the rising cost of health care, employees frequently have to forego pay raises and pay higher deductibles (out-of-pocket expenditures for health care) to maintain their health benefits. In the past 10 years, after controlling for inflation, wages and salaries increased only 1 percent, whereas the amount that employers pay for health benefits rose 163 percent. Employer-sponsored health insurance has several ramifications for business, covered in the following sections.

■ Costs of Employer-Sponsored Health Insurance Affects International Trade

The cost of employer-sponsored health insurance for employees and retirees is passed on to consumers as a cost of production for many goods and services. The United States must compete in a global economy with nations whose employers do not have to pay for health insurance or with nations whose health care systems are more "efficient" or less comprehensive.

Thus, rising health care costs directly affect American business' ability to compete internationally. When the price of their goods and services, driven by high health insurance, is higher than their competition, American companies are at a disadvantage. Consequently, industry is the biggest force behind health care cost reform.

Improving the health status of their employee population is a priority of all competitive businesses. For instance, The National Business Coalition on Health is one of the premier stakeholders that represents the interest of businesses and their priority of maintaining the health status of their employee populations. It represents 52 coalitions across the United States, with thousands of employers and millions of employees. The goal of the coalition is to provide employees with tools and incentives to purchase high-quality health care as well as improve the quality of care delivered by providers to employees.

■ Employer Strategies to Decrease Health Care Fringe Benefit Costs

Faced with increasing premiums for health insurance for their employees, employers use various strategies to decrease their share of the health care cost burden. First, employers shift employees into managed care plans such as preferred provider organizations (PPO), point-of-service (POS) plans, and health maintenance organizations (HMO). See Figure 10–5 for an illustration of the shift away from enrollment in conventional indemnity plans to enrollment in managed care plans for covered workers.

Second, employers reduce the number of health insurance companies with whom they do business, to concentrate their purchasing power and maximize their advantage. Third, employers transfer an increasing share of health care costs to employees. Employers require employees to pay a higher percentage of health insurance premiums as well as higher deductibles, copayments, and coinsurance.

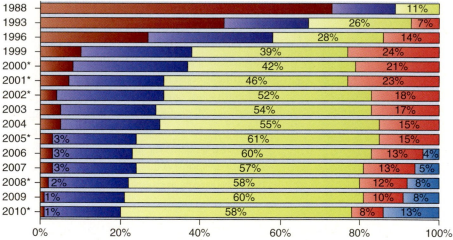

* Distribution is statistically different from the previous year shown (p<.05). No statistical tests were conducted for years prior to 1999. No statistical tests are conducted between 2005 and 2006 due to the addition of HDHP/SO as a new plan type in 2006.

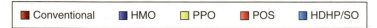

Figure 10–5 Distribution of health plan enrollment for covered workers, by plan type, 1988–2010.

Source: Kaiser Family Foundation. (2010a). Employer health benefits 2010 annual survey. Menlo Park, CA: Author.

Note: Information was not obtained for POS plans in 1988. A portion of the change in plan type enrollment for 2005 is likely attributable to incorporating more recent Census Bureau estimates of the number of state and local government workers and removing federal workers from the weights. See the Survey Design and Methods section from the 2005 Kaiser/HRET Survey of Employer-Sponsored Health Benefits for additional information.

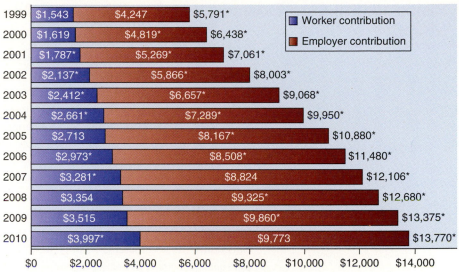

	Worker contribution	Employer contribution	Total
1999	$1,543	$4,247	$5,791*
2000	$1,619	$4,819*	$6,438*
2001	$1,787*	$5,269*	$7,061*
2002	$2,137*	$5,866*	$8,003*
2003	$2,412*	$6,657*	$9,068*
2004	$2,661*	$7,289*	$9,950*
2005	$2,713	$8,167*	$10,880*
2006	$2,973*	$8,508*	$11,480*
2007	$3,281*	$8,824	$12,106*
2008	$3,354	$9,325*	$12,680*
2009	$3,515	$9,860*	$13,375*
2010	$3,997*	$9,773	$13,770*

* Estimate is statistically different from estimate for the previous year shown ($p<.05$).

Figure 10–6 Average annual worker and employer contributions to premiums and total premiums for family coverage, 1999–2010.
Source: Kaiser Family Foundation. (2010a). Employer health benefits 2010 annual survey. Menlo Park, CA: Author.

Fourth, employees must pay an increasing portion of the cost for dependent care. See Figure 10–6 for a graphical description of the increases in the average worker contribution to his or her family health insurance coverage.

Fifth, employers have added utilization review to employees' health insurance to better control access to expensive care. In sum, all of these measures act to increase the out-of-pocket health care expenses for individuals.

Health insurance premiums, even for employer-sponsored health insurance, continue to rise, which forces some employees to choose between keeping their employer-sponsored health insurance and paying for other necessities. Many employees earn low wages and cannot afford to have any extra deductions from their paychecks for their employer-sponsored health insurance. Even though they have the choice of enrolling in employer-sponsored health insurance, they choose not to and therefore join the ranks of the uninsured. Their resultant out-of-pocket expenses may include all the costs of prescription medications and treatment that are required should they become ill.

A recent survey of employers indicated that among the different options for containing costs, most employers choose to increase the employees' share of health care costs. Employers also provide financial incentives to their employees to be prudent purchasers of health care. Few employees have the option of switching to a health plan that may provide higher quality care or offer more member-centered service. Employees are often locked into a health insurance plan while they are employed, such as a managed care plan, and express their discontent in health care surveys that ultimately have adversely affected the public's perception of managed care.

▪ Rising Health Care Expenditures Are Affected by Medical Malpractice Suits

The United State has become a highly litigious society with many trial lawyers who earn high incomes by suing physicians and hospitals for malpractice or negligence. **Medical malpractice** is the improper treatment of patients by physicians and other providers. To protect their assets from litigation, clinicians obtain malpractice insurance. When a settlement is reached and a patient receives compensation, these costs are passed on to society. Medical malpractice lawsuits cause increases in liability insurance premiums, which are passed on to patients, employers, and taxpayers, in the form of increased costs of care, increased health insurance premiums, or higher taxes. Some of the most frequent malpractice claims arise from surgical and post-operative complications, failure to diagnose cancer, an inadvertent surgical act, or an adverse birth outcome.

Specialties most vulnerable to suits are OB-GYN, orthopedics, and neurosurgery. These specialists are at increased risk of being sued during their career. Fear of a medical malpractice lawsuit has an adverse effect on physician morale, with some physicians leaving states that have high malpractice premiums or eliminating from their practice procedures that have a high risk of litigation. In that regard, there has been a significant increase in the number of verdicts won by plaintiffs in surgery-related and childbirth-related cases.

The increase in medical malpractice suits has a variety of causes. Most patients see multiple providers for different conditions and often lack a primary care clinician who coordinates their care. Frequently, patients see several providers for the same condition. This fragmentation in the delivery of care, exacerbated by the increase in specialization among physicians, has produced a breakdown in the communication between clinician and patient. In addition, as a highly mobile society, we continually develop new clinician–patient relationships that often have not had sufficient time to develop the level of trust needed to avoid miscommunications. We are less likely to sue a clinician we know well and trust, and increasingly, patients do not have close relationships with their clinicians.

In addition, patients have become more skeptical of and less confident in the health care professions. The media and the Internet among other societal factors have contributed to this perception by increasing our expectations of what health care can actually accomplish—often unrealistically.

Attorneys that promise to charge fees only if they recover money for their patients provide incentives to sue clinicians. Clinicians are human and make mistakes. As medical procedures have become more complex, the likelihood that mistakes will injure patients has increased, producing more suits. The factors that contribute to increases in litigation heighten an environment of resentment over skyrocketing health care costs and physicians' high incomes. As a result, many states are facing medical malpractice crises.

Malpractice premiums more than doubled between 2000 and 2006 (American Association of Justice (AAJ, 2011)). These increases contribute to rising health care costs that are often passed on to the patient in the form of higher prices and premiums. The increase in malpractice lawsuits has encouraged the practice of unnecessary "defensive medicine." Defensive medicine entails the ordering of more tests, procedures, and consultations than are medically necessary, with the hope of decreasing the likelihood of a lawsuit.

Policy makers have proposed solutions to the malpractice crisis. Some politicians have proposed tort law reform, whereas others call for elimination or reduction of the contingency payment system for lawyers. The contingency system stimulates malpractice claims because it enables individuals who cannot afford lawyers to be able to retain them without up-front fees. Attorneys receive a percentage of the awards from successful lawsuits.

Other proposals include sanctions for lawyers who bring frivolous suits and no fault insurance or maloccurrence insurance. Shorter statutes of limitation between the time of the injury and the medical malpractice lawsuit have been proposed to limit suits that involve pediatric injury during birth. One of the most popular proposals is a $250,000 cap on **"pain and suffering"** awards for patients. Such a cap would not preclude the patient from recovering compensation for ongoing health care bills, lost wages, and future health care treatments. Others have proposed mandatory arbitration between the patient and clinician in lieu of a jury trial to curb suits. Ultimately, improved quality control is the best strategy to limit malpractice claims.

Vignette

PATIENT WITH HEADACHE RECEIVES MRI, CT, AND OTHER TESTS—IS THIS DEFENSIVE MEDICINE OR GOOD MEDICINE?

Background

Medical imaging through use of CT scans and MRIs is one of the fastest sources of health care cost increases. The use of medical imaging and its associated increases in costs far outpaces other medical procedures and tests. Several factors have been identified as causes for this rapid rise. Medical imaging tests are ordered out of physician habit or based on antidotal evidence of their effectiveness (Hillman & Goldsmith, 2010). Although medical imaging use has dramatically increased, it is unknown whether additional use of such tests improves overall health. In other words, although use of medical imaging has increased, the accuracy of physicians' disease diagnosis has not (Hillman & Goldsmith, 2010).

Direct-to-consumer marketing, as well as information on the Internet, has led to consumers demanding the latest diagnostic tests despite their costs. Physicians also have incentive to provide the tests whenever they are performed in their own offices. Hundreds of thousands of dollars have been invested in the health care technology, and additional imaging tests provide revenue to pay for the investment (Hillman & Goldsmith, 2010). Physicians also train in hospitals were the sickest cases are referred and where treatment typically requires multiple diagnostic testing. Physicians carry habits learned in training with them to their private practices, where the severity and frequency of complicated diseases is lower. However, old habits of ordering the tests and the associated comfort level remains with the physician.

Another driver of the overuse of medical imaging is physician fear of medical malpractice claims from patients. Physicians are concerned about missing a possible serious diagnosis, and a simple order for a CT scan or MRI enables them to mitigate the threat. The consequences for a physician in missing a serious diagnosis due to omitting a "routine" test can be severe in our litigious society. Although the actual costs of defensive medicine are difficult to quantify, estimates range from a high of $650 billion to a low of about $56 billion (Mello et al., 2010). However, on a personal level, a malpractice lawsuit is a life-changing event in the life of a physician. Facing liability risk represents a palpable horror that is mitigated through simply checking a box and transmitting an order.

Perhaps equally as fearful for a physician is the dreaded scenario of standing before his or her peers in a morbidity and mortality conference and defending his or her clinical decisions. Perhaps these decisions ended in the death of a patient, and the physician is called upon to give an accounting of his or her decisions. Failure to order a necessary diagnostic imaging test is a mistake the physician will avoid at all costs in the future. This behavior may lead to future overuse of the test when faced with cases where a CT scan is borderline unnecessary.

Overuse of medical imaging is not without its consequences. CT scans expose patients to significant amounts of radiation, which are cumulative and increase patients' risks of cancer. (Brenner & Hall, 2007; Fazel et al., 2009). More use of imaging also raises the risk of patients receiving additional tests to clarify the previous ones and unnecessary invasive procedures if the tests are false positives (Fazel et al., 2009).

The Scenario

Gretchen Carlson, a former Miss America, has a very stressful job as well as small children to care for. Over the last several months, she has experienced random headaches during various times of the day. At first, she thought her headaches might be due to lack of sleep, giving up coffee and soda, or the stress of her job. She had a high pain threshold and tried to ignore the distraction that the headache pain caused her. She treated her symptoms with increasing dosages of ibuprofen and relaxation techniques she had learned when competing in the Miss America pageant. She had never suffered migraines and did not have a family history of debilitating headaches.

Eventually, Gretchen visited her primary care physician, who performed a complete physical but could not find the cause of the headaches. She referred Gretchen to a neurologist, who also preformed a battery of diagnostic tests in an attempt to identify the cause of the headaches. The neurologist had just heard of a colleague who had been sued for medical malpractice after he had failed to order a CT scan for a patient with a headache who had later that night died of a ruptured aneurism. She remembered another colleague who was sued for medical malpractice by the parents of a child who had hit his head while snowboarding. After the physician sent the child home from the ER, the child later complained of dizziness and headaches and grew unresponsive. The child later died, and the ER physician was sued for medical malpractice by the child's parents. The neurologist had never known of her colleagues being sued for overuse of the CT scanner.

However, the neurologist had received notices from Gretchen's HMO quality-control officer not to order diagnostic tests and procedures without medical necessity, in order to control costs. The neurologist also did not want to waste money on unnecessary testing if there were other less costly methods of reaching a diagnosis on the cause of Gretchen's headaches. She performed careful research on the topic and decided to leave no stone unturned in identifying the most likely cause of the headaches and confirming it with the greatest possible certainty.

She ordered the CT scan for Gretchen, which came back negative for any abnormality. She was not satisfied and contemplated ordering an MRI for further assessment. She then remembered that a possible cause of headaches is food allergies. She closely assessed Ms. Carlson's diet and had her keep a food intake journal. An allergist was able to identify several foods that were possible causes of the headaches. Once Gretchen stopped eating the flagged food items, her headaches gradually disappeared.

1. Do you ever question the necessity of CT scans or MRI when the tests have been ordered for you or your loved ones?

2. As a patient, do you think it would make you feel reassured that your physician was thoroughly assessing your complaint if he or she ordered more diagnostic tests?

3. Do you keep any records of the number of diagnostic imaging tests you have undergone since you were a child or teenager?

4. Are you aware of any of the dangers of overexposure to radiation through diagnostic imaging?

▪ Variation in Per Capita Health Expenditures

Health care use and resultant costs are not spread equally over any population. For every 50 people, 33 percent of all expenditures, on average, can be attributed to just one person who is critically ill. In addition, many patients demand and use unnecessary health care services. Also, how health care is practiced varies from state to state. The services patients receive may be more a function of the region of the country in which they live than the services they actually need.

Researchers and policy makers debate whether patients are over- or underserved based on the availability of hospital beds in the area. Data show that as the number of hospital beds increase, so do admissions to hospitals to fill those beds, after controlling for other factors that would contribute to the increase. The phenomenon of increasing hospital capacity by constructing more rooms and then admitting more patients is an example of **Roemer's law** (Roemer, 1961). That is, when there are more hospital beds, there are more patients to fill those beds and therefore reimbursement for providers. This rule assumes that the population is insured and that physicians influence their patients to demand more services through induced demand (Roemer, 1961).

The use of procedures also varies greatly by region and clinician. According to Wennberg (2005), the frequency of back surgeries depends on the supply of orthopedists and hospital beds. This variation is fostered by a general disagreement regarding what surgeries are clinically effective. The data also show that 30 percent of the variation in where people die is attributed to the number of hospital beds per capita in the area; the more hospital beds in an area, the greater the likelihood of dying in a hospital bed (Wennberg, 2005). These results demonstrate unnecessary utilization that adds to the rising costs of health care, and is further proof of Roemer's law.

In sum, the sources of variation in health care expenditures are scientific uncertainty, substitutability among various health care interventions, intrinsic differences in illness patterns, and clinician practice style—all of which are different from the actual need for care.

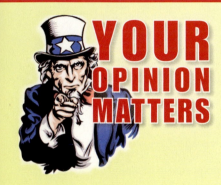

Should the United States Adopt a Medical Savings Account Plan?

Background: What Are Medical Savings Accounts?

Medical savings accounts (MSAs) have been one of the most contentious health care reform proposals debated in recent years. Persons who qualify for MSAs must also have a high deductible health insurance plan—referred to as catastrophic coverage—in the event that expenses exceed the available funds in the account. The account owner may use the funds to pay for medical and health expenses not covered by a health insurance policy. Proponents argue that MSAs will help to address rising costs and improve quality and access in the health care system. Opponents maintain that MSAs are not likely to contain costs, may result in owners foregoing necessary care, and can have an adverse effect on the insurance market by segmenting risk. We assess these arguments in more detail below.

Yes

The major benefits of MSAs include placing the first-dollar payment for health care expenses on consumers. This move significantly affects their purchasing behavior, which is likely to decrease the unnecessary use of services. Second, MSA year-end balances can be rolled over or used for nonhealth care expenses provided relevant taxes are paid. Clearly, consumers, not government, know what is best for themselves, especially with the advice from one or more providers. MSAs are tantamount to removing the inherent paternalistic nature of the current third-party fee-for-service system.

Consumer Choice

Proponents of the free market as the appropriate tool to allocate health care services argue that individuals should have more control over the spending of their health care dollars. MSAs offer beneficiaries a tool to choose freely among providers and hospitals that deliver the highest quality care, a viable alternative to the managed care plans that currently cover many employees. Managed care plans have attempted to reduce costs with strategies that have angered their members, such as denying claims, reducing member choices among providers, limiting coverage for experimental tests and procedures, and managing doctors' services.

Supporters further assert that MSAs will give patients more freedom to choose among providers and obtain their preferred mix of services. As a result, patients will have increased access to services because providers will not be limited to the service restrictions imposed by managed care. The patient, as a rational consumer, will seek care from providers based on the quality and value they receive, and is not constrained by the limitations of his or her managed care network.

Increased Access to Health Insurance

MSA holders must also be members of high-deductible health insurance policies that typically have lower premiums than traditional health insurance plans. With traditional plans, members have higher premiums but must remember that they must cover copayments and deductibles out of pocket. Many people do not budget or save in anticipation of such expenses and as a result either drop their coverage or incur heavy indebtedness. Currently, many employees are at risk of losing their employer-sponsored health insurance when businesses try to cut costs. With MSAs and high-deductible health plans at far lower premiums, more people would be able to afford health care insurance and have more choices among providers.

Administrative Cost Reduction

Paying an insurance claim with a commercial company is a costly process and often fraught with delays. Many companies deny claims, request verification documentation, or require time-consuming resubmissions. With MSAs, these administrative costs will be reduced because individuals will use their MSAs to pay for most of their health care expenses and therefore will not make insurance claims. In fact, annual health care expenses for many consumers may fall within the deductible levels of high-deductible policies and not even trigger an insurance claim. When this phenomenon happened, insurance carriers would not be part of the process, thus minimizing the costs of the overall process of paying claims for many health care expenses.

MSAs Encourage Informed Consumption of Services

When patients purchase health care services with funds from MSAs, they bear more of the actual costs of the services. Under a traditional health insurance plan with minimal copayments and lower deductibles, the impact of purchase

(*Continued*)

decisions is indirect, with limited incentives to carefully select providers and services. When the impact of the purchase decision is minimized, consumers often over-consume services that may not be beneficial or necessary. Over-consumption of services reduces access for others who are actually in need yet are unable to afford care.

Over-consumption also increases overall health care spending levels. Over-spending reduces funds available for long-term investment in capital projects necessary to produce durable goods, machines, schools, and hospitals, investments that are necessary to grow the economy as a whole.

MSA Tax Advantages

Money deposited into MSA accounts is exempt from federal income tax and in some states, from the state tax. Employers may contribute toward MSAs, and employee contributions are on a pre-tax basis or may be deducted from their taxable income (U.S. Department of the Treasury [DOT], 2011). In 2010, the maximum amount of contributions an individual could make was $3,050 and for families, was $6,150. If older than age 55, the contribution amount could be increased by $1,000 (DOT, 2011). Also, patient withdrawals to cover copayments, deductibles, and other health care expenses are tax exempt. When owners change jobs, they can take their MSAs with them. The money that remains in the account earns interest that is also not taxed. In addition, when account holders reach the age of 64, they can withdraw the funds for any reason (DOT, 2011).

No

Fiscal Restrictions and Tax Disadvantages

Money in MSAs not used to purchase health care services is added to gross income for tax purposes. If the MSA account holder withdraws funds for non-health care expenses, taxes must be paid on those dollars. Moreover, if the account owner is under 65 years of age, a 10 percent penalty must be paid (DOT, 2011). The MSA account holder must always purchase a high deductible health insurance policy, with a minimum deductible of $1,000 for single coverage and $2,000 for family coverage. The insurance policy must stipulate out-of-pocket expenses of no more than $5,000 for individuals and $10,000 for families (DOT, 2011).

MSAs and Preventive Health Care

MSA account holders must pay for services such as preventive care, diagnostic tests and procedures, and other health care expenses out of their MSA account. Account holders may reduce their health care spending and eliminate essential preventive health care services that are critical to maintaining their health. This avoidance may ultimately cost the health care system more if it has to treat MSA owners for serious health care problems. In other words, consumers using MSAs to pay for routine health care may not be better consumers who are more informed about procedures, alternative treatments, and medications. Furthermore, they may not be able to judge the advice given by their provider any better than non-MSA users. Modern medicine is highly technical and complex, and new advancements occur routinely. Most consumers do not have the experience, information, or the time to be fully informed. Even though they are paying for their care directly, they may not have the ability to determine whether a health care service is suitable or needed. As a result, consumers may not be rational, and the free market may not efficiently determine the optimal levels of cost, access, and quality of care.

MSAs Attract Only Healthy Consumers

Opponents argue that the elderly and sick will not be able to save enough in their MSAs to cover the quantity of services they consume. As a result, segmentation of the risk pool will result in higher premiums for those who remain in traditional insurance plans. Opponents argue that MSAs will appeal to young and healthy consumers with low health care costs and with sufficient disposable income to contribute to their MSAs. The elderly and the sick, whose health care expenses are much higher, will not use MSAs. Those who remain in the traditional insurance pool will face higher premiums when substantial numbers of the young and the healthy use MSAs. MSA opponents argue that premiums should be affordable for everyone, and the only mechanism to maintain lower premium levels is to spread risks among as many people as possible, with healthy members contributing to the costs of those who are sick (Remler & Glied, 2006).

MSA opponents further state that those who are uninsured and sick will likely not have the financial resources to contribute to an MSA. The uninsured do not have sufficient funding to purchase either employer-sponsored or individual insurance, so they likely would not have the resources to contribute to an MSA and pay the premiums for high deductible health insurance policies. Therefore, MSAs will have a minimal impact on reducing the number of uninsured.

MSAs Will Not Reduce Wasteful Health Care Spending

MSA opponents argue that savings from MSA use is overestimated. The wasteful spending that does occur from the present overuse of services does not represent a significant portion of overall health care spending. Thus, the amount of wasteful spending reduced by MSAs will be minimal compared with all of the other sources of wasteful spending in the health care system.

(Continued)

You decide:

1. Which side of the MSA argument do you think is more persuasive?

2. What type of information do you require to make a decision regarding the benefits and costs of MSAs?

3. Does your predisposition toward capitalism and free-market principles or your predisposition to health care as a common good influence your evaluation of the pro and con arguments?

4. Would MSAs be an option for providing insurance to persons currently uninsured?

5. Would MSAs be an option for providing insurance to persons who reach the age of 65 and find that Medicare is no longer able to provide them with necessary benefits because of a lack of funding?

■ Reasons for Increased Demand Despite Prices Rising Sharply

Health care inflation contributes to rising prices as well as increases in the quality of care. The demand for health care services has increased despite the rising prices for those services. Increased demand is fostered by increased competition among providers and increased expectations from consumers. The availability of health insurance and prepayment has stimulated consumer demand for services that has contributed to price inflation. Price inflation is the primary driver of increased spending on health care services each year. Inflation occurs when demand for health care services exceeds the supply. The increase in health care prices is significantly higher than increases in all other consumer prices. Improved technology and increased quality, combined with the increase in the perceived effectiveness of health care, drive demand higher.

Two major types of health care price inflation are **demand–pull inflation** and **cost–push inflation**. Demand–pull inflation occurs when consumer's willingness to purchase services is greater than the supply offered. Demand–pull inflation is enabled by health insurance, as it increases consumers' buying power and removes price sensitivity or cost consciousness. Other causes of demand–pull inflation include aging of the population, higher incomes, overuse of services, population growth, and higher expectations for care.

Cost–push inflation results in higher production costs for the provider of services. Cost–push inflation may stem from new technology, increased wages of health care personnel, duplication of health care services, unionization or threat of unionization, and inappropriate use of health care such as defensive medicine and inexperienced providers using services inefficiently.

Experts measure inflation with the Consumer Price Index (CPI), an index of the cost of living. The CPI is an index of the purchasing power of the dollar. The CPI is a monthly measure of average changes in price paid by urban consumers for a fixed market basket of a sample of approximately 400 goods and services that are representative of what urban consumers purchase. Health care is one of the eight major groups of consumer items within the CPI. The health care component of CPI produces trends in health care prices based on specific indicators of hospital, health care, dental, and drug prices. When calculating the CPI, the items are weighted based on the percentage of income spent on each item, with a base year selected as a reference point.

The CPI is not the perfect measure of inflation in health care. It does not include changes in prices due to changes in quality. New items are not always included, such as prescription drugs, and the index may include old/obsolete drugs. Manufacturers do not increase the prices of obsolete products; otherwise, they would not be able to sell them. In addition, with the length of hospital stays decreasing, hospitals have had to pack more services into a shorter period—this increases costs. Changes in amenities are also not measured.

For the past 25 years, the CPI for health care has outstripped the rest of consumer price movements (Bureau of Labor Statistics [BLS], 2010). The current decrease during the past decade in health care inflation simply reflects a decrease in overall inflation. Historically, hospital services and prices have inflated at a higher level than other health care items (BLS, 2010).

■ Strategies to Deal with Cost

Third-party payers have led efforts to control health care costs. Cost-cutting strategies have focused on hospital payments, inputs used by hospitals, alternative delivery systems, and hospital utilization. These strategies have been largely unsuccessful because the continued aging of the population and advancements in health care technology have been the major driving factors in increases in costs and expenditures. Cost-cutting policies cannot address some of these factors, but they are already aiming at what is considered inflationary "sacred cows." Such "sacred cows" include medically uneducated and insufficiently price-sensitive consumers, because their behavior can be altered by increased use of copayments, coinsurance, and deductibles.

The highly fragmented insurance industry, with little expertise in health care management, has also contributed to cost increases. The industry uses enrollment in managed care organizations to try to control such costs by containing the overuse of physician specialists. However, higher costs come from excess hospital capacity exacerbated by the many procedures now performed on an outpatient basis, as well as varying health care practice standards. Policy makers and practitioners are employing clinical guidelines and care protocols to reduce variation and thus cut costs.

Higher health care costs also result from the focus on acute rather than preventive care. The lack of health care outcome data increases costs with the use of expensive technologies that many times do not have demonstrable efficacy. **Quality improvement (QI) initiatives** emphasizing patient-centered care and clinical outcomes have been proposed to help reign in these costs.

▪ Summary

Rising health care costs not only affect the health care industry but also the entire U.S. economy. These rising costs are primarily driven by the presence of third-party payers and the explosive growth of high-cost health care technology with the subsequent use of this technology to provide care for patients. Uncontrolled rising health care costs affect access to health care, its quality, and the growth in the **national deficit** and federal debt. These costs are driven by the significant use of resources to delay inevitable death, increased malpractice lawsuits and unnecessary defensive medicine, and variations in practice patterns.

The highly fragmented insurance industry, with little expertise in health care management, leads to cost increases. Managed care organizations are used in an effort to contain such costs. However, higher costs stem from excess hospital capacity, the growth of many procedures performed on an outpatient basis, and the variations in health care practice standards. Clinical guidelines and care protocols are being employed to cut these costs.

Regarding the heroic attempts to save lives, and the malpractice fears, it is important to note that in 1932, the *Final Report of the Committee on the Costs of Medical Care* expressed the same cost-access-quality concerns as we are addressing today (Committee on the Costs of Medical Care [CCMC], 1932). Some would argue that little progress has been achieved since that era.

▪ Review Questions

1. What is the chief driver for the increase in health care costs during the last 10 years?

2. Why do patients and their families desire the most extensive interventions to take place when they are sick despite their impact on the cost of care?

3. What types of changes has the government put into place to control costs in the health care industry?

4. How do increases in costs in the delivery of health care impact health insurance premiums, copayments, and deductibles for those with health insurance?

5. How do increases in costs in the delivery of health care impact employers as they provide health insurance for their employees?

6. How do increases in health care costs impact the amount of money that is spent by the federal government on Medicare and Medicaid?

7. How has moral hazard affected the increases in cost in the health care industry?

8. How is health care reform legislation that was passed in 2010 projected to impact cost increases in the health care industry?

9. How does the cost of health care borne by providers, payers, and patients differ, and why?

10. What would you suggest as the top three means in which health care costs could be reduced, and what would the impact be on access and quality of health care?

▪ Additional Resources

American Health Insurance Plans: http://www.ahip.org/

California Healthcare Foundation: http://www.chcf.org/

CATO Institute: http://www.cato.org/

Centers for Medicare and Medicaid Services: https://www.cms.gov/

Congressional Research Service: http://www.loc.gov/crsinfo/

Freakonomics: The Hidden Side of Everything: http://www.freakonomics.com/

HealthCare.gov: http://www.healthcare.gov/

Kaiser Family Foundation: http://www.kff.org/insurance/index.cfm

National Federation of Independent Business: http://www.nfib.com/

Office of Management and Budget: http://www.whitehouse.gov/omb

Social Security Administration: http://www.ssa.gov/

UC Atlas of Inequality: http://ucatlas.ucsc.edu/index.php

▪ References

American Association for Justice (AAJ) (2011, February). Medical negligence: The role of America's civil justice system in protecting patients' rights: Retrieved November 1, 2011, from http://www.justice.org/resources/Medical_Negligence_Primer.pdf.

Brenner, D., & Hall, E. (2007). Computed tomography—An increasing source of radiation exposure. *New England Journal of Medicine, 357,* 2277–2284.

Bureau of Labor Statistics (BLS), U.S. Department of Labor. (2010). *Consumer price index.* Washington, DC: U.S. Department of Labor.

California Healthcare Foundation. (2007). *Snapshot: Health care costs 101.* Oakland, CA: Author.

Centers for Medicare and Medicaid Services (CMS). (2010). National health expenditures 2010 edition. Retrieved November 1, 2011, from https://www.cms.gov/DataCompendium/14_2010_Data_Compendium.asp.

Committee on the Costs of Medical Care (CCMC). (1932). Medical care for the American people. Report No. 28. Chicago: University of Chicago Press.

Fazel, R., Krumholz, H., Wang, Y., Ross, J., Chen, J., Ting, H., et al. (2009). Exposure to low-dose ionizing radiation from medical imaging procedures. *New England Journal of Medicine, 361,* 849–857.

Hillman, B., & Goldsmith, J. (2010, July 1). The uncritical use of high-tech medical imaging. *New England Journal of Medicine, 363*(1): 4–6.

Kaiser Family Foundation (KFF). (2009, March). *Health care costs: A primer*. Menlo Park, CA: Author. Retrieved November 1, 2011, from http://facts.kff.org/results .aspx?view=slides&detail=29.

Kaiser Family Foundation (KFF). (2010a). Employer health benefits 2010 annual survey. Menlo Park, CA: Author. Retrieved November 1, 2011, from http://www .kff.org/insurance/ehbs-archives.cfm.

Kaiser Family Foundation (KFF). (2010b). Health tracking poll. Conducted June 17–22, 2010. September 21. Menlo Park, CA: Author. Retreived November 1, 2011, from http://facts.kff.org/chart.aspx?ch=840.

Kaiser Family Foundation (KFF). (2010c). Kaiser Slides. Per capita total current health care expenditures, U.S. and selected countries, 2008. Menlo Park, CA: Retrieved November 1, 2011, from http://facts.kff.org/results .aspx?view=slides&topic=3.

Mello, M., Chandra, A., Gawande, A., & Studdert, D. (2010). National costs of the medical liability system. *Health Affairs*, *29*(9), 1569–1577.

Norman, J. (2010, February 8). Washington Health Policy Week in review: National health expenditures now grab 17.3 percent of GDP. Commonwealth Fund. Retrieved November 1, 2011, from http://www.commonwealthfund.org/ Newsletters/Washington-Health-Policy-in-Review/2010/Feb/February-8-2010/ National-Health-Expenditures-Now-Grab-173-Percent-of-GDP-Study-Projects .aspx.

Office of Management and Budget (OMB). (2010). *The federal budget deficit*. Washington, DC: Author.

Remler, D., & Glied, S. (2006). How much more cost sharing will health savings accounts bring? *Health Affairs, 25*(4), 1070–1078.

Roemer, M. (1961). Bed supply and hospital utilization: A natural experiment. *Hospitals*, *35*, 36–42.

U.S. Census Bureau. (2010). *Historical estimates of the U.S. population*. Washington, DC: Census Bureau, Department of Commerce.

U.S. Department of the Treasury (U.S. DOT). (2011). Publication 969: Health savings accounts (HSAs) and other tax-favored health plans. Washington, DC: Author.

Wennberg, J. (2005). *Variation in use of Medicare services among regions and selected academic medical centers: Is more better?* Washington, DC: The Commonwealth Fund.

White, C. (2007). Health care spending growth: How different is the United States from the rest of the OECD? *Health Affairs, 26*(1):154–161.

Health Care Financing

Key Terms

adverse selection

capitation

classic principles of insurance

coinsurance

community rating

copayment

deductible

disparities

fee-for-service

health (medical) savings accounts (HSAs)

healthy worker effect

individual, or differential, rating

moral hazard

underinsured

uninsured

Learning Objectives

- Identify current macro trends in financing of health care services.

- Identify reimbursement methods for physicians.

- Identify reimbursement methods for hospitals and other providers.

- Weigh the pros and cons of reimbursement based on tests and procedures versus time spent with patients.

- Understand the influence of financing of health care on the delivery of services and practice patterns of physicians.

- Understand the implications of moral hazard and adverse selection.

- Differentiate between community rating and individual rating for health insurance.

▪ Introduction

The study of health care financing is an assessment of how patients pay for the services they receive and how providers are paid for the services they deliver. Reimbursement for care affects utilization of services and the quality of care delivered by providers. The manner in which the consumer pays for health care may be different from how a physician is reimbursed for delivering health care services.

Health care financing is important because care is expensive, and in certain instances the life and death of the consumer hangs in the balance. **Disparities** in access to care are a concern, as is the fact that many people cannot pay for their care, even though they are sick and require care services. The United States consumed $2.5 trillion of health care services in 2009 (Truffer et al., 2010). Although it is not deemed per se in our

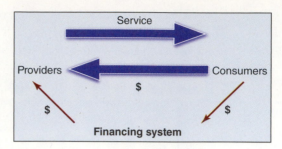

Figure 11–1 Model for financing health services.
© *Cengage Learning 2013*

federal Constitution, some believe that citizens deserve care when needed regardless of ability to pay. Many think that health care is a right, but hospitals and other providers pass the expense of those who cannot pay for their care to the rest of the population.

Health care reimbursement is based on the following key assumptions. First, providers of care must be reimbursed for the care delivered. They have invested significant resources and years in their training, they are highly skilled, and delivering care is their profession. Second, the general public who consumes health care is the final payer. We cannot assume that costs for health care can be passed on to government and business without any consequences. The government will increase taxes, and business will pass the cost on to the customer, or their employees will receive fewer raises, benefits, or bonuses. The real question is, to what extent should the costs of health care be born directly or indirectly by the consumer?

Figure 11–1 illustrates the interrelationships between providers, consumers, and the financing system.

This model demonstrates that in certain instances consumers pay providers such as pharmacists, dentists, and physicians directly for services. However, most often care is reimbursed through a health care financing system. Consumers pay health insurance premiums, and in exchange, the financing system pays the provider for the care that the consumer receives. An insurance company will reimburse the physician, hospital, or nursing home. Therefore, at the time the consumer receives the service, the consumer is not paying for that service.

Under the traditional **fee-for-service** reimbursement, an employer or individual pays a premium to the insurance company. The patient then seeks care as needed, and the provider sends the insurance company a bill. Once the patient has paid his or her portion in the form of a **deductible**, the insurance company then reimburses the provider for the price of the care. Often, the patient is responsible for paying a portion of the **coinsurance**, which may be 20 percent of the cost of care after the deductible amount has been met.

Under managed care and prospective payment systems, this reimbursement scenario is modified. The gatekeeper, or a primary care physician (PCP), limits access to specialists and other forms of costly services. The role of the PCP is to provide comprehensive care to patients and manage their health. Under managed care, patients typically pay more in the form of copayments and deductibles, while the providers are reimbursed at a lower level than traditional fee-for-service.

Under the traditional fee-for-service reimbursement arrangement to the provider, there are few incentives to save money or be efficient; the more services provided, the higher the income for the provider. With the traditional insurance model, there is little consumer cost-consciousness because patients pay such a small fraction of the total cost of their care at the time of use. Managed care uses the PCP as a gatekeeper, as well as increases the share paid by the patient, to spread the financial risk to create cost-consciousness. However, under this system providers may have an incentive to withhold needed care.

▪ Developments in Health Care Financing

Spending on health care is divided roughly evenly between public or government sources and private sources such as insurance companies and out-of-pocket sources (KFF, 2009). The most important trend in health care financing has been the shift to third-party payers through private insurance, Medicare, and Medicaid and away from direct or out-of-pocket payment by patients. Out-of-pocket payments, in the form of cash, check, and consumer credit for health care services account for only about 22 percent of private health care spending (KFF, 2009). There has been an increase in the coverage levels of private health insurance since 1940s and a corresponding increase in the share paid by private insurers and the share paid by government.

▪ Health Care Spending Trends

Spending on health care is becoming an increasing larger percentage of the United States GDP (KFF, 2009). Spending as a percentage of GDP was approximately 17.3 percent in 2009 and is projected to continue to grow throughout the next decade to 19.3 percent by 2019 (CMS, 2010). Medicare spending at 8.1 percent of GDP in 2009 is projected to average a 6.9 percent increase per year over the next decade. On a national basis, the US spent over $2.5 trillion on health care services in 2009, or $8160 per capita (CMS, 2010).

During 2010, health care spending grew at an historic low, with fewer people demanding health care services due to lost insurance coverage from unemployment. At this time, the United States was suffering through an economic recession that officially lasted from 2007 through 2009, the longest of all recessions since World War II (Martin et al., 2011). The amount of health care spending as a percentage of GDP (17.6%) remained relatively constant in 2010 due to increases in both the GDP and health care spending.

During the period of 2011–2013, health care spending is projected to increase by 4.9 percent as more consumers will be covered by employer-sponsored health insurance during an economic recovery (Keehan et al., 2011). Additional health care reforms are expected to be enacted throughout this period, including coverage for dependents age 26 years old and younger and for persons with preexisting conditions (Keehan et al., 2011).

In 2014, it is estimated that there will be 22.9 million new people who are able to purchase health insurance through plans established by the Patient Protection and Affordable Care Act of 2010 (PPACA) (Keehan et al., 2011). National health care spending is projected to grow rapidly during this period and jump from a 5.5 percent rate in 2013 to an 8.3 percent rate in 2014. The newly insured are expected to consume more physician services and prescription drugs because of lower copayments for these services.

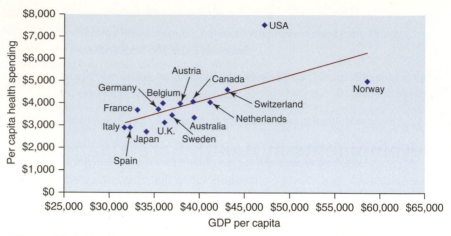

Figure 11–2 Total health expenditure per capita and GDP per capita, United States and selected countries, 2008.

Source: Organization for Economic Co-operation and Development (2010), "OECD Health Data", OECD Health Statistics *(database). doi: 10.1787/data-00350-en (Accessed on 14 February 2011).*

Notes: Data from Australia and Japan are 2007 data. Figures for Belgium, Canada, Netherlands, Norway and Switzerland, are OECD estimates.

Throughout 2015–2020, health care spending is expected to grow at approximately 6.2 percent per year (Keehan et al., 2011). During this period, it is expected that employers who hire low-wage workers are going to stop providing insurance coverage, as paying the penalty mandated by the PPACA is more economical. Another provision of the act will afford incentives to employers to offer plans with lower premiums and higher cost-sharing requirements.

Increases in health care spending are important to track because they should result in a commensurate improvement in the health status of the United States population. For instance, if on average our society is spending $8,160 per person on health care, the health status of the population should reflect such high spending. The United States spends more per person than any other similar country in the world (OECD, 2010).

Most of the health care spending is for hospital and physician services, with payment for prescription drugs as the next largest category (KFF, 2009). Figure 11–2 provides a graphical description of the spending per capita by the United States as compared with other developed countries.

Figure 11–3 provides an illustration of the historical and projected growth of health care spending, per capita, from 1990 to 2018. Based on the data, health care spending per capita is expected to increase above the rate of inflation for the foreseeable future.

▪ Cost-Shifting to Employees for Health Care Insurance

Employees now pay more in premiums and in deductibles for their health insurance compared with 10 years ago. Average annual premiums in 2010 for employees were $5,049 for single coverage and $13,770 for family coverage, an increase of 5 percent and 3 percent from 2009, respectively (Claxton et al., 2010).

Deductibles have also risen for employees from 2009 through 2010. The percentage of workers with a deductible of $1,000 or more rose from 22 percent in 2009 to

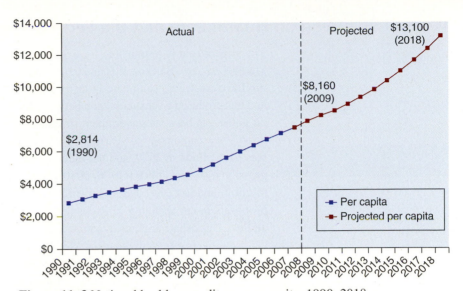

Figure 11–3 National health expenditures per capita, 1990–2018.
Source: Kaiser Family Foundation (KFF). (2009). Trends in health care costs and spending. Menlo Park, CA: Author.

27 percent in 2010. Workers in smaller firms are more likely to have a higher deductible compared with workers in larger companies.

Workers' share of the premium cost has also risen by 47 percent from 2005 through 2010. Insured employees now contribute 19 percent of the premium for single health care insurance plans, an increase from 17 percent in 2009 (Claxton et al., 2010). Insured employees now must pay 30 percent of the premium for family coverage, up from 27 percent in 2009 (Claxton et al., 2010). This increase is notable because employees' share of premiums has remained generally stable over the past decade.

The economic recession that began in 2008 has led more firms to reduce the scope of health benefits or increase cost sharing (Claxton et al., 2010). Firms shift costs to employees by providing them with high-deductible health plans with a savings option. These plans increased significantly from 2009 through 2010, with enrollment rising from 8 percent to 13 percent of insured employees in 2009 (Claxton et al., 2010). This shift increases the out-of-pocket burden for employees, as they must first pay the high-deductible amount before health insurance begins to provide coverage.

The burden that employees will bear for their health care insurance is projected to continue during a time of economic recession, high unemployment, and rising health care costs (Claxton et al., 2010). Employees are generally resistant to measures that would reign in costs, such as restrictive managed care arrangements that limit their choice of physicians, services, and specialists.

Health reform in the PPACA, passed in March 2010, is not likely to alter the amount that covered employees pay for premiums, copays, and deductibles in the short term. Changes in the deductible and limits on out-of-pocket expenses for insured patients do not go into effect until 2014 (Claxton et al., 2010).

▪ Federal Spending on Health Care and the Federal Debt

The government is responsible for over half of all health care spending in the United States (Chernew, Baicker, & Hsu, 2010). The rising levels of federal health care spending have created a health care industry that is tightly linked to government spending and has produced a substantial gap between federal expenditures and revenues. A deficit is the gap between government revenues and government expenditures in a fiscal year. The accumulation of yearly deficits is called the national debt. The federal deficit was $1.4 trillion in 2009, and the federal publically held debt was $7.5 trillion (Congressional Budget Office [CBO], 2010). However, the full national debt has continued to climb and has exceeded $13.6 trillion in 2010. Policy makers have made various proposals to cut spending in exchange for Congressional approval to raise the debt ceiling. This debate remains dynamic and contentious, as policy makers are hesitant to cut spending in either Medicare or Medicaid.

Federal spending on health care is projected to continue to increase throughout the next 40 years. As a percentage of gross domestic product (GDP), it is projected to climb from 5 percent of GDP and 20 percent of all federal spending in 2009 to 12 percent of GDP in 2050 (Chernew et al., 2010). As federal spending on health care increases, the projected deficits and national debt are also projected to increase (CBO, 2010).

There are implications for the continuing increases in the national debt. The federal government issues Treasury bonds as a form of borrowing money from investors. Interest rates are the return investors earn from their bonds, so higher interest rates make government bonds more attractive. However, as interest rates rise, the government is financially responsible to pay lenders more for their bond purchases. Rising interest payments reduce the amount the government has available to fund other priorities such as public education, defense, and health care.

Interest rates for the rest of the economy are tied to the rates paid by the Treasury Department. Rising federal interest rates therefore drive increases in other areas of the economy. Individuals, local governments, and private companies must pay higher interest rates, which siphons money away from other priorities and investments. This phenomenon is called "crowding out" of investing in other capital investments that would increase economic productivity in the long run (CBO, 2010).

High national debt levels also reduce the ability of the federal government to respond to emergency expenditure requirements such as international crisis, industry bailouts, waging war, national disasters, and economic downturns (Chernew et al., 2010). Policy makers may raise tax rates to pay for the increases in the federal deficit and debt. However, this decision may have the unintended consequence of discouraging work, savings by individuals, and overall economic output (CBO, 2010).

In the long term, a national debt that steadily increases is unsustainable for the United States economy (CBO, 2010). If the national debt becomes too large, it increases the probability of a financial crisis, reflected in the confidence of lenders who purchase bonds from the federal government. Federal bonds would lose much of their value if lenders' confidence drops in the government's ability to pay the interest on their bonds. Interest rates would then need to be raised to higher levels to encourage lenders to continue to finance the national debt (CBO, 2010).

■ Increased Purchase of Private Health Insurance

There are several important reasons for the increase in purchasing of private health insurance. Real income, controlling for inflation, has increased over time, and therefore patients have more disposable income to spend on health insurance. Health insurance as a fringe benefit of employment has increased. The employers' cost to provide health insurance to employees is nontaxable, which provides employers with an incentive to provide health insurance to their employees.

Consumers prefer health insurance because it is more convenient than paying out of pocket. Providers also prefer health insurance because they are reimbursed for their services even though they may not agree with the amount the insurance company is paying or with the timeliness of the payment. Finally, consumers prefer the security or peace of mind that health insurance brings them. As real income increases, the desire to protect resources such as health and financial assets also increases.

■ Increase in Financing through Medicare and Medicaid

Medicare covers 47 million elderly and disabled Americans, and finances hospital and physician visits, prescription drugs, and other acute and post-acute services (KFF, 2010a). Medicare spending accounts for a substantial portion of the discretionary spending in the federal budget. For instance, in 2010, Medicare spending absorbed 12 percent of the federal budget (KFF, 2010a). The largest portion of this spending is for hospital services, and overall Medicare spending amounts to 23 percent of national health care spending (KFF, 2010a).

Medicare spending is projected to increase from $519 billion in 2010 to $929 billion in 2020, with an annual growth rate of 5.8 percent. These growth figures account for the changes in Medicare that will be implemented as part of the the PPACA (KFF, 2010b).

Medicare is funded from three primary sources: general revenues, payroll tax contributions, and premiums paid by beneficiaries (KFF, 2010a). The largest source of funding is financing from general revenues. Over time, Medicare spending is projected to comprise an increasing share of federal spending and national health spending (KFF, 2010a). The increases in Medicare spending are driven by many of the same forces that are causing health care costs to increase. For instance, rising prices of services, more utilization of services by beneficiaries, and the reimbursement of care requiring new and expensive technologies are the main causes (KFF, 2010a).

Medicare funding is experiencing other financial pressures. For instance, the elderly population continues to age, and life expectancy continues to increase; yet there are fewer workers available to contribute to pay for the care of beneficiaries (KFF, 2010a).

The government has increased financing for health care for several reasons. During the past half century, our society has shifted from a libertarian perspective emphasizing personal responsibility to an egalitarian view that holds that health care is a right. Such an egalitarian view holds society as a whole responsible, as embodied in Franklin Roosevelt's New Deal legislation. Second, the breakdown in the free-market system of health care delivery adversely affects the less fortunate, who often cannot afford increasingly expensive health care. As a result, government becomes involved for the welfare of its citizens.

Finally, the importance of the immediate and extended family as a source of payment for health care has decreased. Our population is more mobile, and more women are in the workforce. In past decades, women in the family had much more of the care responsibilities for family members. Now, government has taken on some of the responsibilities previously held by the extended and nuclear family.

Health Insurance Trends

Classic Principles of Insurance

It is more likely that Americans will have health insurance that covers hospital, surgical, inpatient medical, and outpatient diagnostic services than other types of health insurance that cover outpatient physician, dental, and prescription services. This phenomenon is explained by the **classic principles of insurance**.

The definition of an insurable event is one where the financial risk is significant. Second, the risk or the probability of occurrence is measurable for a group. Third, the occurrence of the event is infrequent. For example, the probability of an admission to the hospital is far less likely than visiting a physician. Fourth, service is not desirable by the patient. In other words, having insurance should not make the insured demand the service more. Finally, it is beyond the control of patients whether they receive care. For example, patients do not control when they are admitted into the hospital as compared to when they voluntarily see a physician or dentist.

Health insurance began by primarily covering the hospital and surgeon's bill, in keeping with the above principles. Later, companies started providing outpatient physician care, dental care, and pharmaceutical coverage, even though generally they do not fit the principles of insurance. Insurance companies insure against these services for the predictability of expenses and for the convenience of prepayment. Thus, for many health care services we consume, there is little or no cost-consciousness on the part of the patient at the time care is received.

Out-of-Pocket Payments

We pay more for out-of-pocket cost for hospital care than we do for dental care and physician services because the costs are higher for hospital services. However, as a percent of the total cost health care, the out-of-pocket expense is less. Out-of-pocket payments affect the poor the most, as they are a greater percent of their income than they are for those who are wealthier.

Uninsured

The number of people who lacked health insurance at any time during a 12-month period rose from 46.3 million in 2008 to 50.7 million in 2009, while the percentage increased from 15.4 percent to 16.7 percent over the same period (U.S. Census Bureau, 2010).

The lack of health care insurance has profound consequences for those finding themselves in such a position. The uninsured are more likely to encounter barriers to both receiving care and paying for it. Others at risk are not included in uninsured totals, such as the **underinsured** who have health insurance coverage but do not have comprehensive coverage. The **uninsured** and the underinsured are a concern because without the resources to pay for their health care, they are often unable to obtain services. If they do receive health care, they are unable to pay, and providers lose money after delivering services, often called uncompensated care. Providing care for patients who are uninsured frequently results in shifting the cost to privately insured patients. Hospitals also write off millions of dollars every year in uncompensated care as bad debt or charity care (Weissman, 2005). Incurring unsustainable levels of bad debt can lead to hospital closure.

The impact of lack of insurance on access to care affects the behavior of consumers. Those who lack insurance typically do not have a usual source of care (USOC); that is, they do not typically have a primary care clinician from whom they seek care on an annual basis (Hadley, 2003). They may also postpone care because they cannot afford it. Care postponed may include visiting a physician's office to diagnose a problem or not taking or filling their prescriptions. These choices have long-term consequences for patients, including forgoing the benefits of early detection and prevention, diagnosing illnesses at later stages, developing complications in conditions that are easily treatable, and loss of years of life (Ayanian et al., 2000). These risks are profound among smokers, obese patients, binge drinkers, and for those with other major health risks (Ayanian et al., 2000).

Employers provide most health insurance in the United States for their employees (KFF, 2009). Because federal law froze wages during World War II, employers competed for employees by offering attractive fringe benefit packages, including health insurance. As mentioned in Chapter 10: Cost of Health Care Services, health insurance premiums for employers have steadily increased over the last decade. These costs have been passed on to consumers as costs of operations. A smaller percentage of the population receives its insurance from Medicaid or other governmental sources (KFF, 2009).

Some experts debate the accuracy of the estimate of the uninsured. Surveys that count persons uninsured at some point during the year, as used by the Census Bureau, produce higher estimates by 40–50 percent over those that define uninsured as persons without insurance for the entire year (Robert Wood Johnson Foundation [RWJF], 2008). This number also increases whenever people are counted as uninsured even though they have obtained insurance through Medicaid.

In addition, many uninsured are young adults who elect to spend their income on other goods and services and accept the risk of not being insured (RWJF, 2008). Over 9 million uninsured in 2006 were ages 19–23, nearly half of all young adults in this age group. Apparently, uninsured status is a common characteristic of young adults (Agency for Healthcare Research and Quality [AHRQ], 2009). This choice may be due to multiple factors, including recent graduation from college and working for an employer that does not offer health insurance. Young adults may also be among the healthiest of individuals and may not perceive the need for health insurance (Callahan & Cooper, 2005). However, there are risks to being young and uninsured. The young uninsured are at significantly higher risk for delaying or missing care, forgoing taking prescribed pharmaceuticals, having no contact with a health provider, and having no usual source of primary care (Callahan & Cooper, 2005).

Vignette

NECESSARY MEDICINE OR DEFENSIVE MEDICINE?

Susan Webster, a sophomore at Yale University, had been experiencing mild abdominal discomfort late in the fall semester. Susan had a lot on her mind, with studying for final exams and making a travel schedule for her winter break. She concluded that her symptoms were a function of her current stress level and used an over-the-counter pain medication to cope with the pain and help her sleep. After a week of persistent pain, she decided to visit her local emergency department.

After more than 3 hours in the waiting room, the nurse on duty called her into one of the exam rooms. The nurse took her vital signs, with no abnormalities, and then immediately scheduled Susan for a computed tomography (CAT) scan. One hour later, and still in significant discomfort, the CAT scan results revealed the presence of an ovarian cyst. The ER physician prescribed a pain medication and scheduled another visit to examine the size of the cyst and verify that the pain medication was eliminating the persistent discomfort. Later, the hospital billed her insurance company for $8,500, of which Susan was responsible for a small deductible and a 20 percent copayment.

Unknown to the hospital emergency room staff, Susan's father was a physician and medical director of a local group practice. After reviewing the case, her father concluded that a history, pelvic examination, and an ultrasound would have been adequate and is considered standard practice in cases like Susan's. Such a process would have been far less costly, with a CAT scan only used as a further measure if the less extensive actions proved inconclusive. According to Dr. Webster, the hospital could not justify the use of the CAT scan because they did not perform the lower level procedures first.

The hospital defended the CAT scan, claiming that an ultrasound might have missed something more serious, such as appendicitis or a kidney stone. Although her father agreed, he argued that the hospital should have started with the ultrasound and undertaken the CAT scan only if necessary. He then contacted the national media, accusing the hospital of trying to cover the costs of expensive equipment and performing defensive medicine unnecessarily.

1. Do you think it was possible that the hospital staff was practicing unnecessary defensive medicine in order to cover the costs of expensive CAT scan equipment?

2. Based on your experiences as a patient, do you think that the lower level tests would have revealed the ovarian cyst?

3. Is this a case of 20/20 hindsight and judgment after the fact, or did the ER circumvent quality care for financial reasons and protection from litigation?

4. Have you ever questioned whether a diagnostic test or procedure was necessary as a patient?

5. Do you think that there is an imbalance of information between health professionals and patients that causes patients to accept the need for the diagnostic tests and procedures that are ordered for them?

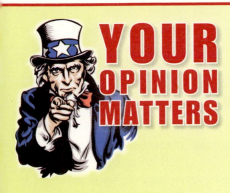
YOUR OPINION MATTERS

Should We Insure the Uninsured?

Background

Over 46 million people in the United States are uninsured. This figure has been growing in number and percentage. Despite the federal programs such as Medicaid and the Child Health Insurance Program, many people who do not meet the poverty eligibility for these federal programs remain uninsured. However, a significant percentage of the uninsured are young and healthy and elect to spend their hard-earned income on other necessities. In other words, many people choose to remain uninsured instead of paying for health insurance even though they are healthy. Younger people who are healthy and who have never had large health care expenses may elect not to purchase their employer-sponsored health insurance in favor of having a larger paycheck. Self-employed persons may elect not to purchase insurance and instead reinvest their business profits back into their company. Persons who have lost their jobs and whose unemployment benefits have expired may choose not to purchase individual health insurance and deplete their personal savings account.

Yes

Insuring the uninsured would reduce and perhaps even end the filing for medical bankruptcies. In addition, the newly insured would seek care in a timely fashion and thus improve public health. By seeking care early and avoiding late-stage intervention, insuring the uninsured would also reduce overall health care spending. How can the richest nation on the planet leave such a large percentage of its population without health care?

Proponents argue that the lack of guaranteed health care for all Americans has resulted in Americans having relatively poor health compared to other developed nations. Of a group of 27 comparable high-income democracies (members of the Organization for Economic Cooperation and Development [OECD]), the United States tied with Hungary and Slovakia as having the highest infant mortality rate and ranked 23rd in life expectancy at birth (OECD, 2011). The United States is one of the few developed nations in the world that does not guarantee universal health coverage for its citizens (OECD, 2011). Out of the 193 member states of the World Health Organization, the United States ranked first in per capita health care expenditures, number 31 in life expectancy, and number 152 in infant mortality rate (OECD, 2011).

No

Opponents argue that using tax revenue to provide health care to all Americans amounts to socialism. In a capitalist free-market system, citizens have the

(Continued)

right to choose to remain uninsured. Nowhere in the Constitution or any other document of law in the United States does it say that the federal government is responsible for guaranteeing health coverage. Many point to the phrase "promote the general welfare" in the Declaration of Independence as the intention to guarantee health coverage, but such a phrase is broadly general and says "promotion" not "guarantee."

Moreover, guaranteeing all Americans health care will decrease the quality and availability of health care in the United States. The United States is estimated to have the highest prostate and breast cancer survival rates in the world. According to the Institute of Medicine, the United States health care system is the "most responsive" in the world to nonhealth aspects of care, including patient confidentiality, consumer preference, and short wait time for elective procedures, and it also ranks high in health care technology availability (Institute of Medicine [IOM], 2001). Currently, United States law prohibits hospitals from turning patients with life-threatening conditions away because of inability to pay.

Clearly, having insurance does not guarantee access to care. The nation already suffers from a shortage of generalist providers and nurses. Even with insurance, many Americans are not physically close enough to essential primary care practitioners. By insuring the uninsured and increasing the demand for care, the shortages would only be exacerbated, increasing waiting times and access to essential services for those who really need the care. Are we prepared to lose our premier ranking in the world for short wait times by insuring the uninsured, many of whom elect to be uninsured?

Finally, the relatively low national rankings on some health indicators are not necessarily explained by lack of insurance. The U.S. indicators are low because a significant proportion of the population has third-world levels on these indicators, and most are eligible for and are beneficiaries of Medicaid. Improving access to care and raising health indicator levels require a focus on other health industry policies such as increasing supply of providers and patient education. Attention to insuring the uninsured only diverts our energies from attacking the real problems.

You decide:

1. Is health insurance a right in a free democracy?

2. Is insurance the cure to access and health status problems, or is it something else?

3. Does insurance result in seeking preventive care and reducing late-stage, expensive interventions?

4. Because hospitals cannot turn anyone away, don't we already have a mechanism for the uninsured to obtain care?

A better measure of the uninsured would be one that distinguishes between the chronically uninsured and others who lack health insurance periodically. Poverty status is a strong predictor of insurance status (Hadley, 2003). Minorities are disproportionately without health insurance because minorities are disproportionately poor. The primary reason why uninsured persons report that they are uninsured is the expense of health insurance (Hadley, 2003). A majority of the uninsured are poor, but over one-third are not poor (Hadley, 2003).

Employment Status

Most of the uninsured are employed either full-time or part-time (Gilmer & Kronick, 2005). Small employers, those with less than 10 employees, are less likely to offer health insurance than larger employers (Gilmer & Kronick, 2005).

Small firms may not offer health insurance for any of the following reasons: premiums are too high; they cannot qualify for group rates; they fear that they will have to take the benefit away in the future due to downturns in business; premium increases are too uncertain; health insurance is not needed to attract workers; workers prefer higher wages to health insurance; workers are covered by their spouse's health insurance; they wish to avoid administrative hassles; and employee turnover is too high to offer health insurance benefits. Companies often avoid offering health benefits by hiring temporary or part-time employees.

The current trend is for large, higher wage firms to offer health insurance for their employees. Smaller firms with lower wages are more likely not to offer health insurance benefits for their employees.

▪ Reimbursement by Health Care Consumers

This section provides an overview of the types of reimbursement for health care services. It provides a description of how clinicians are paid for their services by consumers of care. The trend in health care insurance is for more third-party reimbursement and less out-of-pocket reimbursement directly from patients.

▪ Direct Reimbursement

Direct payment is payment at the time service is delivered to the consumer and is in the form of cash, check, or credit card. Direct payment accounts for only about 22 percent of health care spending (KFF, 2009). Direct payment is often on a fee-for-service basis and can be in the form of uniform fees, for instance, the same fee charged for everyone.

Alternatively, direct reimbursement can be in the form of price discrimination or a sliding scale where the fee is based on the income of the patient. Common examples of price discrimination include different prices charged based on senior citizen discounts, student discounts, and in-state or out-of-state tuition. Essentially, price discrimination is charging different prices to different people.

Price discrimination is a method to maximize profits by charging each group the most they can pay. The public tolerates price discrimination because some groups "deserve a break." Physicians argue that reimbursement on a sliding scale is altruistic, although economists tend not to agree.

▪ Third-Party Reimbursement

Reimbursement to providers from third parties accounts for a large percentage of health care spending; specifically spending by commercial health insurance comprises 64 percent of private health expenditures (KFF, 2009).

A brief introduction to terms used in health care reimbursement might be helpful. The first party is the patient or the person responsible for the patient who received health care services. The second party is the provider who delivers the health care services, such as the physician, hospital, nursing home, clinic, or dentist. The third party is the health insurance company from which the patient has purchased insurance and with which the provider has a contract for reimbursement. The third party can also be called a payer.

Payment can be in the form of reimbursement for services, where the payer will pay up to a specified amount for each service. Prepayment can also be in the form of service benefits, such as when the payer pays for a specified number of physician visits per year. Another example of service benefits is payment for services for a specified period, for example 300 days of hospital each year, with no dollar amount defined or limitation set.

Community and Differential Ratings

Third-party reimbursement is based on payment of health insurance premiums by the insured. Health insurance premiums are set through two premium-setting methods. **Community rating** is coverage of different groups in a defined service area or community at the same cost. **Individual or differential rating** is based on the risk factor of the individual groups. Differential rating is good for low-risk groups, but difficult for high-risk groups with preexisting conditions or with unhealthy behaviors such as smoking. Differential ratings drive up costs for high-risk groups such as smokers, the elderly, or individuals with serious preexisting medical conditions. Conversely, individuals who are younger, do not smoke, and are generally healthy will pay lower premiums under differential rating. Proponents of community rating argue that these inequities balance out over the life cycle. To the extent we can manage our health, this phenomenon argues in favor of differential rating. To the extent that our health status is "luck of the draw," community rating appears to be fairer.

There are two main types of insurance with indirect payment schemes. In one case, participation is optional or considered voluntary insurance. This form insures people of similar risk and pays benefits only to those participating. Under compulsory insurance, participation in the group is required to maintain discounted group rates. This form of participation requires all members to pay premiums regardless of consumption, which spreads the risk across all members of varying risk levels.

From both a payer and a patient perspective, a group policy is the most economical. A group policy encompasses a large number of persons and covers all members of the group. Employment-based groups are the most common type of group, but they can also be a professional organization or community group. A group policy spreads the risk and costs of illness among all the members, making it less expensive to insure members of a group relative to individuals. Furthermore, insurers prefer to sell to employed groups to reduce adverse selection. Providing health insurance to an employed group takes advantage of the **healthy worker effect**. Health care costs are lower for an employed group of individuals because working individuals are more likely to be in good health simply because they are able to work.

An individual policy is more expensive because the probability or risk is more difficult to determine. Data such as age, gender, and preexisting conditions are all used to determine the cost of an individual policy. Adverse selection may also be present with an individual policy because sicker individuals typically enroll in such policies. Administrative costs are higher with an individual policy, so insurance companies charge a higher amount for individual policies as compared to group policies.

▪ Health Care Savings Accounts

Health (medical) savings accounts (HSAs) are employer deposits and other dollars set aside to insure against a catastrophic illness. The employee can write a check out of this account to cover the costs of necessary health care services. If the account is depleted after covering health care costs, an insurance policy can cover the balance of the health care services. If there is money remaining in the HSA at the end of the year, it can be rolled over to the next year or used as disposable income. Any amount used as income would be taxed at the employee's tax bracket. The goal of the HSA is to instill cost consciousness on the part of the employee when purchasing health care.

Self-insurance is an approach used by employers who are large enough to assume the financial responsibility for the health care costs of their workers. Typically, only very large companies or organizations have a sufficient number of employees to be self-insured. Self-insured plans are exempt from state-mandated benefit laws, state premium taxes, and state insurance reserves. Small companies are the least likely to be self-insured. Self-insured companies hire fiscal intermediaries (insurance companies) to process claims, reimburse providers, and perform utilization review.

▪ Moral Hazard

Moral hazard is a term first coined by Pauly (1968) to describe a phenomenon where individuals who have health insurance tend to use more health services than those who do not. The following hypothetical example describes this phenomenon:

> Suppose car insurance paid half the price of purchasing a car—"Car Purchase Insurance." What would happen to the number of people purchasing cars? Obviously, people would increase their purchase of automobiles significantly, and sale of luxury cars would likely increase. In the United States, we have decided that everyone is entitled to some level of medical care. As a result, health insurance has become less of what has traditionally been defined as insurance, such as underwriting against a catastrophic fire or flood, and more subsidized consumption, as in the car insurance example. (Pauly, 1968)

▪ Cost Shifting to Patients

Insurance companies attempt to shift the cost of care to patients and protect against moral hazard through several means. First, insurance plans have deductibles, or a dollar amount paid by the insured before insurance begins to pay for the services. The deductible usually is based on a calendar year, such as $200 to $1,000 per year. Thus, for example, patients will pay the first $1,000 out of pocket, and thereafter their policy will cover a percentage of the health care costs. The percentage paid by the insurance company after the patient pays the deductible amount out of pocket is roughly 50–80 percent. This sharing of expenses after the deductible is called coinsurance.

Second, insurance plans employ copayments. A **copayment** is a fixed dollar amount paid by the insured for each type of service. For example, a copayment may be $20 per physician visit, $10 per prescription, or $100 for each day in the hospital. Third, health insurance plans have coinsurance, which is the percentage of the cost of each health service that the insured pays, with the remaining portion paid by the insurance company. Coinsurance is commonly 80/20. The patient pays 20 percent after meeting the deductible.

Finally, health insurance plans have exclusions for such services as cosmetic surgery other than to repair damage from an illness or an accident. There are also exclusions for preexisting medical conditions. Preexisting conditions are illnesses that existed, such as cancer, before the purchase of the insurance.

Deductibles, copayments, and coinsurance all are attempts to make the consumer more conscious of health care costs and thus limit any unnecessary consumption of health care services. The impact is based on the amount of individual or family financial resources. Out-of-pocket payments affect the poor more than the wealthy. Some individuals purchase policies to cover all or part of the deductibles, coinsurance, or copayments. A common example of this extra coverage occurs with Medicare recipients, called "gap policies." As real income increases, people want to protect what they have, so they will purchase more insurance that is supplemental.

The 1984 Rand health insurance experiment demonstrated that price does matter and that individuals will actually decrease their consumption of health care if they have to pay for a greater porportion of the direct cost up front (Brook et al., 1984). Deductibles, copayments, and coinsurance all derive their utility from the results of the RAND study that supports the argument that making the consumer more price-sensitive limits the extent of the effects of moral hazard (Brook et al., 1984). Increased out-of-pocket expenses for patients usually mean decreased utilization of health care services (Brook et al., 1984).

▪ Adverse Selection

Adverse selection is a problem where the high-risk enrollees with high health care costs drive out the low-risk persons, or those with low health care costs. Insurers are entrepreneurs; they are in the business to make a profit. Insurance companies acquire profits by insuring a large pool of individuals who pay premiums. In return, the insurer pays for health care in the event it is needed.

Ideally, from a profit-making standpoint, the insurer wants to limit the amount it pays out. The best cases for insurers are when their revenues, or premiums, are greater than their costs or health care claims paid. If the costs of paying all the health care claims exceed the sum of all the premiums paid by enrollees, then the insurer will experience a loss.

When an insurer offers health insurance, it attracts sick as well as healthy enrollees. Sick enrollees are more costly, and more costs mean that insurers will raise premiums to cover their costs and ensure reasonable profits. The result is that insurers raise premiums and/or reduce benefit packages in the face of escalating payouts.

However, some healthy enrollees do not find it worthwhile to retain health insurance. Even if only a small number of healthy enrollees leave, insurers will find that their source of revenues is diminishing. As a result, they have to raise premiums, causing more healthy enrollees to depart, until mostly sick enrollees retain insurance because they find it worthwhile to have health insurance. This selection process of sick enrollees drives out healthy enrollees and is called adverse selection.

However, if enrollment is a requirement of employment, then the resulting enrolled group, such as university faculty and staff, will have numerous healthy individuals to balance the cost of caring for the minority who are really sick. This phenomenon is the reason why individual insurance premiums are much higher than group premiums.

■ Reimbursement Methods for Providers

This section covers reimbursement methods for providers, or how providers are paid for delivering health care services. Reimbursement for providers may differ depending on whether the provider is a hospital, clinic, or physician. Providers are typically not paid directly by a patient, but through a third-party financial intermediary.

■ Reimbursement Models

Self-Pay

Self-pay is paying a specific amount for each service by the patient or those responsible for the patient (Casto & Layman, 2006). Self-pay may be in the form of the cash or electronic reimbursement to the provider hospital, physician, or clinic. Patients may then submit their receipts for expenses to an insurance company for reimbursement or absorb the full cost themselves. Among private sources of spending on health care, private out-of-pocket expenditures account for approximately 22 percent of spending.

Payment from a patient may result from lack of insurance or a choice to pay out of pocket for health care. Self-insurance, a form of self-pay, is when a group or company is large enough to cover the health care expenses of its employees. The employer is able to cut administration costs by eliminating the health insurance company as a third-party (Casto & Layman, 2006). The company or professional organization bears the full risk of the health care costs of its employees and pays for their health care costs (Casto & Layman, 2006).

Retrospective Reimbursement

This payment method reimburses the provider after health care services have been delivered to the consumer. It is a form of fee-for-service, and payment is based on the charges that are submitted by the provider (Casto & Layman, 2006).

Reimbursing hospitals on a cost basis creates problems. First, the purchaser does not know how much the service costs beforehand. Second, the provider is retrospectively paid. This process creates incentive to raise prices, waste resources, and provide unnecessary services. The result is longer length of stay, more tests, and higher rates of admissions.

The proponents of cost reimbursement argue that cost-based reimbursement provides incentives to deliver the best care, as there is no incentive to withhold necessary care. Opponents argue that it provides an incentive to provide unnecessary services.

Fee-for-Service

Physicians each set their own fee-for-service (FFS) rates as reimbursement for the services they provided. The fee is a specific payment for each health care service rendered by the provider. The provider charges a fee for each service, and the payer reimburses the provider based on a contractual agreement. The fee that is charged by the provider may also be known as charges.

The provider sends a claim to the payer in which each of the tests or procedures is listed with its associated fee. Based on the pre-negotiated contractual rates, the provider is reimbursed when the payer pays the claim. Most physicians in the United States are reimbursed through a fee-for-service system (Casto & Layman, 2006). In a FFS model, reimbursement may be based on negotiated fee schedules or discounted rates.

Fee Schedule.

A fee schedule is a contractual arrangement between the provider and the payer regarding reimbursement for services. The provider and the payer agree to a list of services for which the payer will reimburse at a set amount. The fees are called allowable fees and are the maximum that the payer will reimburse for the services rendered (Casto & Layman, 2006).

Discounted Fee-for-Service Schedule.

Payers negotiated discounted FFS schedules in an attempt to control the increases in the costs of care. The negotiated rates may be referred to as usual, customary, and reasonable, or UCR, rates. In other words, the rates that are agreed to between the provider and the payer are typical for the provider, the community, and the diagnosis of the patient (Casto & Layman, 2006).

A second form of discounted FFS schedule is the resource-based relative value scale (RBRVS). Medicare provides negotiated fee-for-service reimbursement based on a resource-based relative value scale (RBRVS) or usual, customary, and reasonable (UCR) rates.

Customary, Prevailing, Reasonable (CPR). The customary, prevailing, reasonable (CPR) method is used to determine reimbursement rates for physicians. Payers base the "customary" rate on physician clinical history, such as what the physician charged for diagnoses over the past 6 to 12 months. The "prevailing or usual" criterion is based on the average physician practice patterns for similar physicians in the community. The carrier determines the "reasonable" criterion. The payer reimburses the physician at the lesser of the "customary," "prevailing or usual," and "reasonable" rates. A physician can profit financially in this system by "gaming the system." In other words, all the physicians in the community could continue to raise their prices and thus receive higher reimbursements.

Under the CPR method, there is no incentive to hold down cost or decrease utilization. Medicare no longer uses CPR because of all the "gaming" taking place. Instead, the RBRVS system was set up to counter the "gaming." The Omnibus Reconciliation Act of 1989 changed Medicare physician payments from physician charges to relative value of service and is now the national fee schedule.

Resource-Based Relative Value Scale (RBRVS). The Health Care Financing Administration (HCFA), the predecessor of CMS, developed the resource-based relative value scale (RBRVS) in 1991. The RBRVS is Medicare's physician fee schedule. RBRVS is a reimbursement system that attempts to appropriate payments for both health care management and surgical or procedural intervention. A RBRVS reimbursement system rewards cognitive and procedural skills, such as surgery, in a more equal fashion. For example, procedural skills may include when a cardiologist treats a myocardial infarction or a surgeon performs surgery. RBRVS began to be phased into Medicare reimbursement formulas in the early 1990s.

The primary purpose of RBRVS is to reevaluate all procedure codes and set payment levels, while accounting for practice costs, the value of work performed, the cost of training, malpractice insurance costs, and geographic differences. Previously, payers reimbursed procedures, such as invasive surgery, more than cognitive skills. The solution was to also reimburse for such activities as time spent with the patient, researching the diagnosis or treatment, and training. It is the choice of physicians to participate or not participate since they can just refuse to accept Medicare patients.

RBRVS assigns a value of one relative value unit (RVU) to a reference service, such as an annual physical. Other services are compared to the reference service. Services are compared on the basis of physician and personnel time and effort to perform the procedure, geographic differences in cost of living, cost of liability insurance, equipment cost, and malpractice cost.

If the RBRVS system deems a service to require three times the resources as the reference service, three times the amount of the reference service would be reimbursed. The RBRVS attempts to reduce the variation in reimbursement among as well as within physicians. Many private insurers are following Medicare's lead in adopting RBRVS. Insurers such as Blue Cross and Blue Shield, and Medicaid, use RBRVS as a way to decrease payments to providers, therefore saving money.

"Unbundling" is a strategy by which physicians can "game" the reimbursement system. "Unbundling" entails charging separately for each component of care. For example, a physician could bill separately for each component of service provided in an annual physical office visit. Another way to raise income is to discontinue telephone consultation and require patients to come to the physician's office so the visit can be billed as an office visit and be reimbursed.

Target income is a notion that physicians work to maintain a set income; they use the "gray area" in health care to manipulate their income through providing more services. Evidence shows that physicians maintain their incomes despite changes due to economic cycles.

The proponents of FFS reimbursement note that it gives incentive to provide patients with all the necessary services. Persons that have insurance that reimburses providers through a fee-for-service arrangement have more choices among physicians and specialists than those with other types of health plans (Casto & Layman, 2006). Patients are responsible for making the most of their own health care decisions regarding which physicians to visit and which types of treatments to seek.

Opponents of FFS argue that it provides incentive to over-serve, or provide patients with unneeded services. There are also disadvantages for patients as they have higher copayments or deductibles than other types of plans (Casto & Layman, 2006). Health insurance plans also assume more risk because they cannot predict costs and future expenditures as reliably as they are able to do so with other plans (Casto & Layman, 2006). Under FFS, costs will continue to increase for health insurance companies if patients demand more services, providers increase their prices, or the covered members of the plan become sicker at higher rates (Casto & Layman, 2006).

Reimbursement Based on Negotiated Rates

Negotiated rates may be based on a per-patient-day basis, which creates incentive to keep patients in hospitals as long as possible. The rates also may be based on the type of diagnosis with diagnosis-related groups (DRGs). In 1983, the government established DRGs or a prospective payment system in which the payer guarantees the provider reimbursement for providing service to a patient with a particular diagnosis. If the provider incurs costs that are above the DRG reimbursement amount, the hospital loses money. If hospital costs are under the DRG amount, the hospital will have a surplus.

The incentive with DRGs is still to admit patients. However, DRGs affect length of stay because hospitals can and do discharge patients to their home or long-term care (LTC) "quicker and sicker." Other incentives created by the system are to provide fewer diagnostic tests and other ancillary services. Because DRGs in and of themselves do not affect admission rates, third-party payers employ other strategies in conjunction with DRGs. Strategies include professional review organizations (PRO), which have stringent standards for admission.

Proponents of DRG-based reimbursement argue that it provides incentive to give only necessary services. Opponents argue that DRGs provide incentive to withhold care and discharge patients too early.

Capitation

Capitation payment is a set amount of money given to physicians for each person who enrolls in their practice prior to the provision of any care, usually used with primary care physicians. In return, the physician is responsible for providing specified services for a designated period of time. Thus, if physicians do not see some patients at all during the designated time period, they will be reimbursed the same amount as if they had seen patients many times.

Proponents of reimbursement based on capitation argue that it provides a physician with incentive to be efficient, keep the patient healthy, and offer more preventive services. However, opponents of capitation argue that there is also an incentive to withhold services.

Lump Sum Transfer

A lump sum transfer is a defined amount of reimbursement for a defined number of people for all their services for a specified amount of time. The provider is reimbursed up front. Lump sum transfer may be in the form of capitation payment or a global budget. The Veteran's Hospital Administration (VA) uses a global budget. The VA hospitals provide care for a specified period for a specified population. However, once the hospital expends its money, it is out of money. Other providers, such as mental hospitals and local health departments, also use such a system.

Another example is Medicare payment to a home health agency for their services. All of the services that were used to treat a patient at home are consolidated into one payment for the agency. The services may include rehabilitative therapy, changing of dressings and administering of medication, and health care supplies (Casto & Layman, 2006).

The incentive in a lump sum transfer system is to lower admissions, length of stay, and discharge patients quickly. Proponents of this reimbursement system argue that hospitals only provide needed services. Opponents argue providers have incentives to withhold necessary care.

Salary

A physician receives a salary when he or she is an employee of a hospital system, a member of a group practice, or an employee in a government-owned hospital. Proponents of reimbursement by salary argue that physicians do not need to worry about reimbursement because they are on a salary. In other words, the physician can provide whatever is necessary to treat the patient without worrying about reimbursement.

Opponents of salary reimbursement argue that physicians have incentive to be lazy and work only a minimum of 40 hours per week. Further, even though a physician receives a salary, the physician's employer may put pressure on him or her to change their practice style by decreasing admissions and length of stay (LOS) and prescribing fewer diagnostic tests. Salaried physicians may have incentive to reduce costs by under-serving patients.

Share of Profits

Physicians who share profits also typically receive a salary, and they receive a percentage of the profits of the department or organization. Examples of such departments include hospital departments of radiology and pathology.

■ Prospective Payment Model

Prospective payment reimbursement is based on rates that are linked to pre-negotiated rates with providers. The payment does not change even if the costs of the care for the patient are above or below the level of reimbursement. The level of reimbursement is based on the average cost of care for the average patient over either a set period of time or upon a given diagnosis. Reimbursement based on the average patient during a given time period is called per diem payment and reimbursement based on diagnosis is called case-based reimbursement (Casto & Layman, 2006).

The goal of prospective payment models is to control costs by giving incentives to providers to control costs. Providers receive a predetermined amount of reimbursement regardless of increases in costs of the patient care. Providers have incentives to manage the care of patients rigorously, invest in new technologies to reduce the costs of care, and to limit inpatient admissions for patients (Mayes & Berenson, 2006).

Per Diem Prospective Payment

Per diem prospective payment system is based on reimbursing the provider at a fixed rate for each day of care that is delivered (Casto & Layman, 2006). Historical cost, length of stay, utilization of services, and severity of illness data are used to determine the typical cost of care for a patient.

There are downsides to using historical data to base future reimbursement rates. For instance, providers have incentives to drive up costs through admitting patients and increasing the length of stay. Higher costs will be incurred and subsequently used to calculate future reimbursement rates. This form of payment results in rising prices for the third-party payer to reimburse.

Case-Based Prospective Payment

Diagnosis-Related Groups (DRG). Medicare initially used DRGs for the payment of inpatient hospital bills. DRGs work by reimbursing providers based on primary diagnosis. Medicare compares the resources that clinicians use to provide care to patients with a particular DRG and compares them to the resources used in other DRGs. The DRG payment is composed of an initial payment fee multiplied by a DRG weight. Medicare assigns each DRG a weight relative to a standard weight of 1.00. A hospital is assigned a basic fee for standard care. The DRG weight is adjusted for location, such as urban or rural; hospital type, such as teaching or non-teaching; size of the hospital, such as small or large; and patient mix. The final payment is the basic fee multiplied by the DRG weight (Figure 11–4).

Other third-party payers such as state Medicaid programs and insurers like Blue Cross and Blue Shield have been using DRG or prospective payment mechanisms to cover hospital services. Third-party payers are moving away from cost-based reimbursement to prospective-based reimbursement.

Over the past two decades, DRGs and the prospective payment system (PPS) have been associated with hospital closures and a decline in profit margins. DRGs and PPS have contributed to a decrease in inpatient admissions and an increase in outpatient care as well as increases in the use of other sites of inpatient care such as nursing homes. The problem with DRGs and PPS is that there is an incentive to under-serve the patient. Employers and many third-party payers also continue to negotiate lower reimbursement rates from providers, especially those with a surplus of hospital beds. Eventually providers may lose the incentive to further improve their efficiency as reimbursement rates fall. There are limits to gains in efficiency, and thereafter, quality and access will suffer significantly.

In its early stages of adoption between 1989 and 2003, DRGs had a negative effect on hospital operating margins because they were increasing as little as 1 percent per year, not keeping pace with the inflation rate (Rosenberg and Browne, 2002). DRGs have had a significant impact on the health care practice of physicians. As early as 1989, according to a physician opinion poll, 81 percent of physicians reported that DRGs had a significant impact on health care. They reported that time spent with patients was reduced, and they tended to code office visits at higher levels of complexity than what

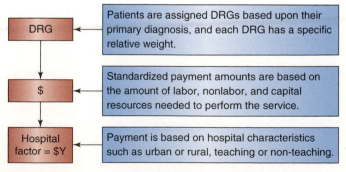

Figure 11–4 Medicare prospective payment rate determination.
© Cengage Learning 2013

had occurred (Seiber, 2007). Quality was affected, and hospitals that could not keep pace with the changes were closed.

A hospital closure greatly affects the local community, with the loss of jobs and decreased access to hospital care. Positive operating margins are important because such funds are used to fund uncompensated care, buy new equipment, pay shareholders if the hospital is for-profit, and expand facilities. DRGs have had a significant impact on decreasing length of stay. Although not necessarily a negative impact, in some cases a shorter length of stay is not beneficial for patients.

DRGs provide incentives for providers to embellish the diagnosis to move patients to a higher paying DRG, attract more profitable cases through marketing, discontinue services that lose money for the hospital, and discharge patients prematurely. These trends have led to decreasing length of stay (LOS), increasing the number of hospital closures, and shifting patients from inpatient to outpatient care.

Proponents argue that DRGs provide incentive to not over-serve, a concern that increased nationally after the passage of Medicare and Medicaid. However, since 1983, with the passage of prospective payment systems there has been a growing concern about under-service.

Summary and Implications of Our Financing Systems

The respective systems of financing affect the solvency and performance of the health care system. Rising costs are affecting all consumers of care, but particularly those who may be uninsured or underinsured who are not able to pay for the cost of their care, and more so for those who are very sick. Some care is ultimately delivered to these individuals, usually in emergency rooms, in the form of uncompensated care. In a fee-for-service system, patients absorb all the costs and insurance spreads the risk across a group. A community rating system spreads this risk more broadly because everyone in the community pays the same amount for insurance. Opponents of the community rating system argue: Why should individuals who take care of their health pay more because others are ill or have not cared for themselves? And such a system provides disincentives for individuals to assume responsibility for their health. An insurance system that uses differential rating, or rates based on risk factors, partially spreads the cost of care, with those at higher risk paying more.

These cost and financing issues raise questions about what is right, just, and fair. To the extent individuals control their health status, a differential rating would be appropriate. To the extent individuals' health status is not under their control, a community rating would be appropriate. It is simple to determine the impact of various financing schemes on utilization; however, it is difficult to determine what is fair or just.

In response to rising national debt levels, Barack Obama campaigned on a platform of health care reform and reducing the national debt (Obama, 2008). The health reform proposals that were enacted were based on three main principles. First, Americans should have access to high-quality affordable health care. Second, waste, fraud, and abuse should be eliminated in the health care system. Third, public health should be modernized to prevent disease and improve health (Obama, 2008).

Our systems of health care financing affect utilization, quantity of and access to services, and quality. By understanding and assessing the financial incentives, it is possible to predict the behavior of consumers and providers. These tools inform the health care reform debate and determine the future cost burden of proposed and enacted legislation. Does the recently passed Patient Protection and Affordable Care Act (March 2010) encompass an appropriate balance of these financial incentives and disincentives in its composition, and what impact will it have in the years to come?

▪ Review Questions

1. What are the implications for the delivery of health care when providers are reimbursed based on a prospective payment system?

2. What are the implications for the delivery of health care when providers are reimbursed based on a fee-for-service system?

3. Why is the individual market for health insurance so much more expensive than buying insurance as part of a group?

4. What are several trends in health care insurance and reimbursement, and how are they affecting the delivery of care for patients?

5. Is health care insurance a right that is guaranteed by the United States Constitution?

6. If you were a health care provider delivering care to a healthy patient population, would you prefer to be reimbursed based on a fee-for-service system or a prospective payment system (PPS)?

7. How has the change from fee-for-service reimbursement to PPS influenced the average length of stay (ALOS) for patients receiving care in hospitals?

8. If you were a shareholder of a major for-profit health insurance company, would you prefer to have more or fewer sick persons covered by an insurance product sold by the company?

9. How has health care reform influenced the health insurance market for patients with preexisting conditions?

▪ Additional Resources

Centers for Medicare & Medicaid Services (CMS): http://www.cms.gov/

Healthcare Finance News: http://www.healthcarefinancenews.com/

Healthcare Financial Management Association (HFMA): http://www.hfma.org/

Medicare.gov: http://www.Medicare.gov.

State Children's Health Insurance Program (SCHIP): http://www.cms.gov/home/chip.asp

U.S. Department of Veterans Affairs Health Care Financing & Economics (HCFE): http://www.hcfe.research.va.gov/index.asp

World Health Organization (WHO): http://www.who.int/health_financing/en/

References

Agency for Healthcare Research and Quality (AHRQ). (2009). Characteristics of uninsured young adults: Estimates for the U.S. civilian noninstitutionalized population, 19–23 Years of Age, 2006. Statistical Brief No. 246. June.

Ayanian, J., Weissman, J., Schneider, E., Ginsburg, J., & Zaslavsky, A. (2000). Unmet health needs of uninsured adults in the United States. *Journal of the American Medical Association, 284*(16), 2061–2069.

Brook, R., Ware, J., Rogers, W., Keeler, E., Davies, A., et al. (1984). *The effect of coinsurance on the health of adults.* Santa Monica: Rand Corporation.

Callahan, T., & Cooper, W. (2005). Uninsurance and health care access among young adults in the United States. *Pediatrics, 116*(1), 88–95.

Casto, A., & Layman, E. (2006). *Principles of healthcare reimbursement.* Chicago: American Health Information Management Association.

Congressional Budget Office (CBO). (2010). *Federal debt and the risk of a fiscal crisis.* Washington: Author.

Chernew, M., Baicker, K., & Hsu, J. (2010). The specter of financial armageddon— Health care and the federal debt in the United States. *New England Journal of Medicine, 362*, 1166–1168.

Claxton, G., DiJulio, B., Whitmore, H., Pickreign, J., McHugh, M., et al. (2010). Health benefits in 2010: Premiums rise modestly, workers pay more toward coverage. *Health Affairs, 29*(10), 1–9.

Centers for Medicare and Medicaid Services. (CMS). (2010, June 29). *NHE Fact Sheet.* Retrieved September 23, 2010, from Center for Medicare and Medicaid Services: www.cms.gov/NationalHealthExpendData/25_NHE_Fact_Sheet .asp#TopOfPage.

Gilmer, T., & Kronick, R. (2005). It's the premiums, stupid: Projections of the uninsured through 2013. *Health Affairs*, W5-143–W5-151.

Hadley, J. (2003). Sicker and poorer—The consequences of being uninsured: A review of the research on the relationship between health insurance, medical care use, health, work, and income. *Medical Care Research and Review*, *60*(2), 3S–75S.

Institute of Medicine (IOM). (2001). *Crossing the quality chasm: A new health system for the 21st century.* Washington, DC: Author.

Kaiser Family Foundation (KFF). (2009). *Trends in health care costs and spending.* Washington: Author.

Kaiser Family Foundation (KFF). (2010a). *Medicare Spending and Financing.* Menlo Park, CA: Author.

Kaiser Family Foundation (KFF). (2010b). *Summary of the New Health Reform Law.* Menlo Park, CA: Author.

Keehan, S., Sisko, A., Truffer, C., Poisal, J., Cuckler, G., et al. (2011). National health spending projections through 2020: Economic recovery and reform drive faster spending growth. *Health Affairs, 30*(8), W1–W12.

Martin, A., Lassman, D., Whittle, L., Catlin, A., & Team, N. H. (2011). Recession contributes to slowest annual rate of increase in health spending in five decades. *Health Affairs, 30*(1), 11–22.

Mayes, R., & Berenson, R. (2006). *Medicare prospective payment and the shaping of U.S. health care.* Baltimore: Johns Hopkins University Press.

Obama, B. (2008). Modern health care for all Americans. *New England Journal of Medicine, 359*, 1537–1541.

Organization for Economic Co-operation and Development (OECD) (2010). OECD Health Data. *OECD Health Statistics* (database). doi: 10.1787/data-00350-en (Accessed on 14 February 2011).

Organization for Economic Cooperation and Development (OECD). (2011). *OECD Health Data 2011: How does the United States compare.* OECD. Retrieved November 15, 2011, from http://www.oecd.org/dataoecd/46/2/38980580.pdf.

Pauly, M. (1968). The economics of moral hazard: Comment. *The American Economic Review, 58*(3), 531–537.

Robert Wood Johnson Foundation (RWJ). (2008). *Comparing federal government surveys that count uninsured people in America.* Princeton, NJ: Author.

Rosenberg, M., & Browne, M. (2002). The impact of prospective payment system and DRGs. *North American Actuarial Journal, 5*(4), 84–94.

Seiber, E. (2007). Physician code creep: Evidence in Medicaid and state employee health insurance billing. *Health Care Financing Review, 28*(4), 83–93.

Truffer, C., Keehan, S., Smith, S., Cylus, J., Sisko, A., et al. (2010). Health spending projections through 2019: The recession's impact continues. *Health Affairs, 29*(3), 1–8.

U.S. Census Bureau. (2010, September 20). *Income, poverty and health insurance coverage in the United States: 2009.* Retrieved September 23, 2010, from http://www.census.gov/newsroom/releases/archives/income_wealth/cb10-144.html.

Weissman, J. (2005). The trouble with uncompensated hospital care. *New England Journal of Medicine, 352*(12), 1171–1173.

Managed Care

Key Terms

adverse selection

closed panel

discounted fee-for-service

gatekeeper

group model HMO

HMO Act of 1973

independent practice association (IPA)

integrated delivery system (IDS)

Kaiser Permanente

managed care

managed indemnity plans

network model HMO

open panel

per member per month (PMPM)

physician hospital organization (PHO)

staff model HMO

Learning Objectives

- Identify and understand managed care models.

- Understand how providers are reimbursed in the respective managed care models, and the pros and cons of each reimbursement schedule.

- Identify the various HMO models and their benefits for providers and patients.

- Understand the distribution of risk between provider and managed care company through different forms of reimbursement.

- Understand the differences among capitation, fee-for-service, and discounted fee-for-service.

- Identify the unintended consequences of providing patients with affordable HMO plans.

- Identify the major milestones of managed care.

- Understand how HMOs developed and the role played by the HMO Act of 1973 and the American Medical Association.

▪ Introduction

Managed care is a term used to describe a spectrum of approaches used to integrate the delivery and financing of health care. **Managed care** is a system of health care delivery that monitors the cost, quality, and access to health care; a set of comprehensive health services that emphasizes preventive services and primary care to contain costs, improve quality, expand access, and reduce the need for more expensive specialty services.

A managed care company contracts with providers to serve on its panel or in its network. The panel is dominated by a variety of primary care providers who tend to operate more efficiently by serving as a patient's regular and usual source of care, which historically results in admitting fewer patients to the hospitals and ordering fewer laboratory and diagnostic tests. Managed care companies usually have explicit selection criteria for the panel of providers that include checking to see whether they have a history of keeping the cost of services low.

Managed care companies have formal quality assurance and utilization review programs. Quality assurance programs can be retrospective, concurrent, and prospective (see Chapter 14). Employers use the results and ratings of these quality assurance programs to determine which plans they will offer to their employees.

Managed care companies have a process of utilization review to address high costs. After the passage of Medicare and Medicaid and the resultant skyrocketing of health care costs, managed care organizations focused on the growing concern about over-serving patients. With the growth of managed care companies and their attempts to keep costs low, some have argued that managed care organizations have under-served their patients to control spending.

A managed care plan also has financial incentives to use providers associated with the plan by limiting benefits to members/patients who use noncontracted providers unless they obtain preauthorization to do so. Managed care plans also employ these authorization systems before visiting a specialist for care.

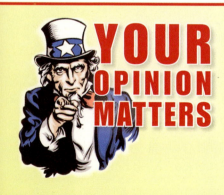

YOUR OPINION MATTERS

Should Americans Be Required to Purchase Health Care Insurance?

Background

As part of the Patient Protection and Affordable Care Act, passed by Congress and signed by the president in March 2010, it is projected that by 2019 approximately 32 million more people will be provided access to health care through health insurance coverage (Galewitz, 2010). The provisions of the legislation will be phased in over the next 17 years. Previously, health insurance plans could reject coverage to an applicant having a preexisting health care condition and could drop members if they became sick due to a preexisting condition. Dependent children of parents were also dropped from their parent's health insurance plans on reaching a certain age or upon graduation from college (Galewitz, 2010).

As part of the health reform legislation, health insurance plans will be required to provide coverage for dependent children until they are 26 years old if their parents are members of the plan. Persons that become ill while on a health insurance plan will no longer be dropped due to their preexisting medical conditions (Galewitz, 2010).

In 2014, the government will provide subsidies for families earning up to 400 percent of poverty level, currently about $88,000 a year, to purchase health insurance (Appleby & Steadman, 2010). The legislation requires most employers to provide coverage or face penalties, and most people as well will have to obtain coverage or face penalties.

By the time the bill is fully in effect in 2019, the government will be spending an additional $212 billion a year for expanding Medicaid and subsidizing private insurance for families who work at jobs without coverage (Goozner, 2010). About $400 billion of the $940 billion, 10-year price tag on the bill will come from tax increases, primarily on upper-income households, and efficiencies in Medicare will pay for the rest (Appleby & Steadman, 2010). The Congressional Budget Office analysis showed the federal deficit would actually decrease by more than $130 billion over the bill's first decade (Goozner, 2010).

In 2014, the Patient Protection and Affordable Care Act will require most people to obtain health insurance coverage or face penalties (Galewitz, 2010). The penalty would start at $95 for individuals, or up to 1 percent of income, whichever is greater, and rise to $695, or 2.5 percent of income, by 2016. Families have a limit of $2,085 (Galewitz, 2010).

Yes

Supporters of the individual mandate argue that Congress has the authority to pass legislation that falls within the powers enumerated in the United States Constitution. Two of those powers include the authority to pass legislation for taxation and regulation of interstate commerce. The individual mandate is argued to be a tax, as it penalizes those who choose not to purchase health care insurance (Balkin, 2010). The question is whether such a tax promotes the general welfare of the United States (Balkin, 2010).

Proponents argue that the mandate easily passes the "general welfare" test established by the Constitution (Balkin, 2010). The mandate is part of legislation that insures more people and prevents patients from being denied coverage due to their preexisting conditions. The success of the reform legislation depends on people who were previously uninsured signing up for insurance and joining the risk pool of all patients. Spreading the risk among millions of newly insured persons, most of whom are expected to be young and healthy, will lower the cost of health insurance premiums for everybody (Balkin, 2010).

Supporters of the mandate emphasize that the tax is necessary to pay for the costs of the reform regulations. Substantial taxpayer money will be

(*Continued*)

required to enact all of the provisions of the legislation. There are varying estimates, depending on which assumptions are made, but the reforms are expected to cost approximately $940 billion over 10 years (Goozner, 2010). It is estimated that $212 billion a year will be spent on expanding Medicaid and subsidizing private insurance for families who work at jobs without coverage (Appleby & Steadman, 2010).

Supporters of the mandate counter arguments made by the opposition who say that people who do not purchase insurance are being penalized for doing nothing. Supporters argue that when the uninsured become ill, they substitute family financial support, over-the-counter-remedies, and consumption of emergency services for purchasing health insurance (Balkin, 2010). All of these activities cumulatively affect interstate commerce, which Congress has the power to regulate with the Commerce Clause of the United States Constitution.

Therefore, the uninsured are not just doing nothing when choosing not to purchase insurance, but they are also hindering reform legislation that Congress has enacted. Congress has determined that in order for health care reform to be successful, the uninsured need to purchase insurance and spread more of the risk among the young and healthy (Balkin, 2010).

No

Those who argue against the individual mandate say that it will be ineffective in solving the problem of paying for the health care of those who refuse to purchase health insurance. These individuals will choose not to purchase health insurance, but will expect society to pay for their health care expenses. The cost of health insurance premiums will be much greater than the penalty for many people and they will simply choose to pay the penalty rather than pay the monthly premium cost. Such persons must be provided care if they present at a hospital emergency room with a life-threatening condition. Many people use hospital emergency services as their sole source of care and providers pass this cost on to insured consumers.

Opposers of the mandate argue that it will not affect the actual cost of health care services. Physicians and hospitals will still be motivated to charge competitive prices that allow them to earn a profit as well as cover their costs. Increasing costs of medical technology, prescription drugs, and consumer demand drive costs higher and push health care insurance premiums higher. A mandate that people purchase health insurance will not reduce health insurance premiums and costs.

Inability to enforce the mandate effectively is also a source of opposition. The difficulty of enforcing the health insurance mandate is so pronounced that it severely limits the effectiveness of the mandate. The mandate is rendered ineffective if even a small percentage of uninsured choose to pay the penalty rather than purchase insurance (Whitman, 2007). Moreover, even if the mandate could be enforced successfully, the amount of health care that previously was uncompensated (due to lack of health insurance) is so small that it would not make a significant difference in private insurance premiums (Whitman, 2007).

Those who oppose the individual mandate argue that reform efforts should be focused on addressing escalating health care prices and insurance premiums (Whitman, 2007). For instance, patients pay substantially higher out-of-pocket prices when they seek care outside of their managed care network. Patients seek care from high-quality specialists they determine are able to provide them with appropriate care, but pay a substantially higher price for seeking quality care. Moreover, insurance premiums are too high for many people, and the individual mandate is ineffective in addressing this issue. Many uninsured persons are hardworking, employed individuals who must decide between paying their mortgage and groceries and paying a health insurance premium. For many families, keeping a roof over their heads and food on their table has priority over paying a premium for insurance they may never need (Whitman, 2007).

Further, those who oppose the individual mandate argue that as citizens of the United States, Americans should not be forced to purchase a product from a private company. They argue that health care is not the same as driving a car on a state or federal highway and being required to purchase automobile insurance. A person living in the United States does not engage in any specific licensed action when choosing whether to purchase an insurance product. He or she can choose not to drive and not to purchase a car, and this person would not be penalized by the government (Frieden, 2011).

You decide:

1. Which groups of people will gain the most from this reform legislation?

2. Do you support the measures that have been passed in this legislation?

3. Should uninsured Americans be forced to purchase health insurance?

4. Can you think of other convincing arguments both for and against the individual mandate to purchase health care insurance?

▪ History of Managed Care

The history of the managed care industry includes the following important milestones:

- **1933:** Dr. Sidney Garfield (1906–1984) provided health care services to construction workers in the desert on the Los Angeles aqueduct in exchange for a prepaid, per capita amount deducted from their paychecks.

- **1937:** The Group Health Association in Washington, D.C., for federal workers was formed. The medical community opposed all prepaid health plans at that time, by denying participating physicians access to hospital privileges. This strategy was fought in court (see following).

- **1938:** During the construction of the Grand Coulee Dam in Washington state, Dr. Sidney Garfield (1906–1984) recreated his prepaid health plan for workers on the dam and their dependents, which eventually led to the formation in 1942 of Permanente Foundation, an example of a group model health maintenance organization (HMO). Today, the **Kaiser Permanente** health insurance company has the highest HMO enrollment in the United States.

- **1943:** The United States Supreme Court found the AMA and Medical Society of the District of Columbia guilty of restricting trade due to a violation of the Sherman Anti-Trust Act (1890). Before this ruling, to obtain hospital privileges physicians had to be in good standing with the AMA and the local medical society. Because the AMA and the local medical society held that group practice was unethical, they were able to constrain the growth of prepaid group practices.

- **1973:** The HMO Act of 1973 is enacted.

- **1990–2000:** In this decade, there was a growth in the number of HMO enrollees.

▪ The HMO Act of 1973

During the first Nixon administration from 1968–1972, health care costs escalated rapidly. Policy makers were faced with the decision to either regulate the health care industry and improve its efficiency or use competition to control costs. The Republicans and President Nixon resisted further regulation of the health care industry and instead introduced prepaid group practices as an option for controlling costs and utilization.

The President's advisors demonstrated that prepaid group practices offered comparable health care at 15–20% lower cost through reduced hospital admissions and increased use of ambulatory care. Dr. Paul Elwood coined the term *health maintenance organization (HMO)* to describe prepaid group practices. President Richard Nixon, in a nationwide television address in the early 1970s, proposed to "blanket" the United States with HMOs by the end of the decade.

The American Medical Association (AMA) strongly disapproved of prepaid group practices, holding to solo practices using fee-for-service (FFS) financing as acceptable for the large majority of physicians. Specifically, the AMA objected to its members being forced into group practices and opposed being paid on a capitated basis. The AMA lobbied to maintain the traditional FFS system and spent large sums on political campaigns. With its influence, the AMA managed to scale back the HMO Act of 1973 to only an "experiment." They also successfully lobbied for **independent practice associations (IPAs)**, a hybrid form of HMO, which allows physicians to provide services in their solo offices and bill the IPA a fee. In turn, the IPA was prepaid by the patient.

The **HMO Act of 1973** provided grants and loans for the establishment of HMOs. To receive funds, the Act required that critical health care services be provided and that employers offer a dual choice in health plans. This provision mandated that organizations with 25 or more employees offer an HMO option and contribute an equal amount to traditional insurance and HMO premiums. Although the Act contributed to an increase in the number of HMOs, during the same period the growth of nongovernment-subsidized HMOs was substantially greater, driven by the private industry's desire to control health costs.

▪ Essential Managed Care Terms

The following are commonly used managed care terms:

- **HMO:** An organization that provides a wide range of comprehensive health care services for a specified group of subscribers for a fixed, prenegotiated, periodic rate, normally a PMPM capitation rate.

- **Gatekeeper:** usually a primary care physician (PCP), who must authorize specialty care before any is rendered.

- **Closed panel:** a managed care plan that contracts with physicians and other primary care clinicians on an exclusive basis for services; the clinicians do not treat any other patients other than those who are members of the plan.

- **Open panel:** a managed care plan that contracts with private clinicians to deliver care; however, the clinicians may see other patients not in the plan.

- **Capitation:** a set amount of money paid per enrollee for a predetermined set of benefits to be rendered if medically necessary. Capitation is based on membership rather than on services delivered. A common capitation measure is dollars **per member per month (PMPM)**.

- **Copayment:** portion of a claim or health care expense that a member must pay out-of-pocket at the time of treatment; usually a fixed amount (such as approximately $10 per provider visit, $5 per prescription).

▪ Basic Characteristics of an HMO

A health maintenance organization (HMO) has several important characteristics. It assumes contractual responsibility to arrange for a comprehensive package of health care services. The members are voluntarily enrolled for a specified period. The HMO receives a fixed, periodic payment, usually from the enrollees' employers, independent of the volume of services provided to each enrollee for the coverage for that enrollee. In other words, the financial plan provides services on a prepaid basis. It arranges for provider organizations to bear financial risk through reimbursement based on capitation. An HMO contracts with providers to deliver care to its patients. Consequently, as an administrative entity, the HMO assumes legal, financial, public and professional accountability (Kongstvedt, 2001).

In an HMO, patients are "locked" in to the system so that if they seek care from an outside provider without approval, they are responsible for up to the full cost of the service. HMOs have formal quality assurance procedures and utilization review programs to control costs and offer financial incentives for its member to use providers associated with the plans.

Common HMO Models

Staff Model

A **staff model HMO** employs providers to deliver care to enrollees at their facilities. Physicians on staff are paid on a salary basis and may also receive a bonus based on their efficiency and productivity (Kongstvedt, 2001). The staff model must employ all high-demand specialists and subcontract for specialists that are used less frequently. Staff model HMOs are also referred to as closed panel as all of the physicians are employees and providers in the local market who are not employees do not participate (Kongstvedt, 2001).

Staff model HMOs typically operate out of large freestanding ambulatory centers in which they provide a wide range of patient services. The ambulatory center may include services such as pharmacy, diagnostic imaging, laboratory, rehabilitation, and business office personnel. This model offers ease of service for enrollees as it provides all of the necessary nonhospital services that are required for patient care. Local hospitals are also contracted to provide inpatient services to the HMO enrollees (Kongstvedt, 2001).

This type of HMO has several advantages for clinicians over other models. There is limited monetary investment in the practice, limited legal risk for its employees, and limited financial risk to providers because they are salaried and have regular working hours.

However, there are disadvantages for providers in being an employee of a staff model HMO. Clinicians have limited input into management decisions, limited income potential, greater oversight of clinical practice decisions; they must oversee cost containment measures, with utilization review, and undergo peer review of clinical decisions. Therefore, they have less autonomy.

Group Model

The **group model HMO** contracts with an established medical group for the provision of health care services, instead of individual clinicians. The physicians are employed by the group practice and not by the HMO. The physicians are permitted to still provide services to non-HMO patients. The clinicians operate their own medical practices; they function as a separate group and share support providers, staff, facilities, information technology, and billing and scheduling staff.

The physician group may be reimbursed on a capitated basis to provide all necessary physician services to the HMO members. The group may also be reimbursed based on a fee-for-services basis to provide care to HMO members (Kongstvedt, 2001).

Vignette

WHO DETERMINES MEDICAL NECESSITY?

Ann Baker, a 45-year-old accountant, has been a member of a national health maintenance organization (HMO) for 20 years. She has obtained care from the HMO primary care providers on a regular basis. In addition, she has never failed to pay her monthly premiums over that 20-year period.

After experiencing persistent headaches that she could not contain with over-the-counter medications, she visited her primary care provider at the HMO. Following a thorough physical examination and blood tests, finding nothing significant, the doctor prescribed medication for the headache. Ms. Baker returned a week later with no improvement. With no neurologist on the HMO physician panel, the primary care provider referred Ms. Baker to a well-known neurologist in the urban area near the HMO.

After reading her chart results, the neurologist recommended that Ms. Baker undergo a CT scan, which ultimately revealed an abnormality in the brain. The neurologist then recommended a magnetic resonance arteriogram, which required a one-night stay in the hospital. Ultimately, Ms. Baker underwent surgery which relieved the arterial pressure in her brain and after several weeks of recovery, her headaches abated.

While recuperating, Ms. Baker received the bill from the HMO for her treatment with the neurologist. She was surprised to learn that although the HMO reimbursed the neurologist for the surgery, it denied payment for the magnetic resonance arteriogram on the grounds that the test was investigative. Ms. Baker called the neurologist and he answered the patient in writing with a copy to the HMO. The doctor argued that despite the HMO's denial, he still considered the magnetic resonance arteriogram a medically necessary procedure in her case. The HMO medical director not only did not reconsider reimbursement, but wrote the neurologist directly saying that she considered the doctor's letter to the member to be significantly inflammatory, and that he should be aware that a persistent pattern of pitting the HMO against its members may place her relationship with the HMO in jeopardy.

Faced with paying the neurologist for the expensive test, Ms. Baker repeatedly used the HMO grievance procedure, and after two years of persistent denials, the HMO finally reconsidered and reimbursed for the test.

1. Who determines medical necessity? Ms. Baker's HMO contract states clearly that ultimately it is the HMO that decides.

2. Should HMO members get pre-approval for specialist tests from the HMO?

3. Are HMO grievance procedures effective and worth the time and effort?

4. Isn't it clearer to assess medical necessity after the fact?

Network Model

A **network model HMO** contracts with multiple physician groups to deliver health care to members. The network may be a large single multi-specialty group or it may be composed of many small groups of primary care physicians (PCP). The primary care physician group model focuses on providing services such as family practice, internal medicine, pediatrics, and obstetrics/gynecology to members. The primary care groups in the network model are typically reimbursed on a capitated basis to provide all physician services to HMO members who select them as their PCP (Kongstvedt, 2001).

A network model may be either closed or open panel. In a **closed panel**, the HMO will only allow physicians within the network to provide services to the HMO members. In an **open panel**, physicians who are outside of the network may see the HMO's members as long as those physicians meet requirements established by the HMO (Kongstvedt, 2001).

The network model provides members with additional choices among providers and perhaps a wider geographical distribution of providers. However, it does limit physician participation, especially if it is the closed panel model.

Independent Practice Association (IPA)

An independent practice association (IPA) contracts with clinicians to provide care to HMO-enrolled members, usually on a capitated basis. In the original IPA model, clinicians were paid on a fee-for-service basis. However, because of the financial incentives to provide more services and increase costs, many IPAs had to move to capitated payments. Clinicians participating in IPAs retain their right to treat non-HMO patients on a fee-for-service basis, in an open panel HMO, as well as retain their solo practice.

An IPA is a group of physicians that is separate from the HMO. IPA physicians are free to continue to provide services to non-HMO members. A strong IPA is one in which multiple medical specialties are represented in order to minimize referrals to non-IPA physicians. Providing physician services in a wide range of services also makes the IPA more attractive to HMOs to arrange services for their members (Kongstvedt, 2001).

There are several advantages to IPA model HMOs. An IPA requires less financial capital to operate, as it is legally separate from the HMO functions. It can provide HMO members a wider choice among providers who operate their private practices without the constraints of being in a staff or group HMO (Kongstvedt, 2001).

▪ Other Types of Managed Care Models

▪ Preferred Provider Organization (PPO)

A preferred provider organization (PPO) contracts with independent clinicians to provide care services at a discount. The panel is limited in size, and the PPO employs a utilization review system. The PPO identifies physicians, hospitals, and other providers, as preferred, and contracts with these providers at a discounted rate in exchange for a guaranteed patient flow and timely reimbursement for care, which is an advantage for the provider. Preferred providers have favorable practice profiles where their patients typically have lower costs as a result of fewer hospital admissions and fewer tests. In Chapter 10, Figure 10–5 provided a graphical representation of the growing popularity of PPOs relative to other managed care plans since 1998. Figure 10–5 also shows the diminishing prevalence of the conventional fee-for-service plans that were widespread in 1988.

The PPO gives patients a financial incentive to use the preferred providers. In addition, in a PPO patients can see a provider that is not preferred, but it will cost them more in copayments, coinsurance, and deductibles.

A PPO differs from a HMO in that the PPO reimburses providers on a **discounted fee-for-service** basis, so the provider is not at financial risk. PPOs generally cost consumers more than HMOs, but consumers prefer them because they have more freedom to choose among providers.

■ Point-of-Service (POS) Plans

A POS is a managed care model where members are not locked in to a specific group of providers. For an additional premium, and a higher deductible and coinsurance rate, patients obtain care from providers outside of the organization. POS plans have gained popularity in recent years because of the freedom of choice they afford members. Enrollees are willing to pay a higher price for increased choice.

Advantages of point-of-service plans include increased freedom of choice, access to outside clinicians, and low copays and no deductibles when patients seek care within the network. Disadvantages of POS plans include a more costly structure than HMOs, and high copays and deductibles for non-network care; in addition, referrals for specialists may be difficult to obtain.

■ Managed Indemnity

Managed indemnity plans are a lot like a traditional indemnity plan and are the least "managed." What usually makes managed indemnity different is precertification, which means that some of the care members receive is subject to pre-approval. But, like most indemnity plans, members have access to any doctor they choose; they pay a predetermined deductible for care and then a percentage of health care costs (coinsurance); and they get reimbursed for the remaining health care costs after they receive care. By managing care through precertification, costs are usually slightly lower than traditional indemnity plans but are still higher than other managed care plans.

■ Continuum of Managed Care

Figure 12–1 illustrates the continuum of managed care. The continuum, from left to right, depicts an increasing gradient of strictness in rules of coverage and the associated decreasing premiums and costs.

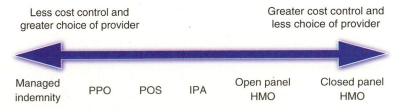

Figure 12–1 Continuum of managed care.

© Cengage Learning 2013

Note: The continuum of managed care, from left to right, depicts an increasing gradient of strictness in rules of coverage but is also usually associated with decreasing premiums and costs.

Other Health Care Delivery Organizations

Other types of health care organizations have emerged that provide care to members of managed care plans. An **integrated delivery system (IDS)** is an organized system of health care providers that spans a broad range of health care services by using vertical integration to contract with a variety of clinicians and health plans.

A **physician hospital organization (PHO)** is a system that bonds clinicians and hospitals together to form an IDS. These models have evolved because of the advantages of contracting with managed care plans, sharing financial risk, contracting directly with employers, and enhancing the quality of care for patients.

The advantages of a PHO are the ability to negotiate with managed care plans, track and use data to manage delivery, and form better relationships between the hospital and the medical staff. The disadvantage of a PHO is that it may not result in improved managed care contracting ability if some clinicians have unfavorable practice patterns.

Economic Concepts Important to Managed Care

Two important concepts are useful to understand when assessing the economics of managed care. **Adverse selection** is the tendency to attract members to the managed care plan who are sicker than the general population. Favorable selection, or "cherry picking" or "cream skimming," is when a managed care plan purposefully seeks out healthy enrollees to reduce costs and increase profits. A managed care plan with healthier enrollees incurs lower costs of care. A managed care plan with sicker enrollees will have higher costs of care and lower profits. Profits are important to health care plans as they are owned by shareholders who wish to ensure their long-term financial viability.

Another key concept affecting cost is that illness and the amount of health care services consumed are not equally distributed among members of managed care plans, or any other group for that matter. A small percentage of people use a disproportionately large share of services. It is not advantageous for a managed care company to provide coverage for sick enrollees from a profit/loss standpoint.

If a plan has a disproportionate share of sick enrollees, its costs are going to be higher, which means that premiums are going to be higher, thus deterring healthy individuals from purchasing health insurance. The concern raised that permeates the entire national health care delivery system is that healthy people self-select into HMOs or that HMOs aggressively seek out healthy enrollees, leaving all the sick people to enroll in FFS, PPO, and POS insurance plans, raising their premiums substantially.

Managed care plans and FFS plans protect themselves from adverse selection through preliminary physical exams, after which coverage may be denied for preexisting conditions; assessing risk factors such as heredity and lifestyle; and insuring groups, not individuals. Managed care plans prefer to insure groups rather than individuals because of the healthy worker effect, which holds that a person must have a certain level of health if he or she is able to remain successfully employed. Consequently, managed care plans and other insurance companies can achieve a better distribution of risk as well as lower administrative costs by insuring groups of employees.

It is important to note that managed care arrangements provide only a one-time cost savings. Increases in costs over time have been similar between managed care and traditional insurance because the factors driving the increase are the same, such as the aging population, technology, and higher consumer expectations.

Selected Empirical Evidence Concerning HMOs

Evidence on HMO performance, studied by Miller and Luft (1993), revealed that prepaid group practice HMOs had lower hospital use and overall costs compared to fee-for-service (FFS) plans, while maintaining a level of quality that was comparable to FFS. There is no reliable evidence to demonstrate that poor-quality managed care plans had lower costs or lower utilization. Nevertheless, it is very difficult to draw comparisons between managed care and FFS because of adverse or favorable selection bias.

More recent evidence on HMO quality found variation in performance among different managed care plans (Miller & Luft, 1997). Therefore, HMO proponents as well as its opponents find support for their positions on quality of managed care, depending on the particular organization model they choose or the particular disease.

However, empirical evidence does not support the fears that HMOs uniformly deliver inferior quality of care; yet expectations that HMOs would increase overall quality of care are not substantiated either (Miller & Luft, 1997). In several instances, Medicare HMO enrollees with chronic conditions received worse quality of care. Miller and Luft (1997) found that such lack of quality uniformity may be due to slow change in practice patterns and poor-quality measurement and reporting. Perhaps managed care providers are better at managing common illnesses, and patients with severe or rare conditions receive better care in managed indemnity, PPO, or POS plans.

Reputation of Managed Care

Over the last 10 to 15 years, the reputation of HMOs among consumers has suffered. Perhaps HMOs save costs by either selecting clinicians willing to provide inexpensive care and who have a history of ordering fewer diagnostic tests (which may not necessarily be an optimal amount of tests), or by limiting the services included in the insurance plan and constructing barriers to accessing care.

In 1998, Brodie, Brady, and Altman found that media attention to managed care changed from 1990 through 1997. Early coverage focused on the economics and business aspects of managed care, but by the mid-1990s attention shifted to patient care and consumer backlash (Brodie, Brady, & Altman, 1998). Although the majority of media coverage is neutral, most attention is paid to negative results that dwell on graphic examples of problems enrollees have had with managed care. The media may be one of many factors influencing people's anxiety about managed care (Brodie et al., 1998).

In the past, if prospective patients were not satisfied with their health plan they had many opportunities to switch plans. Today, employers are limiting plan choice more often, which means that dissatisfied consumers frequently cannot move out of their health plan as easily—or at all. Many employees feel "locked-in," with employers in control. This imbalance has led to a significant shift in customers' satisfaction with managed care. In the 1980s, customer satisfaction with traditional fee-for-service (FFS) and managed care, particularly HMOs, was comparable regarding quality, coverage, and access to service. However, from the mid-1990s on, satisfaction survey

Table 12–1: Fee-For-Service versus Managed Care Characteristics

Fee-For-Service	Managed Care
Focus is on individual services or episodes of illness.	Focus is on managed health over time.
There is little financial incentive for preventive, primary care.	There is an emphasis on preventive/primary care.
Filling inpatient beds is goal. Give patients all they need.	Goal is to reduce system expense over the long run by keeping patients out of hospital, moving patients to other less expensive sites of care.
Maximum income is dependent on high volumes of service.	Maximum income for providers is dependent on effective treatment, or low volumes, of service management.

© Cengage Learning 2013

results have favored traditional or managed indemnity plans or hybrid plans such as POS (Rice et al., 2002). Table 12–1 provides a side-by-side comparison between the major characteristics of FFS and managed care.

Halm, Causino, and Blumenthal (1997) reported that physicians' attitudes toward HMOs were highly negative, and they complained about the paperwork requirements. Physicians perceived HMOs had a negative effect on the physician–patient relationship by limiting time spent with patients, reducing freedom to make clinical decisions, and deterring the ordering of expensive tests/procedures (Halm, Causino, & Blumenthal, 1997).

Physicians also thought HMOs had a negative effect on hospitalizations as well as use of specialists, lab tests, and medication choice. Physicians were concerned that their patients would be denied coverage for the treatments they prescribe and that these refusals would have an adverse impact on the quality of care they provided. However, physicians had a positive view of HMO impact on the knowledge that patients' obtain about their overall care and the frequency of delivery of preventive care services (Halm et al., 1997).

Selected Legislation Enacted in Response to Managed Care

Managed care plans are heavily regulated by both federal and state governments. The federal government has enacted laws that affect maternity stay, ban gag clauses, and require emergency care to be covered. It was not uncommon for an HMO to tell its physicians not to disclose all treatment options available to the patient. In addition, some HMOs required individuals to contact a **gatekeeper** before going to emergency rooms. Now, under federal law, plans must cover ER visits that any prudent individual would deem an emergency.

States regulate managed care plans by enacting regulations that affect information disclosure by requiring clinicians to provide specifics on care and alternative treatments so that patients can make informed choices. Bone marrow transplants are now an option for breast cancer patients, and states regulate utilization review by limiting who can perform them and how.

Summary

Managed care is a term used to describe a spectrum of approaches used to integrate the delivery and financing of health care. Managed care is a system of health care delivery that monitors the cost, quality, and access to health care; a set of comprehensive health services that emphasizes preventive services and primary care to contain costs, improve quality, expand access, and reduce the need for more expensive specialty services.

Throughout the history of managed care, the AMA has been an important stakeholder in lobbying for legislation that benefited physicians. The AMA strongly disapproved of prepaid group practices, holding to solo practices using fee-for-service (FFS) financing as being acceptable to the large majority of physicians. Specifically, the AMA objected to its members being forced into group practices and opposed being paid on a capitated basis. The AMA lobbied to maintain the traditional FFS system and spent large sums on political campaigns.

An HMO has several important characteristics. It assumes contractual responsibility to arrange for a comprehensive package of health care services. The members are voluntarily enrolled for a specified period. The HMO receives a fixed, periodic payment, usually from the enrollees' employers, independent of the volume of services provided to each enrollee for the coverage for that enrollee. In other words, the financial plan provides services on a prepaid basis.

Common HMO models include the staff, group, network, and IPA. Other types of managed care models include the PPO, POS, and managed indemnity. Delivery organizations play a critical role in providing care to the members of HMOs. Integration between provider organizations takes the form of an integrated delivery system (IDS), which is an organized system of health care providers that spans a broad range of health care services by using vertical integration to contract with a variety of clinicians and health plans.

Review Questions

1. How does a managed care company distribute risks to providers so that they have incentive to provide care to maintain the health of their patient population?

2. What is the advantage for a managed care company to reimburse providers based on capitation?

3. What is the advantage for a managed care company to reimburse providers based on discounted fee-for-service?

4. What is the healthy worker effect?

5. What was the position of the American Medical Association regarding the HMO Act of 1973, and why?

6. How has the spread of managed care as a means to deliver care impacted hospitals and their formation of integrated delivery networks and health systems?

7. What is the advantage for providers in joining a managed care network and having patients choose them as their primary care physician?

8. How does the managed care model compare with the fee-for-service model based on cost, access, and quality of care for patients?

9. Do patients who access health care from HMO plans receive more or less quality compared with patients who receive health care from PPO or POS plans?

10. What role does an independent practice association (IPA) play in connecting physicians and a managed care plan?

■ Additional Resources

California Health Advocates: http://www.cahealthadvocates.org/

Children's Health Insurance Program: https://www.cms.gov/home/chip.asp

Health care.gov: http://www.healthcare.gov/

Health insurance reform for consumers: https://www.cms.gov/healthinsreformforconsume/

National Patient Advocate Foundation: http://www.patientadvocate.org/

■ References

Appleby, J., & Steadman, K. (2010, March 22). *The immediate effects of the health reform bill*. Kaiser Health News. Retrieved September 06, 2011, from http://www.kaiserhealthnews.org/Stories/2010/March/22/immediate-effects-health-reform.aspx?utm_source=feedburner&utm_medium=feed&utm_campaign=Feed%3A+Ne.

Balkin, J. (2010). The constitutionality of the individual mandate for health insurance. *New England Journal of Medicine, 362*(6), 482–483.

Brodie, M., Brady, L., & Altman, D. (1998). Media coverage of managed care: Is there a negative bias? *Health Affairs, 17*(1), 9–25.

Frieden, J. (2010). *Should Americans be forced to buy health insurance?* KevinMD .com. Retrieved September 07, 2011, from http://www.kevinmd.com/blog/2010/06/americans-forced-buy-health-insurance.html.

Galewitz, P. (2010, April 13). *Consumers guide to health reform*. Kaiser Health News. Retrieved September 07, 2011, from http://www.kaiserhealthnews.org/Stories/2010/March/22/consumers-guide-health-reform.aspx.

Goozner, M. (2010, March 22). *It's over! Health care is passed. Will it really work?* Kaiser Health News. Retrieved September 06, 2011, from http://www.kaiserhealthnews.org/Columns/2010/March/032210Goozner.aspx?utm_source=feedburner&utm_medium=feed&utm_campaign=Feed%3A+khn+%28All+Kaiser+Health+News%29.

Halm, E., Causino, N., & Blumenthal, D. (1997). Is gatekeeping better than traditional care? *Journal of the American Medical Association, 2789*(20), 1677–1681.

Kongstvedt, P. (ed.). (2001). *The managed health care handbook*, 4th ed. Gaithersburg, MD: Aspen Publishers.

Miller, R., & Luft, H. (1997). Does managed care lead to better or worse quality of care? *Health Affairs*, *16*(5), 7–25.

Miller, R., & Luft, H. (1993). Managed care: Past evidence and potential trends. *Frontiers of Health Services Management*, *9*(3), 3–37.

Rice, T., Gabel, J., Levitt, L., & Hawkins, S. (2002). Workers and their health plans: Free to choose? *Health Affairs, 21*(1), 182–187.

Whitman, G. (2007). Hazards of the individual health care mandate. *Cato Policy Report, 29*(5), 1, 10–112.

13 Utilization of Health Services

Key Terms

Andersen's behavioral model of health services utilization

elasticity of demand

enabling factors

individual determinants

medically underserved areas (MUAs)

predisposing factors

Rosenstock model

societal determinants of utilization

socioeconomic status (SES)

usual source of care (USOC)

Learning Objectives

- Identify the four primary factors that affect the utilization of health care services.

- Identify the major components of Rosenstock's model of utilization.

- Identify the major components of the Andersen model of utilization.

- Identify predisposing determinants of health care utilization.

- Describe enabling factors for health care utilization.

■ Introduction

Interest in the utilization of health care services is driven by the desire to know whether demand for health care equals the need for care. Utilization analysis is used to determine health insurance premiums and assists in the planning and marketing of services. Providers such as hospitals, state and federal governments, and public health officials perform needs and utilization assessments before implementing new service programs. Government agencies assess patient populations to determine whether they are receiving adequate preventive care and coverage for inpatient hospitalizations.

Utilization of health care services is important to examine over time, particularly given the most recent changes in United States health care insurance coverage. By 2019, it is anticipated that many people who were previously uninsured will obtain coverage that may afford them access to health care services. It is projected that 32 million more people will join the rolls of the insured (KFF, 2010). Health insurance, as well as other factors such as the socioeconomic and demographic characteristics of this newly insured population, will likely affect their demand for services (Andersen & Newman, 2005).

■ Characteristics of Utilization of Health Care Services

Utilization assessment often focuses on its predictors. Utilization is measured by demand for care; however, need for care does not always translate into demand, especially among the poor. On the other hand, sometimes the demand for care exceeds need, as is the case with hypochondriacs. Prospective patients' concerns about the cost of care usually affect their utilization patterns when they do not require care immediately, such as with immunizations, preventive dental care, and cosmetic services. When a patient is seriously ill and needs care in a timely fashion, cost is not an issue. The primary predictor of utilization is the level of sickness of the patient (Andersen & Newman, 2005).

■ Factors Characterizing Utilization

There are five major factors that affect the demand for health care services. First, the type of health care provider sought will determine the services utilized, such as physician care, dental care, nursing care, or pharmacy services. Some of these providers are interconnected through the physician office visit where, for example, patients are likely to consume nursing care. The visit may lead to a prescription that will then be filled by a pharmacist. A visit to a primary care clinician may lead to a further consultation with a specialist who may order a battery of tests to provide a diagnosis. A dentist visit may also entail services by a dental hygienist as a well as an X-ray technician. In other words, seeking treatment from one service typically leads to the consumption of additional services.

Second, location or place of residence influences utilization of services. Care may be delivered in a hospital, physician's private office, prison, nursing home, school clinic, factory clinic, or emergency room. Each site generates a unique pattern of demand for services. For instance, a private physician's office may be located in an area that is far from the population that most needs the services, such as a rural population that may be unable to access care because of the challenges with transportation. Likewise, an urban population may not have access to the best primary care clinicians if public transportation is the only means of access and it does not travel near such offices.

Third, the type of health care service affects its utilization. Health care services may be preventive, such as annual physicals or immunizations. Or they may be illness related and may affect the patient's outcome, such as surgery, transplantation, or chemotherapy. Home care is often utilized to stabilize patients in a nursing home or at their own home.

Fourth, frequency of visits, such as the number of times a patient sees a clinician or is admitted to a hospital, will have an impact on the utilization of services. Utilization is also characterized by the regularity of patient visits. Most physician visits are to primary care physicians for general health care examinations (CDC, 2010). In 2006, a typical patient averaged four visits per year to a physician's office, hospital outpatient clinic, or hospital emergency room. Visits have increased 26 percent over the past 10 years. The primary reason for the increase in visits is the aging of the population, because elderly persons utilize physician services more often than the rest of the population (CDC, 2009).

Finally, severity of the patient's illness and the continuity of care that may be required influence utilization of health care services. For example, an episode of illness such as a heart attack or stroke may require a significant number of physician visits to care for that illness. Typically, heart attack patients will require multiple follow-up visits to a physician to monitor their condition and receive physical therapy. Stroke victims may require many follow-up visits to monitor and adjust medications during their recovery. Follow-up speech or physical therapy and medication is frequently prescribed for stoke victims.

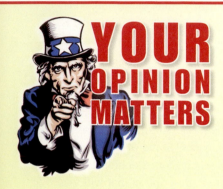

Should Physicians Own Hospitals and Be Permitted to Refer Patients to Them—Will This Lead to Quality Care or Induced Demand?

Background

Physician-owned specialty hospitals are hospitals in which physicians have an ownership stake in the entire facility and where they have staff privileges (GAO, 2006). There are roughly 300 existing specialty hospitals usually located in urban areas with sufficiently large patient populations that can generate high volumes for their services (Weaver, 2010). They typically offer one specialty service such as invasive cardiology, orthopedics, general surgery, plastic surgery, reproductive health services, or endoscopic procedures.

Physician-owned hospitals have grown rapidly, especially in southern and western states, by an estimated 33 percent between 2008 and 2010 (AHA, 2010). They increasingly represent a source of competition for nonprofit community hospitals and have been the target of criticism from those who question the appropriateness of physicians to refer patients to hospitals in which they have a financial interest.

Such special interest groups prevailed upon Congress in 2003 to impose a lengthy freeze on the construction of new doctor-owned hospitals that specialize in cardiac, orthopedics, and other areas (Weaver, 2010). This concern also appeared in the Patient Protection and Affordable Care Act (2010), which mandated a moratorium on new specialty hospitals, and restrictions on the expansion of existing facilities. All new physician-owned hospitals were required to be certified by Medicare by December 31, 2010, or they would be banned from participating in the program. The law further prohibits the existing hospitals from expanding unless they meet stringent conditions.

The politically and financially powerful American Hospital Association (AHA) has also been a vocal opponent of physician-owned specialty hospitals. The AHA claims they focus only on specialized and profitable services and draw patients and revenue away from nonprofit community hospitals that focus on their overall patients' needs (Weaver, 2010).

However, studies have shown that physician-owned hospitals are more efficient, reduce costs, and improve clinical outcomes.

Yes

Supporters of physician-owned specialty hospitals argue that such facilities develop focused processes of care that are tailored to a limited set of conditions, which allows these facilities to provide higher quality care at a lower cost. This principle is consistent with the notion of physician specialization that narrows the scope of practice but produces a better product. Moreover, such facilities increase competition for hospital services and spur innovation in the marketplace, which ultimately raises the quality of care. Ownership by physicians is critical because it gives physicians the freedom and motivation to design the hospital layout and operations in a way that maximizes efficiency and quality. Ultimately, if such facilities do not meet patient demands, they will not succeed in the marketplace.

Some argue that physicians will induce demand beyond what patients need. Although there is some evidence of ineffective health care, little of it can be attributed to physician-induced demand. Research shows that there is enormous variation in the use of care in different areas of the country and across countries, and most of this variation can be attributed to variations in physician practices (Goodman et al., 2011). Differences in practices could be caused by the uncertainty of diagnostic health care and variations in the training and skills of physicians.

The U.S. legal system provides compensation to patients who can prove that they have been victims of medical malpractice, deviations from accepted health care standards of care that cause injury to patients. Even so, the existence of defensive medicine does not necessarily imply excessive or inappropriate health care delivery. In fact, such interventions may result in higher quality care, fewer injuries, or a reduction in the number of high-risk procedures.

No

Physicians will induce unnecessary demand to meet target incomes. Opponents of physician-owned hospitals argue that they select the most profitable patients: those who are healthiest (and hence less costly to treat), who have desirable insurance coverage, and who require profitable services (such as cardiac surgery). This behavior makes it more difficult for general hospitals to cross-subsidize less profitable services (such as burn units and trauma care) and care for poor and uninsured patients. Physician ownership creates a potential conflict of interest between physicians' financial incentives and their patients' clinical needs. This conflict of interest might influence the hospital referral decisions of physicians or might lead to referrals for unnecessary services, thus increasing overall volume.

Physician-induced demand means that a portion of health care purchases may reflect physician preferences in excess of patient needs. It is utilization that is by definition inefficient, that is, the patient either needs no service or another less

(Continued)

costly service (e.g., a telephone interaction instead of another office visit). This demand can occur because of consumers' lack of information about the effectiveness of various health care alternatives. Thus, patients delegate the choice of alternatives to their physicians. Physicians, motivated by the self-interest of increasing income, may prescribe care that provides benefits to the consumer that are less than the costs of providing that care. In some instances, physicians may perform health care procedures to decrease the risk of a malpractice suit rather than because of the benefit such a procedure provides. Physician-induced demand results in the marginal cost of health services exceeding its marginal benefits.

You decide:

1. Can patients discern differences in quality?

2. Are physicians providing services in order to reach a target income or is variation in demand due to other factors?

3. Are specialty hospitals a vehicle for better quality or a means to manipulate patients to produce more income?

4. Is defensive medicine a necessary cost of practice and a quality enhancer, or is this care purely unnecessary?

Models Used to Predict Health Care Utilization

Forecasting models predict utilization based on past experience, analogous to predicting weather patterns. The predictions are usually average patterns, not specific to one individual or event. There are two models for predicting utilization of services, the Rosenstock model and the Andersen model.

Rosenstock Model

The Rosenstock model is based on patients' beliefs regarding their health as a predictor of their preventive health behavior. According to the **Rosenstock model**, four factors predict use of health care services: perceived susceptibility to the disease; perceived threat of the disease and its seriousness; belief in benefit or the efficacy of the health system; and environmental action cues such as billboards and mass media campaigns, social trends such as advice from others and family member with similar illness, and reminders such as postcard reminders from the physician. Figure 13–1 provides a graphical representation of Rosenstock's model and the factors that predict the use of health care services.

One limitation of the Rosenstock model is that it is accurate in predicting preventive health care service use, but it is not good for predicting urgent treatments.

Andersen Model

The Andersen model is used to predict utilization of all health care services. The components of Andersen's (1968) behavioral model of health services utilization include societal determinants, individual factors, and health industry characteristics. Figure 13–2 illustrates the major components of **Andersen's behavioral model of health services utilization**.

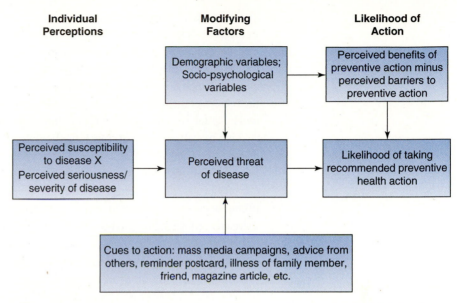

Figure 13–1 The health belief model as predictor of preventive health behavior (Rosenstock's model).

© Cengage Learning 2013

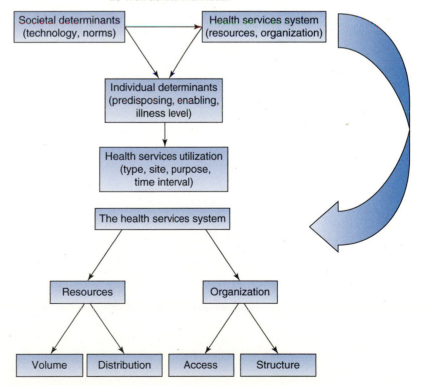

Figure 13–2 Anderson's model of health care utilization.

© Cengage Learning 2013

One societal determinant that affects utilization of health care services is changes in medical technology. For example, a new drug that increases the survival rate of a disease will increase utilization of the drug but may reduce hospital length of stay. On the other hand, the development of a new and highly effective immunization for a disease for which none existed previously increases demand for services associated with the receipt of the immunization but could significantly decrease demand for physician and hospital care associated with the treatment of the disease.

The overall impact of most medical technology developments is to increase utilization of services. For example, in the nineteenth century, anesthesia and asepsis resulted in better outcomes for surgery. As a result, more people consumed surgical services as clinical outcomes improved. With the development of more effective immune system suppressant drugs, the success rate of organ transplants has greatly increased. More mental health services were sought after the introduction of psychotropic drugs.

Societal determinants of utilization are also reflected in a society's norms, which are found in legislation or in the public consensus about health issues. For example, in the United States most babies are born in the hospital, whereas in the Netherlands most births occur at home. Other societal values are reflected in the establishment of the Medicare and Medicaid programs that provide coverage for the elderly, the sick, and the disabled. Laws that limit access to abortion or mandate vaccinations for children before school, as well as sanitation laws and the Americans with Disability Act (1990) are values embedded in legislation that affect utilization.

Technology and societal norms sometimes interact to affect utilization. For example, in the 1950s and 1960s, the development of psychotropic drugs changed society's beliefs about the appropriate care of the mentally ill, which resulted in the removal of many mentally ill patients from institutional settings.

The health service system itself influences utilization of services. For instance, as explained earlier in Roemer's law, the manner in which health resources are organized, including the number of surgeons trained and the number of hospitals and beds created, generates demand for services to a limited but significant extent.

The distribution of health services can alter the use of services. For example, the concentration of clinicians as expressed by the physician–population ratio is greater in cities than in rural areas (Wennberg, 2010). Thus, utilization per capita in rural areas is far lower than in urban areas. Moreover, if services are accessible, then utilization will increase. The distance and travel time to these services, the time in the clinician's waiting room, the time until the next appointment, and the amount paid for these services all affect use. Also, the structure of health care services affects utilization. Whether patients receive care through a point-of-service (POS) plan or a health maintenance organization (HMO) will determine their utilization of services.

Characteristics of the patient are also determinants of utilization. Socioeconomic status of patients, including their income and education, are good predictors of who will use services. Although the poor tend to have lower health status, their use of services is inclined to be lower than those with higher incomes. The aged tend to use more services than the young, and women tend to use more services than men.

There are additional factors that enable individuals to utilize. An enabling condition or characteristic allows or permits patients to convert their access desires into use. Some examples of **enabling factors** include family income, health insurance, and

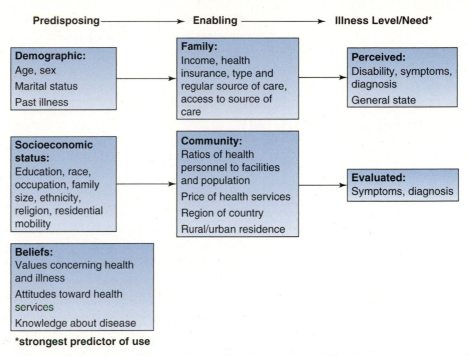

Figure 13–3 Individual determinants of health services utilization.
© Cengage Learning 2013

community resources. The Medicare and Medicaid Acts 1965 enabled the poor and elderly to increase their health care use by giving them additional buying power. According to the Andersen model, individual illness severity and the resultant need, whether perceived or prescribed, is the biggest predictor of health care use. Figure 13–3 illustrates the predisposing demographic and enabling family factors that lead to the perceived need of services.

▪ Trends in Societal Determinants (From Andersen's Model)

Societal norms, beliefs, and standards often are reflected either directly or indirectly in the enactment of laws. For example, the number of abortions performed in 1972 was 13 per 1,000 women ages 15 to 44. By 1996, that number rose to 20 per 1,000 women ages 15 to 44, and by 1999, rose again to 22.9 per 1,000 women. The change in the ruling by the United States Supreme Court in *Roe vs. Wade* (410 US 113, 1973) made abortions more accessible and altered the demand for them.

Immunization levels increased because state laws ordered that for children to register for school, they must first be immunized. These laws had very positive effects, with an increase in immunization rates and a decrease in childhood infectious disease.

Hospitals were reducing lengths of stay after childbirth as a cost-cutting measure. Because of rising health care costs, some third-party payers were limiting their length of stay reimbursement and thus were "pushing" women out of the hospital quickly after vaginal deliveries. Policy makers and clinicians questioned the appropriateness of reduced length of stay and its impact on the health of the mother and child (Weiss et al., 2004). To reflect this concern, Congress passed a law stating that for a vaginal delivery, third-party payers were required to cover a specific minimum number of hours in the hospital.

▪ Trends in Health Industry Characteristics (Andersen's Model)

Studies have demonstrated a positive correlation between surgical rates and surgeons per capita. Some experts argue that the care delivered is required to effectively treat patients. Others argue that this correlation is confirmation of Roemer's law, with physicians in a competitive market performing more surgeries to maintain their target income. Likewise, when there are more physicians per capita, there is a greater likelihood that they initiate additional health care visits. An example of physician-initiated care is the follow-up visit—is it needed, or is it to generate income for the physician in order to obtain a target income?

Studies comparing the United States to other countries tend to confirm Roemer's law. A classic study by Bunker (1970) found four to five times more hysterectomies, tonsillectomies, and hernia and gall bladder procedures performed per capita in the United States compared to England in 1960 and 1970. Perhaps not coincidentally, there were twice the surgeons per capita in the United States at that time (Bunker, 1970).

It is easy to conclude from this study that surgeons in the United States perform excess surgeries, and that this behavior was especially true before DRGs, when there was more of a financial incentive to over-serve. Alternatively, perhaps surgeons in England perform too few surgeries—surgeons in England are salaried.

Health care is practiced differently in different places—there is variation. This trend exists within the United States and within individual states (small area variation). Historically, the Northeast United States has had longer lengths of stay in hospitals (just under 7 days) than the West (just under 5 days) (Wennberg & Gittlesohn, 1973). This difference cannot be explained fully by variation in need, **socioeconomic status (SES)**, or insurance, but rather by the absence of agreement—no "master cookbook"— on how to practice health care.

Short-term hospital admissions dropped significantly in the early 1980s. The institution of DRGs shifted many procedures from inpatient to outpatient locales. In addition, hospital length of stay often depends on patients' insurance coverage.

Advances in health care knowledge affect utilization. Treatment for breast cancer has improved, and the length of hospital stays for surgeries like coronary bypass surgery and hip replacement have decreased. These trends do not necessarily reflect changes in need, but rather changes in health care knowledge many derived from the results of epidemiological clinical trials.

Births in the hospital and types of deliveries are determined by other factors than medical need. In the 1970s, American women were practicing natural birthing, which resulted in fewer C-sections and fewer forceps deliveries. More recently, the rate of C-section deliveries has increased to a level exceeding by two times the rate that is thought to be medically necessary. This rate increase may also be driven by fears of litigation and the practice of defensive medicine as well as increased physician payments for C-sections. See Figure 13–4 for a graphical illustration of the increase in C-sections from 1993 through 2008.

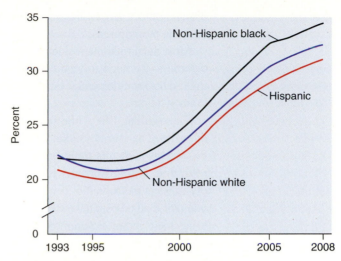

Figure 13–4 Cesarean delivery by race, and Hispanic origin of mother: United States, 1993–2008.
Source: Figure 6 from J. Martin et al., Births: Final data for 2008. National Vital Statistics Report, 59(*1*). *December 8, 2010. Retrieved November 01, 2011, from http://www.cdc.gov/nchs/data/nvsr/nvsr59/ nvsr59_01.pdf.*

The development and use of psychoactive drugs has led to a decline in the number of admissions to long-term mental health care facilities. In addition, the documentation of the deplorable conditions in many mental institutions led to the deinstitutionalization of many patients back into the community to be treated as outpatients or in short-term mental institutions.

Individual Determinants

Individual determinants of utilization include individual characteristics of patients. These individual characteristics can be divided into three major categories: predisposing characteristics, ability to access health care services, and illness severity level (Andersen & Newman, 2005).

Predisposing Factors

Some patients have a propensity to use health care services predicted by their demographic characteristics, social structure, and beliefs (Andersen & Newman, 2005). Some of these traits are **predisposing factors**; that is, they exist prior to use of services and can predict use. Such factors include age, gender, race, education, occupation, marital status, and residence, all of which influence the demand for health care services by the consumer.

Age

Age alone is not necessarily a predictor of demand; however, the very old and the very young use more physician and hospital services and have longer lengths of stay. Older persons have greater rates of hospital admissions and longer lengths of stay primarily because they are sicker. Because they are sicker and may suffer from multiple chronic diseases, older people also use more prescription drugs and are more likely to have multiple prescriptions.

Most nursing home residents are over 85 years of age. The two major factors that determine the need for a nursing home stay are difficulty in activities of daily living (ADLs) and dementia, especially for patients with Alzheimer's disease or organic brain syndrome.

Through the 1980s, the influence of age on frequency of dental visits was the opposite of that for physician visits, with the very young and very old recording fewer visits. However, this trend has stabilized over time because the elderly retain their teeth due to improvements in dental technology and fluoridation of the water supply in most metropolitan centers (Gillcrist, Brumley, & Blackford, 2001). Children younger than 6 years have the fewest visits as they have fewer teeth, but parents may bring their young children to the dentist to acclimate them for the future (Gillcrist et al., 2001).

Gender

Women use more health care services than men, with one exception; men have longer lengths of stay in hospitals. Although it is true that men do not live as long, women use more health services throughout their lifetime. These differences may be explained by women's use of obstetrical services, but even when adjusted for the obstetrical service use, women still have more physician contacts than men. Interestingly, when this same adjustment is made for hospital days, men and women record similar average lengths of stay (LOS).

Women use ambulatory care visits significantly more than men, averaging seven physician visits per year compared to five for men. Women use more dental services and prescriptions, and more women than men are nursing home residents.

Race

Whites use more physician services than blacks and Hispanics (Andersen & Newman, 2005). Blacks are more likely to see a physician in a clinic, hospital outpatient department, or emergency room than non-blacks, partly because blacks disproportionately live in inner-city areas where there are fewer physicians per capita in private practice. Blacks are also less likely to see a specialist.

The evidence of the impact of race on health care utilization is mixed. When education, income, and occupation are controlled, most of the differences between the races disappear. Therefore, differences in utilization can be explained by socioeconomic factors. However, in a number of other studies, even after controlling for education, income, and occupation, differences in utilization by race remain. Some argue that the culture of poverty is still having an effect on the health behavior of even middle-class blacks.

Education

Education is a good predictor of the use of discretionary and preventive care services. Higher education leads to higher utilization. Children of less educated parents have a lower use of preventive care services. Higher educated women are more likely to obtain prenatal care and mammograms than women with less education. Higher educated individuals are more likely to receive preventive dental care.

Occupation

Occupation per se is not a good predictor of utilization of health care unless assessing high-risk occupations such as farming, mining, and construction. Any association between use of health care services and occupation is likely the result of occupation correlated with SES.

Religion

Religious and spiritual dimensions are important for understanding health-related behaviors, attitudes, and beliefs, and are particularly important for those who are ill or consuming health services (Chatters, 2000). Further, several studies indicate that religious belief and participation is associated with better outcomes for persons who are recovering from physical and mental illness (Chatters, 2000). Overall, better physical health status, as measured by a variety of indicators, is associated with patients who consider themselves to be more religious.

Several findings are worth noting regarding the influence of religion on the demand for health care. Among older adults who were hospitalized, it was found that religion does influence their health status. Older hospitalized patients who participate in religious activities and have spiritual experiences are associated with greater social support and better psychological health. These factors contribute to better physical health of the patient (Koenig, George, & Titus, 2004).

Studies have also shown that persons who consider themselves to be highly religious consume more preventive services. Such preventive services include flu shots, cholesterol screening, breast self-exams, mammograms, pap smears, and prostate screening (Benjamins & Brown, 2004). In addition, more religious adolescents were found to engage in lower levels of risky behaviors such as alcohol use and higher levels of healthy behaviors, such as diet and exercise (Chatters, 2000). Religion may play an instrumental role in contributing to the health status of participants due to direct proscription of unhealthy behaviors such as dietary restrictions and smoking and alcohol abuse. It may also play a part in advocating healthy behaviors directly linked to health status such as regular exercise (Chatters, 2000).

The importance of religion for patients is shown in the adoption by several prestigious academic health centers and clinics of a religious component to complement their standard health care treatment (Chatters, 2000). Medical schools and nursing programs also provide future clinicians with an overview of major religions and how religious beliefs influence patient health behaviors. Health education and health promotion also incorporate the influence of religious beliefs in the behaviors and attitudes of patients.

Health Beliefs and Health Education

Attitudes and beliefs about health care, hospitals, physicians, and illness do alter the demand for care. Patients who may have had negative experiences with physicians or nurses may resist seeking care for self-diagnosed minor illnesses. Patients who have had poor experiences in hospital ERs may resist seeking care again without serious cause. Patients may also lack trust in their primary care clinician because of communication or racial/ethnic barriers that illness onset fails to overcome. Conversely, patients who feel that symptoms must be treated immediately either at an ER or physician office may seek care sooner than otherwise (Andersen & Newman, 2005).

Health beliefs and education have significant impact on utilization of preventive care services. A mother's health behavior has an influence on her children's behaviors. A high level of satisfaction with past use of health care services is a good predictor of future use of such services.

Marital Status

People who are divorced or widowed use more health services. Married people have lower morbidity, mortality, and suicide rates; unmarried individuals tend to engage in more risky behaviors than married people do. Married people enjoy better mental and physical health when compared with those who are unmarried, and married men enjoy even greater positive benefits from marriage than do women (Kiecolt-Glaser & Newton, 2001). In addition, those with poor marriages experience negative affects on their health in such forms as depression and health habits, and negative influences on cardiovascular, endocrine, immune, neurosensory, and other physiological symptoms (Kiecolt-Glaser & Newton, 2001).

Health status suffers during bereavement over the death of a spouse or when going through a divorce. Similarly, a dysfunctional marriage is a source of stress for both partners and limits the ability of the spouses to experience the supportive positive benefits from a healthy relationship (Kiecolt-Glaser & Newton, 2001). Dysfunctional marriages are associated with high levels of stress for both parties relative to single unmarried persons. Depression symptoms are associated with persons in dysfunctional marriages with high levels of stress, anger, and conflict. Stress has long-term negative implications for mental health and many bodily systems such as cardiovascular and immune systems (Kiecolt-Glaser & Newton, 2001).

Partners in dysfunctional marriages also exhibit higher levels of hostility that contribute to conflict, arguments, and resentment between partners. These types of behaviors elevate the risk of heart disease and premature death among patients (Kiecolt-Glaser & Newton, 2001). Hostile marital relationships are also associated with depression among married couples, with married husbands exhibiting more severe symptoms when compared with married wives in hostile marriages (Kiecolt-Glaser & Newton, 2001).

Not surprisingly, healthy marriages in which both partners report high levels of satisfaction and happiness are associated with better overall health for both partners. Couples who are satisfied with their marriage engage in more healthy behaviors such as healthy diet, adequate sleep, and adequate exercise (Kiecolt-Glaser & Newton, 2001).

Residence

Patients who reside in **medically underserved areas (MUAs)** or in areas that are economically distressed are at higher risk for poor health. For instance, patients who reside in MUAs are at a higher risk of breast cancer diagnosis at a later stage (Barry & Breen, 2005). This finding is particularly concerning given the high success rate for treatment for breast cancer when detected at an early stage. Those who reside in areas that have poor access to primary care are at increased risk of late detection of breast cancer (Wang et al., 2008). Although inner-city residents may live close to academic health centers and prestigious hospitals, they are more likely to be uninsured and seeking their care from non-physician health providers for their care (Barry & Breen, 2005).

Those who reside in economically distressed communities are also in more danger from the harm of risky and violent behaviors of neighbors, when compared with those who live in areas that are more affluent. For instance, victims of gang violence, drive-by shootings, drug-induced violence, violent assaults, and rape are typically going to reside in less affluent areas. Unfortunately, treatment for injuries from such incidents is typically acute and may be life threatening for the victims.

▪ Enabling Factors

Enabling factors are those conditions that facilitate the fulfillment of demand for health care services. Factors such as wealth, health insurance, location, and supply of providers influence the availability of health care services for patients (Andersen & Newman, 2005). For instance, whenever people are able to be successful in a career that allows them to earn a competitive salary and have health insurance, it influences their demand for health care. Whenever people work for an employer who does not offer health insurance or if they work part-time and are not given the option of health insurance, it affects their health and access to care. Location plays an important role as well in the demand for health care. If an insured consumer resides in an urban area within easy access to prestigious medical centers, they may benefit from the high-quality health care being delivered close to their home.

Wealth

Wealth is a significant determinant of utilization of health care services. The wealth of patients influences the affordability of some very expensive treatment options usually not covered by insurance. Utilization of preventive services is stimulated by patients' desire to anticipate problems occurring in the future. This future orientation is often a function of wealth, with many poor people not inculcating this perspective. Poverty makes getting the next meal and maintaining adequate shelter a priority. National data reveal that poor women are less likely to have an annual mammogram. Children of poor parents are less likely to receive all necessary vaccinations. In addition, poor children use fewer services than wealthy children or children with insurance (NCHS, 2010a).

A **usual source of care (USOC)**, all else constant, results in increased utilization. Yet, poor people are less likely to have a USOC. Also, dental care is less likely to be covered by insurance, so its utilization is highly dependent on level of income because these services often have to be paid for out-of-pocket (Andersen & Newman, 2005). Non-poor use more preventive dental care.

The poor are twice as likely to be admitted to a hospital and also incur longer lengths of stay. Interestingly, a higher percentage of blacks in poverty have a usual source of care than whites in poverty with a usual source of care.

Insurance

The level of health insurance is an enabling factor for patients in their demand of health care services (Andersen & Newman, 2005). During the era before Medicare and Medicaid, the number of physician office visits increased with income. Once Medicare and Medicaid were options for patients, the number of physician visits decreased with income; the poor had a payment mechanism through Medicare and Medicaid programs so their utilization could become more a function of their frequency of illness.

Poor people use more services than non-poor do because they are sicker on average. However, having insurance coverage for illness does not necessarily stimulate healthy behavior. Coverage for illness promotes the seeking of therapeutic services but can be a disincentive to practice healthy behaviors or use preventive services to avoid or postpone illness. All else equal, people with insurance use more services than people without health insurance.

Location

The community in which the patient lives is an enabling factor (Andersen & Newman, 2005). The number of hospitals, clinics, physicians, and walk-in clinics in an area will affect the demand for services in that community. Patients may consume more services if they experience short waiting times for appointments and short waiting periods in a physician's office or in the ER. As travel time increases to hospitals and clinics, there are lower levels of utilization. Yet, patients are more willing to travel for serious health care issues such as cardiac services.

Location is also a function of what region of the country patients live in and whether they are in an urban or rural area. Location influences beliefs and customs about how and when health care services are consumed. Perhaps certain regions of the country have higher consumer expectations that are reflected in their demand for services (Andersen & Newman, 2005).

There is variation in the methods of health care used by clinicians, also known as practice variation, attributed to differences in training and community norms. However, the primary driving force in this variation is uncertainty. Lack of universal standards for practice enables habits and financial incentives to influence the utilization and supply of services.

Physician Supply and Price

Increased physician supply results in increased utilization of health care services. This correlation is an example of Roemer's law in its simplest form, which states that when there are more hospital beds in a community there will be more days spent in those hospital beds (Roemer, 1959). Roemer's law is an example of induced demand, where physicians are able to increase demand for services that would not otherwise be consumed by patients.

Physicians have the ability to generate their own demand to a limited but significant extent. Price elasticity of health care is generally inelastic; however, preventive or elective services are elastic.

$$\text{Elasticity} = \frac{\text{Percentage change in demand}}{\text{Percentage change in price}}$$

Elasticity that is greater than one is elastic demand; elasticity that is less than one is inelastic demand. As price increases, purchasing behavior changes, usually shrinking demand. High **elasticity of demand** means that demand is more responsive to changes in price. Examples of goods and services that have a high elasticity of demand include gasoline; preventive, elective, and dental services; and plastic surgery. Low elasticity of demand means that changes in price do not have a comparable change in demand. Examples of goods and services that are inelastic include cancer treatment, antibiotics for a severe infection, and cardiac thoracic surgery.

▪ Need for Care and Illness Level

The most immediate and most significant factor that predicts demand for health care services is illness severity (Andersen & Newman, 2005). Illness severity can be measured by self-report when patients characterize their health as excellent, good, fair, or poor (Andersen & Newman, 2005). Respondents who rate their perceived health as fair to poor are more likely to utilize physician services than those who rate their health as good or excellent.

Illness severity, either perceived or once diagnosed, is the most important factor in determining utilization of hospital, physician, and dental services (Andersen & Newman, 2005). People who are sicker or have greater disability use more health care services.

Vignette

RECOVERING ALCOHOLIC SEEKS LIVER TRANSPLANT

Bill W., a 35-year-old New Yorker, is recovering from alcoholism by attending Alcoholics Anonymous (AA) meetings and complying with weekly appointments to his Certified Addictions Specialist. He has been sober for five years, but his heavy drinking since his teen years, when his mother and father divorced, has taken its toll on his liver and kidneys, damaging his liver beyond repair. Now that he has been sober for a period of time, he has sought placement on an organ transplant list, along with children who were born with defective organs or people who have illness that prevents normal healthy function of their livers. Some state laws espouse that alcoholism is a disease and that it is inappropriate to differentiate illness caused specifically by an individual's lifestyle choices from genetic abnormalities.

Bill W. has followed the principles of AA by working hard to be a good citizen, a thoughtful parent to his children, and a dedicated husband to his wife. He is a loyal employee and volunteers for charity work in his local community. Bill feels that he deserves a second chance at life and that one mistake should not exclude him from this opportunity. His doctor has informed him that his liver is damaged by cirrhosis, and he has lost 50 percent of his liver function. He has begun to experience fluid retention in his abdominal cavity and persistent pain in his lower left quadrant. He is constantly bruising himself and suffers bleeding as a result. His quality of life has suffered substantially due to the damaged liver and cirrhosis. Bill feels himself slipping into deep bouts of depression due to his loss of quality of life even though he is only 35.

Unbeknownst to Bill, his position on the transplant list was just ahead of a man who also had cirrhosis, but this other man's malfunction was caused by an autoimmune disease, called primary biliary disease, that attacks the bile ducts in the liver and destroys it over time. There is no known cure for primary biliary disease, but in advanced cases a liver transplant provides a chance of improved quality of life.

The transplant center in New York requires that any alcoholic seeking a transplant must be sober for at least six months. Bill W. must prove that he has attended rehabilitation or some type of program where he addresses his alcoholism, specifically why he drank and how to cope with life without drinking. He must also pass an evaluation that includes many medical tests and a psychiatric assessment in which he talks about his alcoholism.

He must be emotionally and physically stable, and understand that he will be taking anti-rejection drugs for the rest of his life. Transplants are lifelong commitments to staying healthy and taking care of oneself. He will also be required to have random drug and alcohol testing done at any time prior to getting a transplant, including during the six months of sobriety that is required. Then a group of doctors will go over all the testing and the psychiatric report, to determine whether Bill will be a good candidate to receive a transplant. They will discuss his alcoholism and what he has done or intends to do to remain sober and get well. They will make the final decision as to whether the transplant will be an option for Bill.

Bill is willing to meet all these requirements and feels he deserves a second chance at life, as he is only 35 and has the rest of his life before him. He feels that he has reformed and wants to be a productive member of society. He knows of a few alcoholics who have had transplants, and they are doing fine today. It is a life-changing experience, and it is his understanding that the number of alcoholics who go back to drinking again after a transplant is extremely low. Bill just wants to live a productive long life.

After waiting two years, Bill was called by the transplant center to receive a liver transplant. He has been increasingly ill, and it has affected his work attendance and responsibilities at home. However, he has remained sober. Bill has been called before the patient with the auto-immune disease, who continues to suffer from his condition while his liver continues to develop more scarring and cirrhosis.

1. Do you believe that Bill should receive the liver transplant before another patient whose liver damage was no fault of his own?

2. Do you believe that Bill has just as much right to an organ transplant, now that he has been sober for seven years, as other patients on the waiting list who may have abused their bodies in other ways such as overeating, smoking, using smokeless tobacco, or by addiction to pain killers?

3. What penalty should Bill experience if he receives an organ transplant but then returns to alcoholism?

4. What would your reaction be if the patient with primary biliary disease who did not receive a transplant were your loved one?

Overall Effect of Individual Determinants

The net effect of the individual components that influence utilization reverberates throughout the health care delivery system. For instance, the ER is an indicator of the health care delivery system's strength and efficiency. Failure in an aspect of the health care system is reflected in ER utilization. For many patients, the ER is the safety net of last resort and is used as the usual source of care for many of the uninsured. Unfortunately, when patients who use the ER as their usual source of care seek care, their condition has become more complicated and more expensive to treat.

The failures of the health care system contribute to overcrowded and strained ERs. Lack of access to other facilities, limited financial access by the poor, and lack of available providers in the area all contribute to overcrowded and inappropriately utilized ERs. Hospital financial shortfalls that have resulted in nursing staff reductions have produced premature discharges that often result in additional ER visits and readmissions. The nation's financial crisis has brought hospital closures that have reduced the supply of ERs and hospital beds. The economic recession has increased unemployment among working-age patients and has led to decreases in health insurance coverage. These factors contribute to a greater numbers of sicker patients using ERs as their primary source of care.

General Trends in Utilization

Physician Visits

Physician visits are provided through private office, hospital clinic and ER, phone, and HMO and private clinics. No longer do physicians make house calls, but phone consultations are on the increase. The physicians' offices are the most common sites for physician visits. About 75 percent of Americans see a physician at least once a year (NCHS 2010b).

Inpatient Surgical Procedures

Inpatient surgical procedures have declined while outpatient surgical procedures have increased. It would seem that as technology has moved many inpatient procedures to the outpatient setting, the severity of hospital admissions would increase and produce greater lengths of stay. However, technology also has made its impact on inpatient care, with average length of stay declining, but it now has stabilized over the past few years. The decline in average length of stay was not only attributable to advances in technology but also to changes in norms, concern over costs, and reimbursement for in-hospital stay. The average length of stay seems to have stabilized at about six days overall and is likely not going to change unless there are major technological advances in practice.

Summary

Utilization of health care services is studied to assure that patients' needs are met. System and personal characteristics serve to facilitate or inhibit utilization. Shortages of providers reduce utilization by generating unmet demand for services. Patients living in remote regions of the country are unable to manifest their need into demand.

Some personal characteristics such as wealth, which can act as a barrier to access, are negated with health insurance, which increases buying power. However, it is unclear whether distancing patients from the price of health care services results in the best outcomes. Although insurance enables sick patients to obtain necessary care that they would otherwise be unable to afford, coverage can stimulate patients to continue risky health behaviors and postpone obtaining valuable preventive care.

Technology has brought reduced costs and better outcomes to patients who obtain health care services. In some cases, expensive hospital procedures are now performed on an outpatient basis. Health care advances have shortened hospital lengths of stay, reduced complications from surgery, and produced better outcomes. However, some technology has been used without full vetting in controlled clinical trials, and hospitals have reduced lengths of stay to cut costs, in some cases jeopardizing outcomes.

Some say that health care is as much art as it is science. This metaphor translates into large variations in the practice for certain illnesses and diseases. Such variation, along with the ambiguity inherent in many outcomes, enables clinicians to generate unnecessary demand for their services, a practice first coined Roemer's law. Recent passage of health care reform legislation, which intends to insure in some capacity nearly 32 million Americans who are currently uninsured, will serve as a modern test of the impact of increased buying power on utilization. The personal characteristics of these newly insured, coupled with apparent shortages of clinicians, will present an interesting formula for assessing the utilization of health services in the future.

▪ Review Questions

1. What is the difference between enabling and predisposing factors that influence utilization of health care services?

2. What are the key differences between the Rosenstock and the Andersen models of health services utilization?

3. What are some practical examples in the lives of the people you know of how the factors in the Rosenstock and Andersen models influence the demand for health care and health status?

4. What is the most important factor from Andersen's model in your life and your demand for health services?

5. Does your health insurance status affect your daily activities, and why?

6. How does the health insurance status of the people in your life influence their daily activities and participation in risky activities, such as participation in contact sports or unhealthy behaviors such as smoking and alcohol abuse?

7. What are examples of Roemer's law mentioned throughout the chapter? Are there similar phenomena that you have observed in the health care system?

8. What is one of the limitations of the Rosenstock model?

9. What is the primary factor that influences your demand for health care services, and how does it fit in the Andersen model?

10. Why does advancement in medical technology lead to increased utilization of services?

▪ Additional Resources

Health, United States, 2010: http://www.cdc.gov/nchs/hus.htm\

Healthy People.gov: http://www.healthypeople.gov/2020/default.aspx

National Center for Health Statistics (NCHS): http://www.cdc.gov/nchs/

▪ References

American Hospital Association (AHA). (2008). Physician ownership and self-referral in hospitals: Research on negative effect grows. Retrieved November 1, 2011 from http://www.aha.org/research/policy/2008.shtml.

American Hospital Association (AHA). (2010). AHA frets over doctor-owned hospital growth. *Health Care Business News*. Retreived on April 3, 2012 from http://www.modernphysician.com/article/20080421/MODERNPHYSICIAN/812011774

Andersen, R. (1968). Behavioral model of families' use of health services. Research Series No. 25, Chicago IL; Center for Health Administration Studies, University of Chicago.

Andersen, R., & Newman, J. (2005). Societal and individual determinants of medical care utilization in the United States. *Milbank Quarterly, 83*(4), 1–28.

Barry, J., & Breen, N. (2005). The importance of place of residence in predicting late-stage diagnosis of breast or cervical cancer. *Health & Place, 11*(1), 15–29.

Benjamins, M., & Brown, C. (2004). Religion and preventative health care utilization among the elderly. *Social Science & Medicine, 58* (1), 109–118.

Bunker, J. (1970). Surgical manpower—A comparison of operations and surgeons in the United States and in England and Wales. *New England Journal of Medicine, 282* (January 15, 1970), 135–144.

Centers for Disease Control and Prevention (CDC). (2009, June 11). *Americans make nearly four medical visits a year on average.* NCHS Press Room. Retrieved December 10, 2010, from http://www.cdc.gov/nchs/pressroom/08newsreleases/visitstodoctor.htm.

Centers for Disease Control and Prevention (CDC). (2010, October 25). *Ambulatory care use and physician visits.* Fast Stats. Retrieved December 10, 2010, from http://www.cdc.gov/nchs/fastats/docvisit.htm.

Chatters, L. (2000). Religion and health: Public health research and practice. *Annual Review of Public Health, 21*, 335–367.

Gillcrist, J., Brumley, D., & Blackford, J. (2001). Community fluoridation status and caries experience in children. *Journal of Public Health Dentistry, 61*(3), 168–171.

Government Accounting Office (GAO). (2006). *General hospitals: Operational and clinical changes largely unaffected by presence of competing specialty hospitals.* Washington, DC: Author.

Goodman, D. (2011, April 18). Dartmouth Atlas Project. A Progress Report. Princeton, NJ: Robert Wood Johnson Foundation.

Kaiser Family Foundation (KFF). (2010). *Summary of the new health reform law.* Menlo Park: Author.

Kiecolt-Glaser, J., & Newton, T. (2001). Marriage and health: His and hers. *Psychological Bulletin, 127*(4), 472–503.

Koenig, H., George, L., & Titus, P. (2004). Religion, spirituality, and health in medically ill hospitalized older patients. *Journal of the American Geriatrics Society, 52*(4), 554–562.

National Center for Health Statistics (NCHS). (2010a). National Health Interview Survey. Washington, DC.

National Center for Health Statistics (NCHS). (2010b). National Ambulatory Medical Care Survey. Washington, DC.

Roemer (1959 April). Hospital costs relate to the supply of beds. *Modern Hospital.* 92(4), 71–73.

Roe vs. Wade. (1973). 410 US 113; United States Supreme Court ruling. Washington, DC.

Wang, F., McLafferty, S., Escamilla, V., & Luo, L. (2008). Late-stage breast cancer diagnosis and health care access in Illinois. *Professional Geographer, 60*(1), 54–69.

Weaver, C. (2010, October 28). *Physician-owned hospitals racing to meet health law deadline.* Kaiser Health News. Retrieved August 21, 2011, from www .kaiserhealthnews.org/Stories/2010/October/28/physician-owned-hospitals.aspx.

Weiss, M., Ryan, P., Lokken, L., & Nelson, M. (2004). Length of stay after vaginal birth: Sociodemographic and readiness-for-discharge factors. *Birth, 31*(2), 93–101.

Wennberg, J. (2010). The Dartmouth Atlas of Health Care. Hanover NH.

Wennberg, J., & Gittelsohn, A. (1973). Small area variations in health care delivery. *Science, 142*, 1102–1108.

Quality 14

Learning Objectives

- Understand the differences between quality assessment and quality assurance.

- Explain the relationships among structure, process, and outcome.

- Describe historical efforts to improve health care quality.

- Understand the impact of medical errors and hospital-acquired infections, and the strategies to combat such dangers in the health care industry.

- Understand recent federal legislation and funding for health care quality.

- Describe the differences between quality evaluation and quality assurance.

- Discuss the major milestones in the development of quality standards.

■ What Is Quality?

Quality of health care measures the outcomes of health care services. However, there is an information and knowledge imbalance between consumer and provider. In other industries, more information is available to the consumer through the use of advertising, objective assessments of products and/or clear results obtained from the purchasing of services, and from comparison-shopping. Health care clinicians provide limited information through advertising, and comparison-shopping between clinicians is inherently difficult. However, the amount of information about the quality of providers is increasing through access to Internet sites such as Healthgrades.com or Leapfrog.org and others. Consumers are also obtaining some comparison information from consumer magazines and advertising.

Many patients assume that the health care they receive is high quality. Patients rely on word-of-mouth referral and referrals by health professionals to guide them through the system. Consumers in other industries are able to return products if they are dissatisfied—not an option for a patient who has just had an appendectomy. Moreover, surgery does not usually come with a warranty. Health care is not an exact science, and often even the best providers, facility, and procedures do not produce a perfect outcome.

The Institute of Medicine of the National Academy of Sciences formed the Committee on Quality of Health Care to address these issues, specifically the issues of overuse, underuse, and misuse of health care that lead to variations in the outcomes (Berwick, 2002). Misuse is the term used to describe failures to execute clinical quality of care plans and procedures properly (Berwick, 2002). **Overuse** describes the use of health care resources and procedures in the absence of healing evidence (Berwick, 2002). **Underuse** describes failures to use evidence-based health care practices that have proven to be beneficial to patients (Berwick, 2002). Such evidence-based practices include the use of beta-blockers in persons with acute myocardial infarction over the age of 65 (Berwick, 2002).

The definition of quality can vary by industry. In the manufacturing and service industries, quality is evaluated in terms of a degree of excellence, or how it "measures up" to the gold standard of value, or conformance to specifications or meeting and exceeding customers' expectations. In health care, we compare the degree of excellence or conformity to established standards and criteria.

Consumer expectations, however, will often differ substantially from professional observers' perspectives. In health care, several questions regarding quality may be asked, such as: What level of quality of care do we, as a nation, wish to ensure for all of our citizens? Is it feasible for all Americans to receive the best quality, or are we seeking to ensure that everyone receives at least a minimum standard of care? What about quality of life and patient well-being? How can we measure, evaluate, or improve quality in health care without a common definition?

■ Reasons for Quality of Care Problems

The health care system is dynamic, extremely complex, and with many stakeholders. The underlying reasons for the problems in quality of care in the United States are as many and unique as the patients that receive care. However, the Institute of Medicine (IOM, 2001a) has identified four key areas that contribute to the overall problems in the levels of quality. First, health care technology is very complex and highly sophisticated, and the pace of change and advancement is faster than clinicians' abilities to deliver care in a safe, effective, and efficient manner (IOM, 2001a). Clinicians are unable to keep up with the pace of change in medical knowledge, biomedical research, and medical devices to deliver care that is evidence based (IOM, 2001a).

Second, physicians must read numerous journal articles on the latest clinical trials and procedures. Clinicians are unable to keep pace with the progress in scientific literature and still provide patients with quality care that is patient centered (IOM, 2001a). The number of drugs, medical devices, and other technology to support care has increased dramatically as health care technology has advanced (IOM, 2001a).

Third, our population is aging, the number of chronic conditions has increased, and cases have become more complicated by the presence of multiple chronic conditions (IOM, 2001a). Care for patients with multiple chronic conditions requires collaboration and coordination among the patient, provider, and the patient's family. Care planning should involve monitoring and management of the condition, with frequent follow-up with the patient and the family. All of these efforts require significant health care resources and increase the complexity of care provided to a large segment of the patient population (IOM, 2001a).

Fourth, care delivery in the United States is highly fragmented and decentralized, causing confusion for patients and breakdowns in communication between patient and provider (IOM, 2001a). There is a lack of integration and coordination between the components of care. For instance, patients with comorbidities may require care from several providers throughout their treatment plan (e.g., primary care provider, hospital, skilled nursing facility, and hospice), and a generalist clinician to oversee and coordinate these treatments. Moreover, throughout the course of treatment there is a lack of standardized evidence-based information regarding what care plans are the most effective and efficient for patients (IOM, 2001a).

The health care system has been slow to adopt the advances in information technology (IOM, 2001a). The Internet has expanded the wealth of information that patients and providers have at their disposal. Patients can obtain enormous amounts of data about their condition via the Internet, and providers can update their knowledge regarding best practices. Information technology has significant potential for improving the delivery and quality of care. However, the health care industry has been slower than other industries to invest in information technology (IOM, 2001a). Significant financial resources are required to use IT appropriately and improve the quality of care patients receive.

Recent Health Care Reform Legislation to Promote Health Care Quality

The Patient Protection and Affordable Care Act was signed into law on March 23, 2010 (KFF, 2010). Legislation effective in 2012 will penalize hospitals with unnecessary readmissions within 30 days of discharge after stays for heart attack, pneumonia, and congestive heart failure (Carrns, 2010). More conditions are expected to be added to the list, and hospitals will face increasing penalties after the first year of enforcement. The legislation creates incentives for hospitals to decrease unnecessary readmission. It may also have the unintended consequence of creating incentives to not readmit patients or to discharge them again prematurely due to the lower reimbursement for their care (Carrns, 2010).

Quality of health care will also be affected by the 32 million additional patients who will be provided health insurance over the next several years (Abelson, 2010). However, many more patients will be enrolled in Medicaid plans that reimburse at levels that do not cover the cost of care (Abelson, 2010). The American Hospital

Association pledged to contribute $155 billion over 10 years to Medicare savings through reductions in the rate of costly hospital-acquired infections, making investments in health information technology, and improving the coordination of care of the chronically ill (Jaffe, 2009). All of these factors will have an impact on the quality of health care.

In 2009, the American Recovery and Reinvestment Act provided $19.2 billion over several years for health information technology (Halamka, 2009). Specifically, the legislation provides incentives for physicians and hospitals to adopt electronic health records (EHRs) (Brailer, 2009). EHRs may enable improvements in patient care, increase patient safety, and simplify compliance for hospitals. They also may enable hospitals to save money, as they would minimize errors and increase productivity and administrative efficiency (Hillestad et al., 2005).

▪ Quality of Health Care as a Priority

In 2001, the Institute of Medicine (IOM) reported that between 44,000 and 98,000 Americans die each year due to medical errors (IOM, 2001b). The current system is "incapable of providing the public with the quality health care it expects and deserves" (IOM, 2001a). This conclusion was a major shift from merely stating that there are thousands of patients who are injured through medical errors in the hospitals and nursing homes (IOM, 2001a). The report further stated that thousands are injured every year due to medical errors and that the current care system is not designed to solve the problem (IOM, 2001b).

Patients are at high risk of injury from systemic characteristics such as reliance on human recollection, poor communication systems, unrealistic expectations for human vigilance, disregard of the dangers of human fatigue, reliance on clinician handwriting in a computer age, and other factors (IOM, 2001a). Reliance on traditionally unreliable systems and processes must end, and new care processes must be formed for the safety of patients (IOM, 2001a).

Patients were more at risk of harm from medical errors in unsafe conditions and with obsolete information technology (IT) systems (IOM, 2001b). Improvement initiatives that are "bold, explicit, uniformly espoused, comprehensive, and patient centered" are necessary to combat the problem of poor quality (Berwick, 2002, p. 82).

Government and industry's expenditures for health care have increased, and there is growing concern over rising costs. What trade-off are we willing to accept between costs and quality? With the rapid advances in medical science, the potential for abuse of new diagnostic and therapeutic modalities increases, and the need for quality controls becomes an imperative.

Health care providers and pharmaceutical companies use quality data to market their products. Yet, 87 percent of hospitals that were surveyed by the Leapfrog Group have not implemented all of the preventive measures for many of the most common hospital-acquired infections (The Leapfrog Group, 2007a). **The Leapfrog Group**, which represents major corporations and purchasers of health insurance, reports that there is an alarmingly low level of full compliance with any of its recommended standards for preventing certain avoidable hospital-acquired infections (The Leapfrog

Group, 2007a). Every hospital should be following protocols and implementing standards to prevent infections, but many are missing the mark. This shortfall presents a serious problem for many of the stakeholders in the health care system, including patients (The Leapfrog Group, 2007a).

■ Hospital-Acquired Infections

One example of poor health care quality is the incidence of hospital-acquired infections (HAI). The incidence rate of HAI is at crisis level in United States hospitals, as they have risen steadily over the last couple of decades (Peng, Kurtz, & Johannes, 2006). Every year, 2 million people contract a hospital-acquired infection, and 90,000 of those who acquire such an infection die. HAIs are very costly for a hospital too. According to the Centers for Disease Control and Prevention's National Nosocomial Infection Surveillance System (NNIS), rates of HAI increased 36 percent between 1975 and 1995 (Peng et al., 2006).

In 2004, there were approximately 12,000 hospital-acquired infections in general acute care hospitals in Pennsylvania, for example (PHC4, 2005). These infections were associated with 1,793 unnecessary patient deaths, 205,000 additional estimated hospital days, and an additional $2 billion in charges (PHC4, 2005). HAIs are a serious problem because they cause unnecessary complications for patients that may result in death, higher costs of care, and economic losses for hospitals. They add over $15,000 to a patient's cost of care and across all patients contribute to $30 billion a year wasted in unnecessary care (Peng et al., 2006).

In 2001, the Institute of Medicine reported that unsafe conditions existed in the delivery of care; however, progress in the elimination of harm has been slow (IOM, 2001b). HAIs are linked to the quality of care that patients receive and their hospital environment, not the preexisting severity of the patient's condition upon admission. Patients with HAI experience increases in mortality, length of stay, and hospital charges (Peng et al., 2006). Patients with HAI have more than four times higher median hospital charges than matched patients who did not suffer from hospital-acquired infections (Peng et al., 2006).

The losses from operations associated with a central line-associated blood-stream infection have been estimated to be $28,885 per patient, totaling a loss of $1,449,306 from operations in the 54 cases studied (Shannon et al., 2006). Surgical-wound infections are one of the most common types of HAI (Hollenbeak et al., 2006). There is a statistically significant association between hospital practices and environments during and after surgery and the risk of acquiring this HAI (Hollenbeak et al., 2006).

HAIs are a critical issue for all hospitals and the communities in which they operate. Hospitals require substantial financial resources to deliver high-quality care and maintain facilities and equipment that reduce the incidence of HAI. However, many community hospitals are struggling financially. Financial strength directly affects a hospital's ability to invest in quality initiatives such as training for their staff, information technology, and facility upgrades to reduce HAI. Nationwide, hospitals face increasing financial pressure from low reimbursement levels from Medicare and Medicaid, price discounts given to managed care plans, and the impact of 47 million uninsured (Encinosa & Bernard, 2005).

Erosion of hospital profitability is associated with the quality of care received by patients. Decreases in profitability margins are associated with increases in rates of adverse patient safety events for both nursing and surgical events (Encinosa & Bernard, 2005). A study of the health outcomes of patients with acute myocardial infarction found that financial pressure on hospitals has an adverse effect on hospital quality (Shen, 2003). Hospitals that are unable to invest sufficient resources in patient care may be placing their patients at higher risk of medical injury and harm (Burstin et al., 1993). Hospital financial performance may therefore impact the rate of HAI acquired by patients in poorly performing hospitals.

The relationship between hospital financial performance and HAI is critical. Decision-makers have proposed reimbursement cuts in Medicare and Medicaid that contribute to the erosion in the financial health of many hospitals (Encinosa & Bernard, 2005; PHC4, 2007). The elimination of preventable HAI is an opportunity to improve clinical outcomes and a significant financial opportunity for hospitals (Shannon et al., 2006). Financial healthy hospitals have the necessary resources to invest in quality initiatives aimed at reducing the factors that contribute to HAI rates. Lives are saved, costs of care decrease, and resources are conserved when fewer patients suffer from HAI.

▪ Health Care Quality Assessment

Quality assessment is the process by which quality of health care is measured at some point in time. Quality assessment does not provide conclusions about quality on a continuous basis. Historically, quality assessment has been used as a means to decrease utilization to save money, and was not necessarily concerned about whether high-quality care was delivered. There are several steps to quality assessment, such as defining how quality is determined or measured. Once the quality standards are identified, measurement variables are defined, data are collected and refined, and then researchers analyze and interpret the results.

There are many reasons why quality assessment is difficult. The health care industry provides clinical treatments where a small variation in quality of care can result in serious long-term harmful effects. Health care involves both empirical assessments as well as personal judgments, and it is sometimes difficult to assess appropriateness of personal judgment. No two patients or their clinical conditions are alike.

Many quality standards reflect current knowledge and region of practice. Quality standards change as knowledge advances and provider responsibilities are redefined. Many clinicians resist self-evaluation to monitor quality, and many physicians do not seek to evaluate clinical outcomes, especially those of non-physicians. A small percentage of physicians are incompetent clinicians and practice "bad" medicine. The challenge in the health care field is to limit the medical errors that virtually all "good" doctors commit at one time or another.

The traditional focus of quality assessment has been on provider performance, the degree of excellence or conformity to established criteria and standards. However, more recently the focus has shifted to include access to care (prenatal screenings and tests), patient compliance, and patient satisfaction.

Vignette

HOW DO WE DETERMINE CARE IS OF HIGH QUALITY?

Amy Smith, a CRNP (certified registered nurse practitioner) works in a busy multi-specialty practice that is affiliated with a large teaching hospital. She used to work in a small rural clinic for many years. Her new practice has clinics around the state and offers an HMO for its Medicare population. She is due for her second-year performance review. Her supervisor tells her that she needs to see more patients per hour, thus spend less time with each patient. He says that she is not productive enough in generating RVU (relative value units, which are the current standard for provider productivity). Amy prefers to listen to her patients and takes thorough histories, which take time. Her thorough histories reveal significant information about her patients and help her eliminate the need for unnecessary and expensive lab tests and imaging studies, as well as unnecessary medications. Her patients also note that she is kind and caring, as reflected in her provider satisfaction scores obtained from her patients on standard follow-up mail surveys (e.g., Press Gainey Survey of patient satisfaction), which are among the highest in the organization.

Her collaborating physician, who is her supervisor, sees almost twice as many patients per day and much more frequently for "return" visits than she does. She recognizes that many of her elderly patients are poor and cannot afford the gas or the copay (which is $20 for some). She uses the organization's electronic medical record system to send herself reminders to call them every three months, although she may only see them in her office once or twice a year.

Recently, Amy was told that she would lose her job unless she started to see more patients. Despite her high patient satisfaction scores, she is not generating enough RVUs to meet the standard.

Amy argues that her care is cost-effective and is not measured by simply counting RVUs. She asserts that the organization needs to measure other indicators like fewer blood tests and MRIs ordered, and fewer meds prescribed, yet her patients are healthy on all indicators. She argues her efficiency and her patient's better health status are not captured through RVU measurements. She asks whether the organization is profiting from the absence of costly unnecessary tests. She contends that the time she spends listening to her patients' health stories significantly reduces health care expenditures and that she is hence a very cost-efficient and high-quality provider.

Imagine that you work for the human resources department and have been asked to resolve this conflict. Amy wants her patient visits to be for 20 minutes, not 10, and wants 45 minutes, not 30, for new patients as well.

1. How would you address the issue of measuring quality when there are several definitions. Is there any credibility to Amy's arguments?

2. What are some of the factors you would address to determine whether Amy is providing quality care? How would you measure the kind of quality she produces?

3. What difference does it make that she is working for an HMO as opposed to a group practice that does not insure its patients?

4. What types of epidemiological data could you use to defend or refute Amy's arguments?

5. Is there any harm associated with unnecessary testing? Can tests lead to more tests and higher costs? Find an example of this.

6. Is there any harm or risk in prescribing unnecessary meds? Can this practice increase health care costs?

7. How does provider-induced demand affect quality and cost?

8. What do data from geographic practice variation research (e.g., the number of providers per person and its impact on demand for services) say about provider-induced demand and health?

Care Evaluation

The focus of quality studies has been on three main areas of care: technical care, the interpersonal aspects of care, and the amenities of care. Assessing technical care focuses on the appropriateness of procedures and the skills of the providers. Assessing interpersonal aspects of care centers on human-level interactions such as the physician–patient relationship and bedside manner. Amenities of care are studied by assessing the place of care and its convenience, decor, quality of its food, and transportation.

Characterization of Quality Assessment Studies

Quality assessment falls into three main categories: retrospective, concurrent, and prospective. Retrospective assessment entails making a decision about quality of care that has already been delivered. This assessment would include reviewing a medical chart to determine the appropriateness of the care delivered. Concurrent assessment analyzes quality of care as it is being provided. Prospective assessment measures quality beforehand; data are collected based on predetermined measures or objectives.

Health Care Quality Assurance

Quality assurance is both an assessment and an improvement effort. It is the process of conducting on-going measurement activities in conjunction with the installation of feedback mechanisms designed for continuous quality improvement. Quality assurance activities were initially implemented mostly out of concern with malpractice, managed care and underutilization. Quality assurance has taken on many different names such as quality improvement (QI), continuous quality improvement (CQI), total quality improvement (TQI), total quality management (TQM), reengineering, Six Sigma, and lean transformation.

■ History of Health Care Quality

The early history of quality assurance included an accounting of outcomes and other measures of the quality of care suggested by noted health care icons such as Florence Nightingale (1820–1910), Dr. Emory W. Groves (1908), Dr. Arthor T. Cabot (1852–1912), and Dr. Ernest A. Codman (1869–1940). However, their suggestions were largely ignored. Florence Nightingale proposed a registry of surgical operations and respective outcomes. Dr. Groves also suggested that a registry of surgical procedures be kept along with their outcomes. Drs. Cabot and Codman proposed that autopsies be performed to determine whether patients succumbed to the diseases they were diagnosed as having.

Quality has played a strong role throughout the history of medical education. In 1872, the Committee on Medical Education was formed to make annual reports to AMA's Council on Medical Education. The Committee's initial report discussed the need for standardization of medical education. In 1910, the **Flexner Report**, delivered to the AMA, severely criticized the nation's medical education institutions, and as a result many proprietary institutions closed and the medical education system was reconstituted based on the Johns Hopkins model of university-based medical education. In 1942, the AMA established the Liaison Committee on Medical Education, which became the official accrediting body for medical schools.

Throughout the 1950s and 1960s several academics, including **Avedis Donabedian** (1919–2000), wrote about quality from a theoretical perspective and proposed various ways to measure it. A few other academicians formulated empirical measures that they used in small-scale studies. There was no significant large-scale quality assessment effort until the Medicare and Medicaid programs were implemented, and expenditures were already rising rapidly. Government programs, under the label of quality assessment, emphasized policing to curb overutilization and costs.

Throughout the 1980s, the quality arena switched to an examination of prospective payment such as capitation and DRG reimbursement, and with these studies came an incentive to withhold services. In addition to over-service, government programs were checking underutilization and its impact on the quality of care and outcomes.

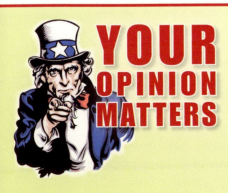

YOUR OPINION MATTERS

Who Should Determine Health Care Quality—The Profession or a Government Oversight Body?

Background

The recent health care reform debate has brought to the surface many of the concerns of both professionals and patients about the decisions of a government body regarding the quantity and quality of care that is appropriate. Some argue that because patients cannot discern care quality and health professionals have incentives to over-treat, an impartial administrative body should be assigned with the task. Others argue that these decisions are very

(Continued)

personal, that patients can discern what they want after discussions with their health providers, and that the decisions about quality and quantity of services should be part of the provider–patient relationship. Both sides of the issue have used scare tactics to convince the voting public.

Yes

Proponents of government intervention argue that patients, unlike other consumers, are not fully knowledgeable about the health care they receive and therefore are not capable of debating health care decisions with their providers. In addition, reimbursement for care remains in the hands of a third party, leaving the patient with little incentive to avoid or postpone care. Fee-for-service reimbursement incentives, moreover, are designed for providers to "un-bundle" their care and deliver more rather than less, which makes these decisions more a function of the provider's target income than necessity.

Government bodies can help contain costs and therefore increase access for many by making critical societal decisions about standards of quality care. Significant practice variations across the nation (Goodman et al., 2011) call for a federal body to take charge to standardize quality. Otherwise, only the rich will have access to critical health care delivery, leaving those in poverty rationed out of the system. That is, rationing is already part of United States health care, based on income of patients rather than their health care needs.

A good example of effective government intervention is the recent Institute of Medicine recommendations to the Department of Health and Human Services for preventive care for women. As a result, DHHS now requires insurance companies to pay for a list of preventive services (IOM, 2011). Implicit in the IOM recommendations is that as a nation we can provide free colonoscopies to women, or we can pay for colon cancer. We can provide free mammograms, or we can pay for advanced breast cancer. We can provide birth control, or we can pay for an unwanted child. We can provide STD and HIV counseling, or we can watch those diseases spread. We can provide domestic abuse counseling or condemn a woman and her children to remain in a violent household.

No

Although improvements are needed in United States health care, many feel strongly that government should remain at "arm's length." The United States system should not emulate either the British or the Canadian systems where government controls more of the delivery and reimbursement of health care. Health care decisions are specific to the individual patient and provider. Also, providers take an oath to do no harm and given the power of word of mouth, providers really have little incentive to deliver unnecessary and potentially harmful care. Government bodies are impersonal and are bound to make rationing decisions.

The British National Health Service (NHS) bases its funding decisions on the recommendations of the quasi-governmental National Institute for Clinical Evaluation and Excellence (NICE), a panel that determines which patients merit preference over others regarding the treatments for which they are eligible, medications they may be given, and how soon they may have access to a doctor. Because of cost considerations, NICE gives preference to young people over older people, and to healthy people over those with chronic disease or with destructive habits such as smoking or alcoholism. The equation is simple: to increase access for all and contain costs, the quality of the health care product must be compromised in some way.

According to the BBC, British patients face an average wait time of 8 months for cataract surgery, 11 months for a hip replacement, 12 months for a knee replacement, 5 months for slipped-disc surgery, and 5 months for a hernia repair (BBC, 2010).

This side argues that Americans enjoy care on demand, and such an asset must not be compromised in any way. In many cases in the British NHS, the condition of patients with diseases that were curable at the time of diagnosis degrades to the point of incurability by the time treatment finally becomes available; other patients become too weak to undergo whatever surgical procedures had originally been recommended for them. Further, most British hospitals are, by American standards, of poor quality. For example, up to 40 percent of NHS patients are undernourished during their hospital stays (BBC, 2010).

You decide:

1. Can provider and patient make quality decisions together, or must a third party intercede?

2. Can government be relied on to tread lightly in quality decisions, or will it take the responsibility completely away from patient and provider?

3. What concessions are Americans willing to make to improve what is ailing about its health care system?

4. Are we sure that the preventive services mandated for coverage by the IOM report are going to result in cost and quality-of-life savings that they are espoused to produce?

■ Approaches to Quality Assessment

In 1966, Avedis Donabedian, known as the father of quality in health care, developed an algorithm for measuring health care quality that contained three components of the delivery of care: structure, process, and outcome. Recently quality assurance in health care has focused on the relationships among structure-process-outcome (SPO). This three-part approach assumes that good structure increases the likelihood of good process, and good process increases the likelihood of a good outcome. The quality assessment is not itself designed to establish the presence of these relationships, but rather to examine their impact. The SPO framework takes into account that quality of care is multidimensional, or comprised of many elements.

■ Structure

Structure focuses on the context of the environment in which services are provided as well as the settings and instrumentalities available and used for care. Structure measures indicate the extent to which providers, facilities, and organizations have adequate capability and capacity to provide the services that they offer.

Assessments of the structural factors in quality make the assumption that "good" structure is known. Examples of structural measures include facility accreditation, compliance with health and safety codes, health care staff appointments and review requirements, staff licensure, and board certification. Structure is the simplest component to measure when assessing quality. Good structure is necessary for good quality, but not sufficient in that good structure does not guarantee good quality.

■ Process

Process is the specific means by which care is provided; the activities of physicians and other health professionals in the management of patients. Process is evaluated against standards and expectations for specific diagnostic categories and procedures. Examples of process in the delivery of health care include taking a patient history, conducting a physical exam, and performing a coronary artery bypass graft.

Process is measured both implicitly and explicitly. The implicit process is subjective, as clinicians base their judgments on their own training, background and, experience. Explicit process evaluation is objective, with a "check list" of appropriate procedures and steps. Quality standards are predetermined and whenever possible based on national criteria. The process assessment assumes that care is useful in promoting health, and the process of care delivery is related to outcomes.

■ Outcomes

Outcomes are the end results of the delivery of health care and include patient satisfaction. These measures provide evidence of whether the standards and process of care produced the desired result. Outcomes are changes in health status and are measured by physical, social, and psychological functioning that can be attributed to receiving health care.

Outcomes research attempts to improve health care decisions by linking the choices of care to their effects on outcomes. Outcomes research can be used to minimize the use of ineffective treatments and to evaluate the implications of choices between cost and quality. Outcomes are not always the best measure of quality because quality care cannot always produce a positive outcome, and many people who receive poor quality care may still regain their health. Examples of outcomes measures include morbidity, mortality, infection rates, complication rates, recovery rates, functional disability, days of work lost, and patient satisfaction.

■ Quality Improvement Methods

There are many methods for improving the quality of health care. This section describes some of the steps the health care industry has undertaken to improve the quality of care delivered to patients and long-term clinical outcomes. The IOM (2001a) provided general guidance for improving quality when it called for future health care to be safe, effective, patient centered, timely, efficient, and equitable. Specifically providers should seek to avoid injuring patients with care that is intended to help. Care should be based on evidence-based practices and provided to all who would receive the most benefit. Care should be guided by patient decisions and reflect the patient's preferences, needs, and values. It should be provided in a timely manner with minimal delays for clinicians and patients. Waste of supplies, equipment, and energy should be avoided. Care should be delivered within uniform quality standards without regard for gender, race, geographic region, and socioeconomic status (IOM, 2001a).

Based on this set of principles, the National Council on Quality Assurance (NCQA) offered the following recommendations to improve the quality of health care (NCQA, 2007b). Health plans and providers should publically report on how their performance compares with quality performance standards. Employers and patients must make choices between health plans and providers based on the publically reported quality information. Access to such information is critical for consumers to make wise decisions for themselves and their families. Despite these principles and assistance from NCQA, more than 100 million people are members of health plans that do not publically report their quality performance information (NCQA, 2007b).

High-quality care should be rewarded by the reimbursement system. The current system rewards clinicians for the volume of services provided to patients. Tests, diagnoses, and procedures are reimbursed regardless of the value to the consumer. Those few health plans that have instituted pay-for-performance systems find them very effective at improving the quality of services and saving consumers money (NCQA, 2007b).

The health care system should focus on maintaining and promoting health (NCQA, 2007b). Our health care system is oriented toward treating patients who are sick or with life-threatening conditions. Although health care delivery should attend to patients across the full continuum of care, maintaining health should be made a priority. Promotion of health and wellness may help to reduce health care costs and increase the quality of life for all patients (NCQA, 2007b). Healthy people are more productive for both employers and for the rest of society.

The following sections provide added detail regarding ongoing quality improvement efforts taking place throughout the health care industry.

▪ Improving the Medical Education Process

The Flexner Report (1910) had the greatest impact on the quality of medical education. It changed medical education into a university-based science model. During the early 1900s, many of the U.S. medical schools were based on an apprentice approach. The report recognized the inherent variability in this training approach and recommended a university-based science model for medical education. John Hopkins Medical School served as the model for this approach, which was recommended for all medical schools.

To improve graduate medical education, the American Medical Association established national bodies to accredit residency programs and board certify physicians in the medical specialties. These bodies develop the length and content of training following medical school. Further, the specialty boards develop national examinations to assure that all physicians completing residency training meet minimum qualifications for practice. Residency programs are largely based in university hospitals where prospective specialists can obtain hands-on training supervised by experts who are already board certified in the specialty of training.

▪ Licensure/Specialty Certification

A physician completing training is licensed by the medical licensing board in the state in which the newly minted physician wishes to practice. For further explanation, see Chapter 5. Specialty boards at the national level deliver exams and certify physicians after they have completed specialty training. Other health professions have state licensure boards and specialty certification procedures.

▪ Continuing Medical Education (CME)

Clinician training does not end with undergraduate and graduate education and training. All clinicians are required to complete some form of continuing education during their practice lives. The specialty boards dictate these requirements for physicians, and other professions determine the criteria for maintaining currency of licensure.

▪ Accreditation/Facility Inspection

The Joint Commission is the most recognized accreditation entity in health care. The Joint Commission is a nongovernmental, not-for-profit system that accredits health care organizations such as hospitals, long-term care facilities, psychiatric hospitals, substance abuse centers, outpatient surgery centers, hospices, and home health agencies. Although health care organizations do not have to have Joint Commission accreditation, they do have to be accredited to participate in programs such as Medicare and Medicaid. Accreditation is important for state licensure and health insurance coverage.

▪ National Practitioner Data Bank

The **National Practitioner Data Bank (NPDB)** was established by the Health Care Quality Improvement Act of 1986. It is designed to impede the movement of incompetent doctors from state to state. Hospitals must check with the data bank before they grant a doctor privileges. The NPDB began operating in 1990, allowing communication across states about licensure issues and any disciplinary action taken. The data bank also contains credentialing and professional society actions. Malpractice insurance companies must report lawsuits to the data bank.

The data bank's information is highly confidential, with only hospital officials and state licensing or accreditation officials having access. Consumers do not have access to this information. However, in California, similar data are available to the public. Some critics of the data bank say that there is an underreporting of out-of-court settlements. On the other hand, those who argue that consumers should not have access to the data bank believe that there is potential for ruined reputations without cause because of the quality and accuracy of the information in the bank.

Many argue that information necessary to judge clinical competency must encompass all facets of education and practice, including education and training, certification (board certification), clinical experience, medical licensure and expertise, and experience with professional liability issues.

Professional Standard Review Organizations (PSRO)

In 1972, Medicare legislation required hospitals to conduct utilization review as a safeguard against unnecessary care or poor quality, with the primary focus on overutilization. The Centers for Medicare and Medicaid Services (CMS) contracted with PSROs to address quality assessment for Medicare and Medicaid. The PSROs delegated their main responsibility to the hospital utilization review departments, which conducted mainly retrospective reviews, with only a few concurrent reviews.

The goal of PSROs was to assure that quality care was delivered to Medicare and Medicaid recipients. PSROs used utilization review to pinpoint unnecessary care, assuring that services were medically necessary and within local standards, and that physicians maintained their documentation. Essentially the peer review process was expanded. If the PSRO found a violation of quality standards, it withheld payment at the hospital level, which gave hospitals some leverage. However, most physicians were independent practitioners, so if hospitals exerted pressure, these physicians just admitted their patients to another hospital.

Quality Improvement Organizations

Quality improvement organizations (QIO) started when diagnostic-related groups (DRGs) were instituted to address quality assessment for Medicare and Medicaid. These organizations are under contract with the federal government to ensure that hospitals and physicians follow Medicare rules. They focus on maintaining quality while controlling cost through utilization review. QIOs work to protect the government from fraud and abuse; conduct admission reviews to determine medical necessity and appropriateness; investigate readmissions and written patient complaints; and emphasize preadmission and concurrent review. QIOs focused on hospital readmissions within 31 days of discharge, and their scope of review expanded in 1987 to include HMOs, nursing homes, and ambulatory care, with additional emphasis on preadmission and concurrent review.

QIOs are an example of an internal process, and the Medicare legislation had limited power to enforce the utilization review or quality standards, so compliance was poor. QIOs were ineffective because evaluators used internalized or implicit standards to make qualitative judgments. Secondly, they were ineffective because there was no rational basis for chart selection that would allow the evaluators to generalize their findings to the rest of the patient population even if deficiencies were identified. Auditors were reluctant to take corrective action against their peers as those colleagues may serve on the QIO next year and take revenge.

State-Funded Health Care Quality Organizations

The Pennsylvania Health Care Cost Containment Council (PHC4) is an example of a state-funded organization that is dedicated to gathering health care quality information. The PHC4 was created in 1986 and publishes risk-adjusted data for hospitals, examines cost and quality data for hospitals, and releases the information to the public (PHC4, 2007).

The purpose of PHC4 was to promote health care cost containment, promote the public interest by encouraging the development of competitive health care services, and ensure that all citizens have reasonable access to quality care, such as by trying to identify providers who provide the best care. PHC4 has information by diagnosis and severity on standards for morbidity and mortality and length of stay; it has actual figures on performance, and compares and releases information to the public (PHC4, 2007).

Pay-for-Performance

The Medicare Modernization Act of 2003 contained a provision for CMS to implement a pay-for-performance program. This program rewarded clinicians who provided superior care to patients. Pay-for-performance (P4P) programs have now grown to 148 nationwide (The Leapfrog Group, 2007b). The primary reason for implementing such programs is to improve clinical outcomes, and the vast majority of programs have achieved that goal with improved clinical performance (The Leapfrog Group, 2007b).

Pay-for-performance programs also save payers and providers money, and many of them will be expanding the scope of the programs and the number of performance measurements that are used. The measurements for such programs are largely based on national standards adopted by Agency for Healthcare Research and Quality (AHRQ), National Committee for Quality Assurance (NCQA), and the Joint Commission, The Leapfrog Group, and others. One of the benefits of P4P is that many of the participants publish the quality measurements and the associated performance levels for consumers to see. This information helps employers and consumers evaluate the quality of services delivered by providers (The Leapfrog Group, 2007b).

National Committee for Quality Assurance (NCQA)

NCQA is a private, nonprofit organization to which health plans report on the quality of care delivered to the members enrolled in their health insurance plans. NCQA's Healthcare Effectiveness Data and Information Set (HEDIS) is the most widely used quality performance tool in the health industry (NCQA, 2007b). According to the NCQA, in 2006 many more Americans were enrolled in health plans that report their quality performance data (NCQA, 2007b), and this figure has risen, yet two-thirds of

Americans remain in unaccountable plans (NCQA, 2010). Many more health plans are reporting their quality information to NCQA as part of accreditation requirements and participation in Medicare. That number has exceeded 1,000 for the first time in 2010 (NCQA, 2010). The increase in participation by plans in reporting their quality performance is a consequence of an increase in the number of preferred provider organizations (PPOs) that are reporting on the quality that was delivered. HMOs and point-of-service (POS) plans have a long history of reporting the quality of the care financed by their members, whereas PPOs have only recently become engaged in the efforts to report quality data to NCQA (NCQA, 2007b).

The results of reporting quality indicators to NCQA indicate that PPOs perform comparably well when compared with their HMO and POS counterparts (NCQA, 2007b). NCQA has determined that many advancements in health care quality have been made as a consequence of publically reporting quality data. Many more heart attack patients now receive beta-blocker drugs to prevent second, often fatal, heart attacks (NCQA, 2007b). This improvement translates into a saving of 4,400 to 5,600 lives over the last six years and improved health for tens of thousands of patients (NCQA, 2007b).

Overall, NCQA reports that quality of care delivered by health plans has improved in the decade, although the rate of improvement has been recently modest (NCQA, 2010). Notably, colorectal cancer screenings, appropriate treatment of beta blockers after heart attack, and eye exams for diabetics improved significantly (NCQA, 2010).

However, there is a great deal of room to improve the quality of health care in the United States. Multiple childhood immunizations dropped for the first time after years of substantial gains (NCQA, 2010). If all patients received the care that is provided to the members of the top health plans, between 35,000 and 75,000 deaths could be avoided annually (NCQA, 2007a). NCQA estimates that 45 million days of lost productivity due to sickness could be avoided and $7.4 billion could be saved (NCQA, 2007a). These figures are not unrealistic goals as improvements in beta-blocker treatment for heart attack patients, cholesterol management, controlling high blood pressure, and improving blood sugar levels for diabetics have been instrumental in saving roughly 125,000 American lives (NCQA, 2007a).

There are key steps that plans can take to improve quality through publically reporting health plan quality data. The process of accreditation, whereby the plan undergoes regular, comprehensive review against a standardized set of quality measurements, is critical to assuring quality care (NCQA, 2007b). The health plan must also allow its quality performance to be publically reported. Health plans that allow their performance data to be publically reported are associated with better quality performance levels (NCQA, 2007b).

▪ Recent Quality Improvement Efforts

Recent quality improvement efforts involve implementing strategies used successfully in other industries and publishing performance data. Following is a summary of these recent efforts:

- Applying philosophies used in manufacturing and other industries to health care (e.g., TQM/CQI, reengineering, Six Sigma, lean transformation)

- Providing consumers with information to make better decisions (e.g., Nursing Home Compare, a site on the Centers for Medicare and Medicaid website that provides information about various quality indicators for all Medicare and Medicaid certified nursing homes)

- Health Plan Employer Data and Information Set (HEDIS)—information for employers to compare health plans

- Quality report cards: provider report cards showing how a physician compares to his or her peers; organizational report cards revealing how health care organizations (hospitals, for example) measure up to their competitors; health plan report cards comparing managed care plans (mostly on HEDIS measures)

- Ranking of hospitals—*U.S. News & World Report*

- CAHPS measures: enrollment or plan coverage, wait times, delivery of unnecessary care, and customer service

- Efforts by health care organizations to increase awareness among medical staff regarding benefits of enhanced quality of care

Summary

Assuring the highest quality health care is critical for a system responsible for saving lives and helping patients manage their chronic conditions. Clinicians have a responsibility to "First, do no harm" to their patients, and most clinicians make that their priority. However, fallible persons implement the processes and systems used to deliver care to patients, so mistakes will happen and medical errors will continue to harm patients. Organizations such as NCQA, Joint Commission, The Leapfrog Group, the Department of Health and Human Services, the American Medical Association, and the American Hospital Association are all committed to improving the quality of care.

Recent legislation in the form of the American Recovery and Reinvestment Act of 2009 and the recently passed the Patient Protection and Affordable Care Act of 2010, have provided substantial funding to improve quality. The economic stimulus bill provided millions for clinicians to invest in electronic health records. Improving quality of care is expensive and time-consuming. It requires additional training in the use of health care technology that may be able to prevent medical errors before they happen. Assuring quality can also be as simple as using a health care checklist for patients before surgery or in the emergency room. The costs of lower quality of care and the associated medical errors and hospital-acquired infections are much higher than implementing preventive measures and establishing methods of quality assessment.

▪ Review Questions

1. What are the primary ways that quality of health care is assessed?

2. What are several ways that quality of health care is measured?

3. Identify several groups that work to assess and improve the quality of health care.

4. Name several early historical quality advocates in the health care industry.

5. How many people contract hospital-acquired infections annually? Approximately how many people die from hospital-acquired infections?

6. What are four key areas that contribute to the overall poor levels of health care quality?

7. What are the three main areas for quality assessments under the Donabedian Model for Quality?

8. What is the most recognized accreditation entity in health care, and what is its role in monitoring the quality of health care?

9. What was the role of the Flexner Report (1910) in changing the quality of health care in America?

10. What is the goal of pay-for-performance programs as they relate to health care quality?

▪ Additional Resources

Agency for Healthcare Research and Quality (AHRQ): http://www.ahrq.gov/

American Hospital Association (AHA): http://www.aha.org/advocacy-issues/quality/index.shtml

Health Plan Employer Data and Information Set (HEDIS): http://www.ncqa.org/tabid/59/Default.aspx

Institute for Health Care Improvement (IHI): http://www.ihi.org/

Institute of Medicine (IOM): http://www.iom.edu/

National Council on Quality Assurance (NCQA): http://www.ncqa.org/

National Practitioner Data Bank (NPDB): http://www.npdb-hipdb.hrsa.gov/

Pennsylvania Health Care Cost Containment Council (PIIC4): http://www.phc4.org/

The Joint Commission http://www.jointcommission.org/

The Leapfrog Group: http://www.leapfroggroup.org/

▪ References

Abelson, R. (2010, March 21). *In health care overhaul, boons for hospitals and drug makers. New York Times.* Retrieved October 1, 2010, from http://www.nytimes.com/2010/03/22/business/22bizhealth.html

Berwick, D. M. (2002). A user's guide for the IOM "Quality Chasm" report. *Health Affairs, 21*(3), 80–90.

Brailer, D. (2009). Presidential leadership and health information technology. *Health Affairs, 28*(2), w392–w398.

British Broadcasting Network (BBC). (2010). British statesman warns America of government health care horrors. http://www.newsrealblog.com.

Burstin, H. R., Lipsitz, S. R., Udvarhelyi, I. S., & Brennan, T.A. (1993). The effect of hospital financial characteristics on quality of care. *Journal of the American Medical Association, 270*(7), 845–849.

Carrns, A. (2010, July 21). Health reform takes aim at hospital readmission rates. *U.S. News and World Report.* Retrieved October 1, 2010, from http://health.usnews.com/health-news/best-hospitals/articles/2010/07/21/health-reform-takes-aim-at-hospital-readmission-rates.

Encinosa, W. E., & Bernard, D.M. (2005). Hospital finances and patient safety outcomes. *Inquiry, 42*(1), 60–72.

Goodman D., Esty A. R., Fisher, E. S., & Chang, C. H. (2011). Trends and variation in end-of-life care for Medicare beneficiaries with severe chronic illness. Report of the Dartmouth Atlas Project. Hanover, NH. April 12.

Halamka, J. (2009). Making smart investments in health information technology: Core principles. *Health Affairs, 28*(2), w385–w389.

Hillestad, R., Bigelow, J., Bower, A., Girosi, F., Meili, R., et al. (2005). Can electronic medical record systems transform health care? Potential health benefits, savings, and costs. *Health Affairs, 24*(5), 1103–1117.

Hollenbeak, C., Lave J., Zetties T., Qanfen, P., Roland, C., & Sun, E. (2006). Factors associated with risk of surgical wound infection. *American Journal of Medical Quality, 21*(6), 29S–34S.

Institute of Medicine (IOM). (2001a). Crossing the quality chasm: A new health system for the twenty-first century. Washington, DC: National Academy Press.

Institute of Medicine (IOM). (2001b). *To err is human: Building a safer health system.* Washington, DC: National Academy Press.

Institute of Medicine (IOM). (2011, July 19). *Clinical preventive services for women: Closing the gap.* Washington, DC: National Academy Press.

Jaffe, S. (2009, August 20). Health policy brief: Key issues in health care reform. *Health Affairs*, 16.

Kaiser Family Foundation (KFF). (2010). *Summary of the new health reform law.* Menlo Park: Author.

The Leapfrog Group. (2007a). Eighty-seven percent of U.S. hospitals do not take recommended steps to prevent avoidable infections. Press release on September 7, 2007. Washington, DC: Author.

The Leapfrog Group. (2007b). Pay for performance programs for providers now total 150. Press release in 2007. Washington, DC: Author.

National Committee for Quality Assurance (2007a). Report: Health care quality continues to improve for 84 million Americans, but more than 100 million in the dark. Washington, DC: Author.

National Committee for Quality Assurance (NCQA). (2007b). The state of health care quality 2007. Washington, DC: Author.

National Committee for Quality Assurance (NCQA). (2010). The state of health care quality 2010. Washington, DC: Author.

Peng, M. M., Kurtz, S., & Johannes, R. S. (2006). Adverse outcomes from hospital-acquired infection in Pennsylvania cannot be attributed to increase risk on admission. *American Journal of Medical Quality, 21*(17), 17S–28S.

Pennsylvania Health Care Cost Containment Council (PHC4). (2005). Hospital-acquired infections in Pennsylvania. Harrisburg, PA: Pennsylvania Health Care Cost Containment Council.

Pennsylvania Health Care Cost Containment Council (PHC4). (2007). Critical condition: The state of health care in Pennsylvania. Harrisburg, PA: Pennsylvania Health Care Cost Containment Council.

Shannon, R.P., Patel, B., Cummins, D., Shannon, A.H., Ganguli, G., Lu, Y. (2006 Nov/Dec) Economics of central-line associated bloodstream infections. *Am J Med Qual*, 21(6 Suppl):7S-16S.

Shen, Y. (2003). The effect of financial pressure on the quality of care in hospitals. *Journal of Health Economics, 22*(2), 243–269.

Key Terms

Certificate of Need

goal

health planning

macro planning

micro planning

objective

reactive planning

regulation

Learning Objectives

- Define and describe health planning and regulation.

- Outline the factors that must be considered in health planning and the goals of health planning.

- Describe the differences between centralized planning and decentralized planning.

- Describe the characteristics of a free market and how market failure leads to regulation.

- Describe the major regulatory theories.

- Discuss planning and regulatory laws that have been enacted in the United States.

▪ What Is Health Planning?

We all plan—formally or informally. Choosing a major or creating a schedule for the next semester are formal plans for your education. Making a "to-do" list or grocery list are informal planning tools to assist you in completing tasks or buying food. **Health planning** is a formal process where organizations or government entities devise strategies and itemize services that promote health or prevent or treat diseases.

Planning entails the following steps:

1. Defining a problem

2. Formulating and evaluating alternatives

3. Implementing the chosen alternative

4. Evaluating the results

Planning is a cyclical process that never really ends. Once the results are evaluated for one program or intervention, we either seek to improve that program or move on to another area of concern. Health planning must always take into account characteristics of the population and projected changes in demographics and social and economic conditions.

Micro versus Macro Planning

Planning can occur at the micro or macro levels. **Micro planning** is planning targeted at the institution or individual. For example, a local hospital might conduct a needs assessment before deciding what types of new services to offer or which services to discontinue. Micro planning is usually decentralized, meaning that no one agency or organization is in charge of planning what services can or should be delivered. **Macro planning** is planning at a national, regional, or state level. Macro planning is often centralized, where a single entity coordinates the planning of services for a large area. For example, some states still have **Certificate of Need** programs, where a state board must approve applications for new facilities, capital improvements, or high-cost equipment. Whether planning at the micro or macro level, objectives and goals must be set to guide the planning process. A **goal** is a long-range statement of an ideal or desired outcome. An **objective** is a specific, measurable target that must be reached within a defined time frame.

Relationships among Need, Demand, and Supply

Health planning attempts to equate units of need with units of demand to units of supply (see Figure 15–1). For example, if 1,000 people per year have a heart attack in a town, health planners would attempt to determine how many hospital beds, pharmaceuticals, cardiac catheterizations and open heart surgeries would be required to treat those 1,000 heart attacks. Health planners would also try to determine how many physicians and other health personnel would be needed to meet the demand for these services. However, not all need translates into demand. People who do not have insurance or live in rural or inner-city areas may have limited access to services, which would leave them with unmet needs. Many people also demand more services than they need. This overuse leads to excess cost to the health care system and may result in harm to the patient. There are some instances where supply and demand do not meet as well. For example, the nation has a surplus of hospital beds in many areas and a shortage of primary care physicians. Most models of health planning, like the one above, are complicated because individuals differ in their needs and demands by age, race, behavior, comorbidities, and other factors. Models of health care utilization, as discussed in Chapter 13, can assist in the planning process, but cannot account for all variables.

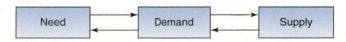

Figure 15–1 Relationships among need, demand, and supply.
© Cengage Learning 2013

▪ What Does Health Planning Involve?

When health planning at the micro and macro levels, the following factors need to be assessed:

1. Health status (measuring need)

2. Use of services (measuring demand)

3. Supply (e.g., facilities, manpower)

4. Organization (can impact supply and use of services)

5. Financing (how services are financed or how providers are paid affects use of services; for example, a person who has full coverage will behave differently from one with limited coverage)

6. Quality issues

7. Cost (can impact supply and use of services)

8. Political issues

9. Legal issues (laws that relate to the organization of practices; laws that relate to licensure of physicians and providers)

All of these factors influence access, quality, and cost, the elements of the Iron Triangle discussed in Chapter 1.

▪ Goals of Health Planning

There are 10 essential goals of health planning:

1. Improving the organization of health services

2. Speeding the development and diffusion of needed new health services

3. Discouraging programs that are not really needed (duplication of services)

4. Improving coordination to facilitate the communication among all clinicians in the continuum of care.

5. Eliminating duplication of services

6. Reducing fragmentation of health care delivery

7. Achieving a better geographic distribution to optimize patients' access to care

8. Identifying health needs and problems and helping to set realistic goals

9. Establishing priorities

10. Integrating health needs into physical, economic, and other areas of planning for community development

What Is Regulation?

Planning (Centralized) + Government (Force of Law) = Regulation

In a broad sense, **regulation** is centralized planning that has the force of law behind it. In the United States, most industries are largely private and operate in a free market, with limited regulation. However, government intervenes in the free market when the health and welfare of the United States citizenry is at stake and there is a breakdown of the free-market system, or a market failure. Finally, government gets involved because of the increasing complexity of the health care marketplace.

There are many reasons for government regulation instead of decentralized private planning in the health care sector. Many people have traditionally been concerned about unmet needs of the population. Government can help provide services that are not provided by the private sector. Also, many believe that health care is a "right." As a result, the federal and state governments provide funding for community health centers where patients receive primary and preventive care regardless of their ability to pay and mandate treatment in emergency departments for patients who do not have insurance.

Since the 1970s, with the growth of both commercial and government insurance coverage, health planners have also been interested in controlling supply of services and limiting overuse. Increased demand for health care services and increased costs and expenditures have raised concern about the ability of the free market to effectively address these issues. In addition, government is concerned that the private sector will invest in expanding services at the expense of assuring quality. To address this issue, government can promulgate minimal standards of licensure or certification to practice to ensure that providers are qualified to deliver care. This form of regulation is often a function of state governments.

Rationale for Regulation

There are several important rationales for government regulation in the health care industry. First, government regulates health care to prevent fraud and abuse. The government will prosecute and fine those who bill for services not provided. Second, government seeks to contain costs and protect the "public's purse" through, for example, using diagnosis-related groups (DRGs) for reimbursement and contracting with quality improvement organizations (QIOs) to conduct utilization review. Third, the government seeks to protect patients. Physicians must be licensed by the state, and prescription medications must be demonstrated to be safe and effective by the Food and Drug Administration before they can be prescribed. Fourth, the government protects employees with regulations that ensure a safe workplace. For example, there are laws that direct the cleaning up of hazardous material spills, working in laboratories, and disposing of used needles.

Competition versus Regulation

Policy makers often debate the merits of a competitive, market-based health care system versus a government-run or government-financed system. There are benefits to both competition and regulation, but it has been an enormously difficult task to strike the appropriate balance, assuming that there can be an appropriate balance.

▪ Benefits of Competition

Competition often promotes innovation and ingenuity. Inventors and scientists are able to profit from new discoveries in a competitive marketplace. Free-market systems also operate using price competition that should result in lower prices. In health care, regulation is not as efficient as in the free market. It is estimated that 20–25 percent of the $1.4 trillion spent on health care in the United States is consumed by regulation (Conover, 2004). The United States has always had a market-based economy and a respect for preserving individual choice in the free marketplace and independence from government intervention. These tenets of American life have led to resistance to government regulation in the health care industry.

▪ Criteria for a Well-Functioning Free-Market System

In general, regulation is not necessary in a well-functioning free-market system. Four major characteristics ensure that the market works properly for the benefit of consumers and producers. In a free market, consumers are well informed about the products they wish to purchase and can judge the relative quality of the products. The individual also pays the full cost and enjoys the full benefits of the product or service at the time of purchase. There are a large number of suppliers from which individuals can choose to purchase a good or service, and the suppliers bear the full cost of production for those items or services.

To the extent that these criteria do not exist, a market failure may occur. Currently, the United States does not have a completely free-market health care delivery system. The government regulates many aspects of the health care industry. However, the United States also is not experiencing a total market failure. For example, through the Internet, U.S. health care consumers can better educate themselves than ever before and learn from the experiences of family and friends. However, consumers still have less information than clinicians. This imbalance in the consumption and delivery of health care produces a partial market failure.

Regarding the second criterion above, enjoying the full benefits depends on the definition of benefits, and the time of purchase may not be easily or clearly identified. These definitions determine whether this criterion is violated. For example, most Americans pay the full cost of care through insurance premiums, out-of-pocket payments, and taxes. However, third-party payment does not allow consumers to experience the full cost of care at the time services are rendered. In addition, some individuals do not pay much for care because other individuals subsidize their care. Although those paying are not receiving the physical benefits of the care delivered, they nevertheless may feel some type of reward for helping other individuals, thus generating a greater benefit, also called externalities. On the other hand, some may feel that subsidizing the care of others leads to irresponsible consumption of care.

The third criterion, which requires a variety of suppliers, depends on the local or regional marketplace. Large cities have multiple hospitals and hospital systems, whereas smaller or rural areas may not have a single facility or may have one small hospital. Moreover, because the large majority of people own a car, including the poor, a large number of hospitals (including major health care centers) are within a four-hour or less drive. However, there are many barriers to substantially increasing the supply of health care providers to meet this criterion. The education of health care professionals,

Competition   Regulation

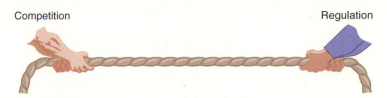

Figure 15–2 The health care tug-of-war between competition and regulation.
© *Cengage Learning 2013*

licensure of professionals and facilities, and Certificate of Need programs limit rather than enhance the supply of new providers and facilities in the market.

The United States also falls short on the fourth criterion because it provides subsidies to suppliers. For example, the Hill-Burton Program gave funding and substantial tax breaks to not-for-profit health care facilities for construction in the 1940s and 1950s. Not-for-profit health facilities receive government support through tax exemptions. Also, medical education and pharmaceutical research are partially subsidized by the government, that is, the taxpayer.

Although free-market criteria are not fully met in the United States, it does not have a nationalized health care system, nor does it have a comprehensive national health insurance program. Because the U.S. health care system only experiences partial market failure, the government intervenes with some regulation, but does not intervene to the extent of creating a national health insurance program like Canada's or creating a national health system like that in the United Kingdom.

These examples of both violation and support for the criteria of a free-market system explain the tug-of-war between competition and regulation in the health care industry (see Figure 15–2).

▪ Characteristics of the Health Care System That Make Regulation Desirable

Although there are many benefits to a free-market system in health care, there are also many characteristics, beyond market failure, that make regulation of the health care sector desirable. Consumers of health care are not rational, especially when the patient or family member is ill. They may not be in an appropriate mental or physical state to seek out health care information or make truly informed choices. They rely on the judgment of health care professionals whose capability is regulated by the government through licensure.

Provision of health care is not a right specified in the Constitution, but it is often viewed as a right. If it is a right, then it must be ensured by the government. Those who cannot pay for care must be subsidized by the government. (This topic will be addressed further in the next chapter as part of the health care reform discussion.) The United States already finances approximately 47 percent of health care costs and expenditures at some level of government. Using taxpayer dollars to support the health care industry requires government oversight to ensure that these funds are wisely spent. The government has a fiduciary responsibility to be as prudent and as effective as possible with the public's money.

Furthermore, competition in some markets may be destructive. Destructive competition exists when there is too little regulation in the market, causing harm to companies, taxpayers, and customers. Competition can become destructive when there is a duplication of services, which can lead to unused capacity and inefficiency or overuse of services. Fixed costs are associated with unused capacity, which ultimately leads to higher insurance premiums and higher taxes. Furthermore, overuse of services has the potential to cause unnecessary harm to the patient.

Some industries, such as utility companies, have government-enforced monopolies. These monopolies work well if they are properly regulated. In these industries, the costs of production are usually too high to allow multiple competitors. However, since the 1970s, many monopolies have been deregulated to the benefit of consumers. For example, the airline and telephone services deregulation resulted in lower prices for consumers (Niskanan, 1989).

There are two questions that should be considered when analyzing whether government should regulate the free-market system: Can government generate prosperity? and, Can government regulation improve the health care marketplace? These highly debated topics will be discussed in the Your Opinion Matters segment.

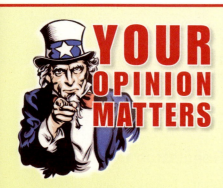

Can Government Regulation Improve the Health Care Marketplace?

Yes

Government regulation improves the health care marketplace in three ways. First, it provides safety nets for those who do not have insurance by funding community health centers and ensuring that patients can get treatment in emergency rooms. Second, regulation helps to lower the cost of health care through price controls. Third, it protects patients from unsafe providers and products. An estimated 46 million people in the United States have no health insurance. If government did not mandate that hospitals care for all who came into the ER, hospitals could refuse to treat the uninsured, leaving them with few alternatives for receiving health care. As we see with the pharmaceutical industry, companies that have little regulation are able to price their products to a level that is prohibitively expensive to some. If government were to increase regulation of the pharmaceutical industry by setting maximum allowable prices, more people would be able to afford medications, which would improve the treatment of diseases, especially chronic diseases. Government regulation also is operating in a variety of the components of the health care system by ensuring minimum standards of quality care. Without licensure of health professionals and drug and device approval by the Food and Drug Administration, anyone would be able to practice health care, and any medicine or device could be sold, regardless of safety or efficacy. Government provisions help patients attain safer, lower cost health care and are necessary to improve the health of the American people.

No

Government regulation is intrusive and is not necessary for the efficient operation of our health care system. In fact, regulation alone drives up health care costs. There are sufficient incentives in the free market to lead to competition on price and quality. Before government intrusion into the health care market beginning in the 1930s and continuing in the 1960s, those who did not have insurance were cared for through pro bono and charitable obligations of physicians and hospitals. Providers had a duty to care for those who were less fortunate and could not afford their services. The passage of Medicare and Medicaid and the favorable tax treatment of health insurance benefits have distorted the market by encouraging over insurance. This subsidizing has induced multiple market failures. For example, patients no longer face the true price of services at the time of service. Comprehensive insurance coverage has led to sky-rocketing costs, which in turn has led to the need for more insurance, which then has led to even more government involvement. Government regulation has also been manipulated in many cases to maintain monopolies for health care providers. The Stark Legislation (Anti-Self-Referral Laws) limits competition by not permitting physicians to refer patients to laboratories and other companies where they hold part ownership. This regulation drives many physicians out of that market. Through licensure, the American Medical Association (AMA) has managed to limit and control chiropractors and other non-MD/DO providers, such as PAs and NPs, from practicing medicine, leading to higher costs for physician care. Finally, the prohibition on physician-owned hospitals has allowed traditional hospitals to maintain a firm hold on the market, which has also resulted in higher costs and potentially lower quality. It is clear that providing more information to prospective patients would make them more discriminating consumers of health care and thus would reduce the need for regulation as a form of protection.

You decide:

1. Can clinicians be relied on to provide pro bono care or does government have to step in?
2. What market factors can restrain price and maintain quality?
3. What are the characteristics of government regulation that make it anti-competitive?
4. What do patients have to know to maintain a safe and competent health care system?

■ Theories That Explain Regulatory Behavior

There are three major theories in political science that explain the behavior of regulatory agencies and the industries that they regulate: The public interest theory, capture theory, and economic theory. These theories are used to explain the relationships among Congress, regulatory agencies, and industry, and the laws that result from these relationships. Congress passes laws that are then promulgated and enforced by executive regulatory agencies. The Department of Health and Human Services is the primary agency responsible for regulating the health care system.

Public Interest

The public interest theory is based on the contention that "We are here to help you." This theory of regulation assumes that disinterested, all-knowing, objective bureaucrats whose desire is to protect the public from monopoly powers (i.e., unscrupulous business people taking advantage of consumer ignorance or market power) conduct regulation. Under this theory, regulation should result in *prices and profits comparable to those that are realized in a highly competitive marketplace.* The lowest prices that can be sustained by suppliers are those in a highly competitive marketplace. Regulation may impose prices that are lower than competitive prices, resulting in suppliers leaving the marketplace (e.g., going out of business). Based on this theory, if there are shortcomings in the regulatory process, they can be rectified by devoting more time and resources to the process.

Capture Theory

The capture theory of regulatory behavior assumes that regulation is proposed, supported, and unduly influenced by the industry being regulated. According to this theory, government power works in favor of the corporation. Protection of monopoly power is the actual goal and result of legislation and regulations. There is no significant counterbalance to a powerful industry's lobbying power. *Thus, the reason for regulation is not in the public interest, but in the interest of those that want to be regulated.* Under this theory, regulation creates a legally enforceable monopoly or cartel that is utilized to prevent other producers from entering the market. Thus, the industry "captures," or controls, the regulatory process. Politicians accept this monopoly or cartel in exchange for campaign contributions as long as the industry does not embarrass the politicians. The politicians retain oversight authority to deal with such an eventuality. Under this model, companies earn high, monopolistic profits, and the prices are higher than in a competitive market.

Economic Theory

Economic theory assumes that regulators, policy makers, and businesses work together to influence the regulatory process, but in an environment with uncertain, expensive, and unbalanced information. Industries and consumer groups demand favorable laws from the suppliers (Congress, regulatory agencies), whereas the market operates on political support rather than price (Feldstein, 2006). However, there are many competing industries and groups in the marketplace, so legislation does not always favor all groups similarly. This theory usually produces competitive or low profits, and consumers experience monopolistic prices because businesses have to comply with regulation. This theory is the one best supported by data and is probably the reason for the *partial* deregulation of some industries (airline, power, and telephone) where the environment is more certain, less expensive, and information is balanced. It is also likely the reason for increasing regulation of other industries (health care) with expensive products and limited information that operate in an uncertain environment.

History of Centralized Non-Governmental Health Planning

There have been several monumental non-governmental planning efforts that have changed the health care system in dramatic ways. These planning accomplishments include the Flexner Report, the Committee on the Cost of Medical Care, and the Commission on Chronic Illness, as well as various disease-specific societies.

The Flexner Report (1910)

The Flexner Report was arguably the most successful act of modern health planning. This report entailed a national, non-governmental, comprehensive study of medical education in the United States, funded by the Carnegie Foundation for the Advancement of Teaching. This report found high levels of incompetence among many proprietary medical schools. Prior to 1910, a majority of medical schools operated under an apprenticeship model. Flexner used the Johns Hopkins model (medical school linked with a medical center and university; two years of science training and two years of clinical training) as the standard by which to judge medical education. Medical schools that adopted the Johns Hopkins model were able to remain open. This report led to the closure of many of medical schools but also set the foundation for the rigorous medical education system that we have today (Flexner, 1910).

Committee on the Cost of Medical Care (1932)

The Committee on the Cost of Medical Care was a self-created, voluntary organization that spent five years surveying and evaluating the organization and cost of the health care system in the United States. It was funded by the Rockefeller and Carnegie Foundations and the Julius Rosenwald and Milbank Memorial Funds. The findings and recommendations of the committee included organizing of physicians into groups, extension of the availability of all public services, and an emphasis on health and prevention of disease in the teaching of physicians. The Committee had historical significance, but did not do much because it had no legal authority; it could make recommendations, but it was not authorized to enforce them (Smith, 1933).

Commission on Chronic Illness (1945)

The Commission on Chronic Illness was formed as the Joint Committee on Chronic Illness by the American Hospital Association, American Medical Association, American Public Health Association and American Public Welfare Association in 1945. By 1949, it was established as an independent commission, and additional membership was sought from outside the four founding interest groups. The Commission constituted 34 members representing areas both within and outside health care, including members of the general public. The purpose of the Commission on Chronic Illness was to define chronic illnesses and help create and coordinate programs for the prevention and treatment of chronic illnesses (Roberts, 1954).

▪ Others

The American Heart Association, National Cancer Society, March of Dimes, Robert Wood Johnson Foundation, the Commonwealth Fund, the Kaiser Family Foundation, and many others support health care research and lobby for particular benefits for the health care system. For example, the March of Dimes played a large role in funding research that ultimately produced a polio vaccine. These efforts at nongovernmental centralized planning tended to have a narrow focus and inadequate funding, were mired in political and territorial disputes, and had no legal authority.

▪ History of Centralized, Governmental Health Planning

Most health planning efforts have been sanctioned or supported by government with proscribed centralized planning goals and objectives. Some of the most important of these activities were the Dawson Report in the United Kingdom, The Social Security Act of 1935; The Hospital Survey and Construction Act of 1946; the Heart Disease, Cancer and Stroke Act of 1965; the Partnership for Health Act of 1966; and the National Health Planning and Resource Development Act of 1974.

▪ The Dawson Report (1920)

The Dawson Report laid the foundation for the creation of a National Health Service in England in 1948. It outlined benefits of a state-coordinated system of care with a regional focus and a single, national authoritative body. This report recommended that most treatment be provided in primary care centers, with referrals to secondary care and medical schools when needed. These secondary services would be regionalized; that is, they would be more spread out than primary care centers and fewer in number.

▪ The Social Security Act of 1935

The Social Security Act of 1935 outlined tuberculosis treatment and planning but restricted intervention in the private practice of medicine. The act contained a clause that stated that state governments should not intervene in the physician–patient relationship, thus rendering the SSA with little impact on individual health care.

▪ Hospital Survey and Construction Act of 1946 (Hill-Burton Act/Program)

The Hill-Burton Act attempted to equalize hospital bed to population ratios across the country. The federal government gave money to build or expand hospitals, with an emphasis on increasing access in rural areas. In return, hospitals had a responsibility to care for all patients, even if they could not pay. However, the sophistication of planning techniques was very poor at the time. The program used bed-to-population ratios of affluent communities as templates, not understanding that these ratios in affluent areas were already too high. The result was over-expansion of hospitals, leading to higher costs and overutilization in the 1960s and 1970s and a surplus of hospital beds, especially in rural areas. Many small, rural hospitals had a daily census of 30–40 percent. After Medicare switched to prospective payment in the 1980s, many of these hospitals closed.

■ The Heart Disease, Cancer, and Stroke Act of 1965

The Heart Disease, Cancer, and Stroke Act of 1965 established regional medical programs (RMPs). The stated purpose of the regional medical programs was "to encourage and assist in the establishment of regional cooperative arrangements among medical schools, research institutions, and hospitals for research and training, including continuing education, and for related demonstration of patient care. ..." RMPs were meant to diffuse "cutting-edge" medical knowledge to community physicians. In reality, it funneled millions of dollars to large medical centers, but little of that money reached community physicians and hospitals where it was intended. These programs led to the expansion of teaching hospitals and medical schools in the United States. The regional medical programs were defunded in 1976.

■ Partnership for Health Act of 1966

This act established the Comprehensive Health Planning Program, *the first example of system-wide (i.e., national) health planning in the United States.* The funding for this program came from both the federal and local levels (75% federally funded, 25% locally funded). The local portion often came from the contributions of hospitals and other providers or facilities. The law divided each state into "B" agencies, often based on county or political boundaries, and named after Part B of the legislation. B agencies were comprised of a local, nonprofit group of planners. In many instances the B agencies' designations "artificially divided" health care market areas.

If a health facility wanted to expand, it had to get permission from the B agency. There were frequent conflicts of interest because the funding for the program usually came from those same providers who were seeking approval to expand. At other times, the behavior of the B agencies was so politically radical that the providers were excluded from the planning process or would not accept the result of the planning. As a consequence, some providers withdrew from the planning process and/or discontinued their financial support.

Also, this law had no "teeth." The B agencies were private entities and could not legally enforce their decisions. Laws without punishment are treated as suggestions. The Comprehensive Health Planning Program was not effective in containing hospital costs and price increases, so government changed this loophole in 1972 to say that the punishment for noncompliance would be that those facilities would not be reimbursed for their new equipment or construction by Medicaid and Medicare. This punitive action was not an effective deterrent because the percent of the hospital's reimbursement for an admission that was cost-accounted to the expanded facility or new equipment was often small and thus frequently ignored.

Overall, this attempt at comprehensive national health planning had little or no impact on cost, expenditures, or duplication of services, for several reasons. First, the planning areas were set within political boundaries and ignored the real health care market and consumer travel patterns to receive health care. Second, some plans ignored providers, whereas others were controlled by providers. Finally, the program did not have legal backing to enforce any of its planning decisions.

■ National Health Planning and Resource Development Act of 1974

The National Health Planning and Resource Development Act of 1974 had several important provisions:

1. For the first time, national goals and objectives were set that were quantitative and measurable.

2. The law had "legal teeth" to enforce planning decisions.

3. The law divided states into health service areas (HSAs)—using actual health care markets and not political boundaries for planning purposes. This act revamped the local planning areas that were previously established and changed them to be more logical and realistic.

4. Each state had to pass a Certificate of Need (CON) law, which stated that before expansion could occur, the facility had to get approval from a state-run planning agency.

Vignette

HOW WELL DOES CERTIFICATE OF NEED OPERATE IN A FREE MARKET?

An owner of a large hospital corporation based in a mid-size city wanted to build a new hospital in a growing and affluent part of town. The Certificate of Need board was not likely to vote to approve the Certificate of Need for a new hospital. The owner then attempted to subvert the CON process. He bribed the governor to give him a seat on the Certificate of Need board so that he could sway the board in his favor. The hospital was built, but not operated. The hospital corporation owner and governor were both convicted of bribery charges.

1. What are the advantages and the disadvantages of having a CON process for the building and expansion of health care facilities and services?

2. Does the CON process lead to too few health care services for needy patient populations?

3. Does the CON process run counter to capitalism and free-market principles where demand determines the supply of goods and services?

If health care facilities did not comply with CON laws, they could lose their license and be shut down. If the local health facility disagreed with the CON board ruling, they could appeal to the state health agency. This CON legislation produced a system of **reactive planning** rather than proactive planning. An additional problem with this law was that those who ran the state health agencies were political appointees of the governor of the state. Thus, the appeals process was most often driven by political and economic considerations because the health care facilities in question were frequently major employers in their community seeking approval to add jobs and increase access to higher quality health care—all wins for local and state politicians. These boards were also prime targets for corruption by health care corporations and politicians through the political appointment process.

Thus, the state health agency would most often acquiesce because government officials want to be reelected. Another option the health care facility had was to appeal a negative decision in the courts. Ironically, the legal fees in this appeals process were considered as "allowable costs" under the Medicare program (i.e., they were reimbursable costs, so the government was paying to be sued). Certificate of Need boards were effective in some states with restricting supply of some services; however, they were not very effective at controlling costs. The federal mandate and funding were repealed in 1987. A number of states have opted out of their CON laws. Only 36 states still had CON laws as of December 2009 (National Council of State Legislators [NCSL], 2011), and most of those that remain are very different from the earlier ones. For example, the "trigger" mechanism (dollar amount mandating review) is set at very high dollar amounts and consequently only covers substantial expansion of facilities and equipment.

▪ Summary

To date, attempts at comprehensive centralized health planning have had little or no effect on stemming the continued growth of health care costs and expenditures. Most planning now occurs at the local or regional levels because resources and needs vary within and among states. Health departments and boards of concerned citizens are often established to set priorities and implement programs. Every 10 years, the Centers for Disease Control and Prevention sets new national priorities for improving the health of the nation in a publication called Healthy People. Communities can adapt the goals and priorities to their own needs and implement programs based on those priorities. The Patient Protection and Affordable Care Act also has resource provisions that may call for more intensive planning in the future.

▪ Review Questions

1. Describe the steps involved in the planning process, and give an example as it relates to health care with each step.

2. Explain the differences in micro and macro planning, and give examples of each.

3. Explain the relationships among need, demand, and supply in health care planning.

4. What factors have to be considered in health planning? Give examples of each.

5. Describe the goals of health planning, and give examples of each.

6. What are some of the reasons for regulation in health care?

7. Describe the benefits of competition, and relate these to the current health care system.

8. What are market failures? Give examples of market failures in health care.

9. Describe the characteristics that make regulation desirable.

10. Describe the theories of regulation in health care and their effect on profit and prices. Give examples of each theory in health care regulation.

11. Describe different nongovernmental centralized planning efforts and their impact on the health care system.

12. Describe different governmental centralized planning efforts and their impact on the health care system.

▪ Additional Resources

American Health Planning Association: http://www.ahpanet.org/

American Public Health Association Community Health Planning and Policy Development Section: http://www.apha.org/membergroups/sections/aphasections/chppd/

Healthy People 2010 Toolkit: A Field Guide for Health Planning: http://www.healthypeople.gov/state/toolkit/

▪ References

Conover, C. J. (2004, October 4). Health care regulation: A $169 billion hidden tax. The Cato Institute. Policy Analysis. Washington, DC.

Feldstein, P. J. (2006). *The politics of health legislation: An economic perspective*, 3rd ed. Chicago: Health Administration Press.

Flexner, A. (1910). *Medical education in the United States and Canada*. Bulletin No. 4. New York, NY: The Carnegie Foundation for the Advancement of Teaching.

National Council of State Legislators (NCSL). (2011, January 28). Certificate of Need: State health laws and programs. Washington, DC: Author.

Niskanan, W. (1989). Economic deregulation in the United States: Lessons for America and China. *Cato Journal, 8*(3) (Winter).

Roberts, D. W. (1954). The Commission on Chronic Illness. *Public Health Rep, 69*(3), 295–299.

Smith, W. H. (1933). The report of the Committee on the Cost of Medical Care. *Canadian Medical Association Journal, 28*(2), 198–199.

Key Terms

disjointed incrementalism

Clinton health reform

Democratic/Normative Reinforcement

Great Depression

Literalism— contemporary

Literalism—historical

Modernism/ Instrumentalism

Originalism/Original intent

Patient Protection and Affordable Care Act (PPACA), 2010

World War I (WWI)

World War II (WWII)

Learning Objectives

- Identify how the government has been involved in the provision and the reimbursement of health care services.

- Describe the progression of national health insurance from its introduction to the most recent reform efforts.

- Describe the different perspectives on interpreting the U.S. Constitution, including Originalism/Original Intent, Modernism/Instrumentalism, Literalism—Historical, Literalism—Contemporary, and Democratic/Normative Reinforcement.

- Describe the major issues when debating health insurance policy.

- Describe the key provisions of the U.S. Constitution and their relationship with health care.

■ Introduction

National health care policy debates in the United States center on the role of government. Conservatives argue that the Constitution and the Declaration of Independence, along with other articles and statutes, do not specifically state that access to health care is a right. Liberals believe just the opposite: that government is responsible for promoting the general welfare, which includes access to health care services. This struggle has lasted for nearly a century, played out in the 1960s with passage of Medicare and Medicaid, and in the 1990s with the Clinton health care plan, and in the **Patient Protection and Affordable Care Act (PPACA) of 2010**.

The role of government in a free society is an unsettling question. In our desire to extend privileges to the poor and elderly, Congress passed Medicaid and Medicare in the mid-1960s. These government programs provide insurance and access to care for millions of Americans. Yet, for the past four and half decades, the nation has struggled with managing the runaway costs of these programs, unable to accurately predict their expenditures, and devouring more and more of the gross domestic product (GDP) each year. How important is access to care for the less fortunate in the richest country in the world? How much are we willing to sacrifice? Can politicians compromise on this increasingly polarizing issue? Do we remain the only developed nation without national health insurance or a national health service? If we determine that access to health care for the less fortunate is a national value, what will that health care system look like in an environment of growing national debt and unbalanced budgets? The history of government involvement in health care, the issues that surround the national health insurance debate, and a discussion of the laws that govern this nation are the foci of this chapter.

National health policy discussed in this chapter will address the role of government in either paying for or actually providing health services. We are focusing on this component of national health policy for several reasons. The cost of health care is rising faster than any other good or service; there are disparities in the geographic distribution of health care personnel and facilities; and there are disparities in access to care and health status among patient populations, depending on social class, place of residence, and age. Some argue that because these factors affect the health status of the nation's population, developing strategies to ameliorate these conditions is an appropriate role of government.

■ Government Has Always Been Involved in the Provision or Financing of Health Services

Government traditionally becomes involved in the health care industry when market forces break down and the health and welfare of the citizenry is at stake. The U.S. national values embrace freedom of choice. So, when government intervenes, we tend to favor voluntary as opposed to compulsory programs. For example, participation in Medicare Part B, as discussed in Chapter 8, is an option for eligible seniors. It is not a requirement that all Medicare beneficiaries sign up for the program. Part D is also voluntary for beneficiaries, and persons eligible for Medicaid are not required to enroll.

In addition, when government intervenes, its programs and strategies can be described as categorical or incremental rather than comprehensive. When national studies revealed that poor children and the elderly had inadequate access to care, the U.S. Congress passed legislation that established the Medicare and Medicaid programs as opposed to instituting a comprehensive national health insurance program like those in Canada and the United Kingdom. Thus, the government's involvement in national health policy can be described best as **disjointed incrementalism** or a "patchwork-quilt" approach. The asset of this approach is that if anything goes wrong with an increment, it does not necessarily burden the entire health care industry, because the problem only affects a portion of the system. However, the liability of this approach is that solutions have a limited impact.

This categorical approach to national health policy can at least partially explain why the United States does not have comprehensive national health insurance similar to Canada or a national health service in the United Kingdom, where government owns the facilities, employs the providers (physicians), and pays for the health care for all of its citizens. However, Medicare is a type of national health insurance, comprehensively covering a defined subpopulation.

▪ History of National Health Policy

- *As early as the U.S. colonial days,* the colonial and state governments provided mental health services. Health care has always been provided to active duty members of the armed services.

- *1848:* In *The Communist Manifesto,* Karl Marx developed the notion that a healthy workforce is a productive workforce. He proposed that investing in the health of the workforce has a payoff in the form of higher productivity.

- *The 1880s:* The Bismarck of Germany inaugurated a system where the government mandated employment-based health insurance or health care provided to the worker.

- *1900–1917:* Government mandated Workmen's Compensation. State governments acknowledged that industry had a responsibility to pay for the health care of work-related injuries. An employer had an obligation to pay for worksite-related illnesses as well as compensate for lost time.

- *1900–1917:* State health insurance plans were proposed by several state legislatures. Most proposals mandated employment-based health insurance. None of the proposals passed because labor unions opposed government health insurance. Unions were suspicious of government because government had supported management (sometimes with army troops) in a number of large, violent strikes. In addition, in **World War I (WWI)** the United States was fighting Germany, which had a similar employment-based insurance system—not a good selling point. We did not want to emulate Germany's social system when we were at war with them!

- *1917:* There was a change in the American Medical Association (AMA) leadership from academic- to community-based physicians that motivated the AMA to act more like a labor union. United States entered World War I in April 1917, and it ended November 1918.

- *The 1920s:* After World War I, a time of general prosperity, politically it was not the time to push for national health insurance because the health care system was working well for those who were not poor ("if it ain't broke, don't fix it"). Furthermore, the poor, historically, "have not counted" in politics because they are less likely to vote and do not contribute to politicians' campaigns.

- *1929–1939:* The **Great Depression** left many people unable to pay medical bills. During this time, private health insurance such as Blue Cross/Blue Shield (BCBS) emerged. The AMA opposed private health insurance because they felt that it intruded into the patient–doctor relationship. Hospitals, however, supported the concept because it helped assure that they would be paid.

- *1932:* President Roosevelt proposed the New Deal program to establish government programs to deal with the suffering of the Great Depression. The Social Security Act (SSA) of 1935, which was signed by Roosevelt, provided benefits to the retired, the disabled, and the poor. A national health insurance plan was part of the initial draft of the SSA, but it was never submitted because Roosevelt knew that the AMA would oppose it, and the passage of the SSA would not be passed because of it.

  - However, **World War II (WWII)**—and *not* the New Deal program—was primarily responsible for raising the United States out of the Great Depression.

- *1939:* The National Health Bill was proposed, which mandated that employers provide comprehensive health insurance to workers. This proposed mandate seemed to open the opportunity for national health insurance. However, the bill was not passed. In September 1939, WWII began and interest in national health insurance was once again tabled.

- *World War II 1939–1945:* The American involvement in World War II focused the nation's attention and resources on winning the war and not on passing a national health care insurance legislation.

- *1946–1952:* President Harry S. Truman gives the first Presidential Health Address to the United States (1946). With President Truman as a proponent of national health insurance, again it appeared that national health insurance was near. At this time, England had adopted its National Health Service, and the United States passed the Hill-Burton Act that supported the construction of hospitals.

  - This period was characterized by a concern about the spread of communism, the McCarthy Era; in addition, the United States entered the Korean War in which the Communist Chinese played a pivotal role. The AMA successfully campaigned against NHI, equating it with socialized medicine and communism.

- *The 1950s:* The 1950s was also a time of prosperity, and the United States was viewed as a "horn of plenty" where sentiment for helping the less fortunate was paramount in our society. Our nation's "social conscience" was directed at the poor and the inequalities in access to health care. The United States initiated the development of social programs to address these issues. The Eisenhower presidency saw the start of these programs, and President Kennedy expanded these efforts particularly for the poor and elderly, but his shortened presidency did not provide sufficient time for substantive legislation to be passed. President Johnson who succeeded President Kennedy envisioned the Great Society. In 1965, Medicare and Medicaid programs were passed into law as part of that Great Society social program.

- *1968–1978:* Many politicians expressed significant interest in national health insurance legislation. The resulting proposals were highly comprehensive in nature. One of which was the National Health Service Act proposed by Congressman Ronald V. Dellums (1935–) in 1977. The National Health Service Act of 1977 was the most liberal/egalitarian program in that it would have established a national health service like the United Kingdom's. This proposal received little support, and most Democrats and labor unions were backing national health insurance based somewhat on the Medicare model.

- The Health Security Act of 1970, supported by Senators Kennedy and Griffith, was proposed, which would have established a single payer system like Canada's and would have eliminated private health insurance. It proposed first-dollar coverage, no copays, deductibles, or coinsurance. This legislation marked the starting point of Senator Ted Kennedy's long time involvement in health policy issues.

  President Nixon countered with a proposal that was endorsed by the AMA, AHA, and the HIAA. It mandated employment-based private health insurance. President Jimmy Carter proposed the nationalization/federalization of Medicaid and a catastrophic coverage plan.

  In 1970 Senators Long and Ribicoff proposed catastrophic health insurance. This type of coverage would deploy after an individual's expenses exceeded some substantial amount. It was intended to save people from financial disaster if they faced a major illness. This proposed coverage was considered the most libertarian or conservative proposal.

  None of the above proposals passed. Not coincidentally, at this time many reevaluated the 1950s perception of the United States as a "horn of plenty" and began to realize that as a nation we could simply not afford to "fix" all social problems. In fact, in the early 1970s, we began to be increasingly concerned about the rapidly exploding cost of a number of the Great Society social programs, including Medicare and Medicaid.

- *1980–1992:* During the Reagan and Bush years, there were no new major health care programs that significantly increased access to care. Instead, these presidents focused on reigning in health care cost and expenditures, especially for Medicare and Medicaid. The philosophy espoused to achieve cost containment was based on encouraging private competition with minimal government involvement (regulation). This policy was implemented in the repeal of federal laws on Certificate of Need (CON). Thus, the Reagan and Bush administrations concentrated on controlling cost and deregulation—not on increased access. *Satisfaction with health care ranked high among the U.S. population during this time.*

- *The early 1990s:* The Pennsylvania Senate race between Harris Wafford and former Pennsylvania Governor Richard (Dick) Thornberg drew national attention. Wafford was the underdog but won the race on a political platform that focused in large part on national health care issues. This Senate win sent a signal to other politicians during the 1992 elections. Moreover, for the first time health care was ranked number one in the top 10 concerns of the public.

  - The Democrats embraced the mantle of reform of the health care system. After his victory, President Clinton proposed a very aggressive plan called the Health Security Act described below. Soon after, substantial concern was voiced from many factions that this legislation would curtail freedom of choice of providers as well as have dire consequences for businesses and employment, especially small businesses, because it would substantially increase the cost of doing business.

The main elements of the Clinton Health Reform Plan:

1. Universal coverage for all citizens and residents

2. Coverage provided through employment-mandated plans

3. Coverage purchased through alliances and subsidies

4. Benefits: federally defined minimum coverage

5. Choice: choice of plan rather than choice of provider; individuals prohibited by law from seeking care outside of their alliance

6. Financing through payroll taxes and employer/employee contributions

7. Other programs eventually incorporated into plan

Problems with the Clinton Health Reform Plan:

1. Limited freedom of choice (provider)—the dominant reason for the proposed plan's failure

2. An estimated minimum of 750,000 lost jobs

3. Substantial costs

4. Increased bureaucracy

5. Soon after its introduction, a sharp drop in public support (as well as political support from Clinton's own party)

- Health care, as an issue, had not been at or near the top 10 concerns of the public until the past decade. Even then, it has consistently ranked below such issues as the economy, crime, education, and more recently, national security. The major health care concern among the American people is its cost. The American public expressed an unwillingness to forego spending on other important issues to pay for comprehensive health care.

  To embark on major change in American society, there needs to be a substantial outcry for such change and a willingness to pay for the change. Although many people indicate (in public opinion polls) that they are not satisfied with the health care system, they generally indicate that they are satisfied with their personal doctor, hospital, and health insurance. A consensus seems to be, "We need to change health care in America, but *my* health care is okay."

- *1996:* Health Insurance Portability and Accountability Act (HIPAA)

  1. HIPAA Health Insurance Reform

  - Title I of the Health Insurance Portability and Accountability Act of 1996 (HIPAA) protects health insurance coverage of workers and their families when they change or lose their jobs.

  2. HIPAA Administrative Simplification

  - The Administrative Simplification provisions of the Health Insurance Portability and Accountability Act of 1996 (HIPAA, Title II) require the

Department of Health and Human Services to establish national standards for electronic health care transactions and national health care markers for providers, health plans, and employers. It also addresses the security and privacy of health data. Adopting these standards will improve the efficiency and effectiveness of the nation's health care system by encouraging the widespread use of electronic data interchange of health information. However, some are concerned that privacy cannot be guaranteed, and the risk of confidential information falling into the wrong hands is markedly increased. In addition, many clinicians are not prepared nor can they afford to capitalize such a transfer of records from paper to paperless. They argue that practices would be disrupted for months. Still others contend that systems are unable to communicate with each other and therefore cannot meet the ultimate objective. A final shortcoming of HIPAA is that it does not help the uninsured and has time-limited exclusions.

■ The Patient Protection and Affordable Care Act, 2010

On March 23, 2010, President Obama signed into law the Patient Protection and Affordable Care Act (PPACA), intended to provide affordable health care for all Americans and reduce the growth in health care costs. The new legislation focused on the health care insurance industry and established requirements of coverage for citizens. It requires most U.S. citizens and legal residents to have health insurance by 2014.

The legislation bars all existing insurance plans from imposing lifetime caps on coverage six months after its passage. Restrictions will also be placed on annual limits on coverage. Insurers can no longer cancel insurance retroactively for reasons other than outright fraud (KFF, 2011). Parents will be allowed to keep their children on their health insurance plan until age 26, unless the child is eligible for coverage through employer-sponsored health insurance. Insurance plans cannot exclude preexisting health care conditions from coverage for children under age 19, although insurers could still reject those children outright for coverage in the individual market until 2014 (KFF, 2011).

■ Health Care Reform by 2014

By 2014, the legislation creates health exchanges for individuals to purchase coverage, with premium and credits available to individuals and families with low incomes. Low-income individuals and families are defined as households with 133–400 percent of the federal poverty level. Specifically, the poverty level is $18,310 for a family of three in 2009 (KFF, 2011).

Health exchanges are created so that small businesses can purchase coverage for their employees. If employees do not receive health insurance from their employer, the employer is required to pay penalties, with exceptions for small employers (KFF, 2011). The legislation also expanded Medicaid to cover citizens whose income and assets were at 133 percent of the federal poverty level (KFF, 2011).

The legislation requires U.S. citizens and legal residents to have qualifying health care insurance or pay a tax by 2014. Exemptions will apply based on financial hardship or religious reasons, but the penalty will steadily increase after 2014 (KFF, 2011). In 2014, employers with more than 50 employees will be required to provide insurance for their employees or pay a fee (KFF, 2011).

The bill expands Medicaid to cover all individuals under age 65, including children, pregnant women, parents, and adults without dependent children, with incomes up to 133% federal poverty level (FPL) (KFF, 2011). Those that are newly eligible for Medicaid coverage will be provided a basic package of essential health benefits, and the federal government will fund the new services. The legislation requires states to continue their current levels of funding for their Children's Health Insurance Program (CHIP) (KFF, 2011). By 2014, most people will be required to have health insurance or face penalties (KFF, 2011).

Tax credits would be provided to small businesses with no more than 25 employees that provide health insurance for their employees. The ultimate goal of the bill is to provide coverage for 32 million more people by 2019 (KFF, 2011).

▪ Benefits for the Uninsured

One of the primary stakeholders in the health industry to be affected by the legislation are the uninsured. Under the legislation, most Americans would have to have insurance by 2014 or pay a penalty. The penalty would start at $95, or up to one percent of income, whichever is greater, and rise to $695, or 2.5 percent of income, by 2016. This cap is an individual limit; families have a limit of $2,085 (KFF, 2011).

However, depending on income levels, the uninsured person may be eligible for Medicaid, the state-federal program for the poor and disabled, which would be expanded beginning in 2014. Low-income adults, including those without children, would be eligible, as long as their incomes did not exceed 133 percent of the federal poverty level, or $14,404 for individuals and $29,326 for a family of four, according to current poverty guidelines (KFF, 2011).

Those persons that did not qualify for Medicaid may be eligible for government subsidies to help pay for private insurance that would be sold in the new state-based insurance marketplaces, called exchanges, to begin operation in 2014. Premium subsidies would be available for individuals and families with incomes between 133 percent and 400 percent of the poverty level, or $14,404 to $43,320 for individuals and $29,326 to $88,200 for a family of four (KFF, 2011).

▪ Benefits for Those with Preexisting Conditions

The PPACA was enacted to address the fact that many people are not able to afford health insurance once they have a health care condition. The legislation makes it easier to purchase health care insurance coverage because insurers would be barred from rejecting applicants based on health status once the exchanges are operating in 2014 (KFF, 2011). In the meantime, temporary high-risk insurance pools have been created for people with health problems who have been rejected by insurers and have been uninsured at least six months (KFF, 2011).

The legislation prohibits insurers from excluding coverage for specific health problems for children with preexisting conditions, lifetime coverage limits for adults and kids are banned. In 2014, annual limits on coverage would be banned (KFF, 2011). New policies sold on the exchanges would be required to cover a range of benefits, including hospitalizations, doctor visits, prescription drugs, maternity care, and certain preventive tests.

In summary, the main elements of the Patient Protection and Affordable Care Act (PPACA) include:

- Expand coverage to 32 million uninsured and establish state-based exchanges for uninsured and self-employed to purchase insurance.

- Expand Medicare Payroll Tax.

- Impose excise tax paid by insurance companies for "Cadillac plans."

- Close Medicare Part D prescription drug "donut hole."

- Insurance companies can no longer deny coverage for preexisting conditions.

- Children can stay on parents' plan until age 26.

- Everyone must purchase insurance or face a fine.

- Illegal immigrants are not permitted to purchase insurance.

- Expand Medicaid by lowering income eligibility level.

Despite its passage in a Democrat-controlled Congress and White House, a sizable percent of citizens are dissatisfied with the plan and a number want it repealed. Several states have attempted to appeal the law's constitutionality in the courts, arguing that the Constitution prohibits forcing Americans to purchase insurance or face a penalty. Others believe that the law did not go far enough, by excluding some uninsured and illegal immigrants.

Problems with PPACA include:

- There is limited freedom of choice of provider.

- Costs would be substantial.

- The plan would increase bureaucracy for national care decision making.

- There is no evidence that Medicare savings are attainable.

- Requiring all to be insured or face penalty may be unconstitutional.

- A sizable portion will remain uninsured.

- Increasing access for 32 million will have a negative impact on cost and quality.

- Care would be rationed.

- Increasing Medicare payroll tax could have consequences for recession recovery.

The outcome of PPACA remains in doubt, with much depending on the 2012 election and also the fact that many of its stipulations do not take effect until 2014. What will happen, few can predict. The preponderance of evidence shows that our current spending trajectory for the entitlement programs of Medicare and Medicaid are unsustainable, and the history of avoiding legislation that modifies these entitlement programs is ending.

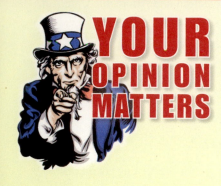

Should the United States Adopt National Health Insurance?

Yes

Franklin Delano Roosevelt first proposed a recognized right to health care in his Economic Bill of Rights. Among the economic rights President Roosevelt proposed was, "The right to adequate medical care and the opportunity to achieve and enjoy good health. . . ." (Roosevelt, 1944). Although the Economic Bill of Rights was never enacted into law, it played a primary role in the development of International law. The Universal Declaration of Human Rights (UDHR), developed by the United Nations with U.S. guidance, was adopted in 1948. Among its provisions are these:

> Everyone has the right to a standard of living adequate for the health and well-being of himself and of his family, including food, clothing, housing, and *medical care* and necessary social services, and the right to security in the event of unemployment, sickness, disability, widowhood, old age or other lack of livelihood in circumstances beyond his control. (Carmalt & Zaidi, 2004, emphasis added)

Some legal scholars argue that this declaration should be legally binding on the United States by virtue of "customary international law or as an authoritative interpretation of the U.N. Charter" (Carmalt & Zaidi, 2004). Although the United States does not officially recognize the right to health care enumerated in the UDHR, all other industrialized nations have established a right to health care and provided systems for universal access to health care. Again, as some believe, as founding nation and member of the United Nations, the United States should do the same.

We should have a right to health care in the United States because access to health care services is essential to keep Americans healthy. No one should be deprived of basic necessities such as food, housing, and health care. Guaranteeing health care for our citizens will result in a healthier, more productive workforce. In addition, it will prove to other nations that we have a commitment to upholding basic human rights. Finally, citizens of the United States agree. Polls have consistently shown overwhelming support for a right to health care since at least 1993.

No

Some national health insurance (NHI) proponents demonize insurance companies and argue that NHI with a single payer would solve these problems. Others contend that it is the current government regulation of insurance companies that has limited their number and that a system with a single payer would make it only worse. It is the free market with a proliferation of insurance companies, where customers could take their business elsewhere, which would guarantee cost-conscious, inexpensive coverage.

In addition, NHI will drive up the costs of health care while decreasing access and quality. By limiting freedom of choice, patients will be forced to ration the care they receive. By providing insurance for a vast number of currently uninsured persons, with the current supply of clinicians, access to care, choice of provider, and choice of procedure will be reduced. If a fixed number of clinicians are required to provide greater access to more patients, then the time and thus the quality of the care they provide will suffer. We know the history of government intervention into health care by observing Medicare and Medicaid. By increasing access to millions, both programs have suffered from runaway cost increases with mounting levels of waste, fraud, and abuse. Asking government to take on a greater share will only exacerbate an already existing crisis in rising health care costs.

Although some polls show that Americans think health care is a right, other polls indicate that most Americans are very happy with the doctor they have and the health care they receive. There is a history of citizens of developed countries with nationalized health care coming to the United States for elective surgery and other procedures. U.S. health care is considered the finest in the world for those looking for the latest treatments. Some argue that nationalizing the U.S. health care system will create long waiting times for treatment and ultimately reduce incentives for innovation.

Health policy analysts have enumerated the problems inherent in national systems like that of the United Kingdom and Canada that Americans would find objectionable. The NHS has been accused of using administrative procedures, like waiting lists, to queue patient care on the basis of clinical need, and patients did in fact suffer health consequences from waiting.

Moreover, the NHS and the Canadian health care system are systems for delivering care, while health care itself is essentially a private matter between doctor and patient. Some criticize the Canadian system as delivering poorer quality care. Access to health care technologies is relatively poor in Canada, and Canadians struggle with a relatively small inventory of health care technologies. At the same time, much of Canada's limited inventory of technologies is old, outdated, and in need of replacement (Esmail & Wrona, 2008).

You decide:

1. Does the "pursuit of happiness" guarantee government health care for everyone, or does it afford the right to obtain health care in any way that free individuals see fit?

2. Do the assets of a free market outweigh its liabilities?

3. What are the assets of the free market approach of the U.S. health care system?

4. What are the cost and access problems of the U.S. health care system?

▪ Reasons for Interest in National Health Insurance

There are several important reasons for contemporary interest in national health insurance. The cost of health care delivery has been increasing every year for the past decade. There continue to be gaps in health insurance coverage for services and sub-populations. The geographical maldistribution of health care personnel and facilities persists. Access to service is determined by a patient's ability to pay, social class, age, and geography. It is argued that national health insurance, or lack thereof, will affect the health status of the nation significantly.

▪ National Health Insurance—the Major Issues

The national health insurance debate is multifaceted; there are no correct or incorrect answers, just political, philosophical, and economic decisions that must be made. Trade-offs between spending on health care versus spending on other issues, coupled with overall reductions in national spending, have to be addressed, which likely will result in compromises from all stakeholders.

Should all persons have a right to health care in this country? Some say no. This question can best be answered by separating it into three questions. Do we (or should we) have a right to health? Do we have a right to the provision of health care services? Do we have a right to health care insurance?

First, do we have a right to health? Some would say yes, or that we at least have the right to the pursuit of health. The Declaration of Independence states, "We hold these truths to be self-evident, that all men are created equal, that they are endowed by their Creator with certain unalienable Rights, that among these are Life, Liberty and the pursuit of Happiness. —That to secure these rights, Governments are instituted among Men, deriving their just powers from the consent of the governed. ..."

Therefore, if we have a right to health, it is because it is an inherent, unalienable right, such as life, liberty, property (recognized in the Constitution and recently hotly debated by the Supreme Court) and the pursuit of happiness. The Declaration of Independence did not name *all* unalienable rights, but it is reasonable to tie the right to the pursuit of health to the right to the pursuit of happiness. The government helps "secure" the right to the pursuit of health largely through its public health efforts (e.g., sanitation and clean water).

However, just as the Declaration of Independence does not guarantee the right to happiness (only the pursuit of it), the government is not bound by the Declaration of Independence to guarantee the right to a minimum level of health. We do have the right to pursue good health in any legal way that we choose. For example, we can seek health care or preventive treatments or many forms of alternative and complementary medicine, but cannot choose to smoke marijuana for pain relief because it is deemed illegal (unless prescribed by a physician and only in some states).

According to the Declaration of Independence and other documents written by the Founding Fathers, governments or republics (as we have in the United States) *do not* bestow rights on their citizens. The government cannot *give* its citizens the right to anything; they either have that right or they do not. It is the role of government to either protect those rights (i.e., secure them) or have no role at all. These rights—life, liberty, property, and the pursuit of happiness—are known as liberty rights "because they protect our right to *act* freely" (Kelley, n.d., author emphasis). Note that the emphasis is on action, as stated by Kelley:

> The wording of the Declaration of Independence is quite precise in this regard. It attributes to us the right to the pursuit of happiness, not to happiness per se. Society can't guarantee us happiness; that's our own responsibility. All it can guarantee is the freedom to pursue it. In the same way, the right to life is the right to act freely for one's self-preservation. It is not a right to be immune from death by natural causes, even an untimely death. And the right to property is the right to act freely in the effort to acquire wealth, the right to buy and sell and keep the fruits of one's labor. It is not a right to expect to be given wealth. (Kelley, n.d.)

So do we have a right to health care? Is obtaining health care equivalent to a pursuit of health? Some may answer no. As stated previously, part of the right to health or pursuit of health, is to be able to choose to seek health care treatment. Nothing bars us from seeking health care, and in the case of life-threatening emergencies, no one can be turned away from a hospital emergency room for inability to pay. In fact, in 2004, $41 billion of the $125 billion spent on personal health care by the uninsured was provided free of charge (KFF, 2004).

Nevertheless, health care is a business, a service that is provided to people by trained professionals to enhance a current level of health or return to a previous state of healthiness. As such, we must and should pay for health care rather than insisting that doctors give care for "free" or that it be paid for by the government. When we pay for health care, among other things, we pay the salaries of those who work in health care, which is about 1 in every 10 people. We pay for the technology used to diagnose and treat.

We pay for training of physicians and other health care providers. We pay for research and development of new health care technologies. Fewer people would have jobs in health care if we did not pay for health care, and such care might not be available when we chose to obtain it. Similarly, part of the right to pursue health is to be able to choose *not* to seek treatment.

In addition, the right to health care is still separate from the right to health insurance. Is health insurance part of the right to the pursuit of health? Health insurance is a mechanism to help pay for health care. This mechanism as it has evolved today is a contributor to rising health care costs. Health insurance is also the primary method we have used to expand access to health care. Medicaid gives the eligible poor a vehicle to pay for health care; Medicare helps the elderly pay for health care.

Arguably, this country did not have a health care cost crisis until the government and employers started providing for health care insurance through companies like Blue Cross/Blue Shield. Health insurance shields the patient from the true price of the purchase of health care services. If patients had to pay the full price, they would only choose those health care services that were necessary. Therefore, the mechanism that we use to expand access to health care leads to an increase in cost, which leads to a greater need for health insurance. Some argue that a government-run national health insurance program would only exacerbate this cycle of spiraling health care costs.

In sum, the Declaration of Independence does bestow the right to the pursuit of health—although the word *health* is not mentioned—and it is our responsibility to maximize our health in ways we see fit. We may choose to engage in healthy behaviors or seek care for acute illnesses. Conversely and perversely, we also have the right to be destructive toward our own health. We can choose to smoke or drink, eat poorly, not exercise, and not wear seat belts. It is our choice. It is the government's duty to protect those choices, not to ensure that everyone obtains a certain amount of health care. When personal destructive behaviors infringe on others, then the government has a duty to protect others from harm. The government has a duty to protect the right to health for others, even though they may impinge on another person's rights. This right is the justification behind laws that make certain drug possession and distribution illegal, or prohibit smoking in public, or impose harsh sentences for driving under the influence.

The question remains, do we—or should we—have a right to health care? Some may answer yes. The Declaration of Independence does not specify all rights, but only minimal rights that the Founding Fathers sought to protect at the time are enumerated. In our nation, and internationally, individuals and countries have recognized that human rights and civil rights exist along with the natural, or liberty, rights enumerated in the Constitution. Human and civil rights have evolved from liberty rights and continue to evolve as society changes. These rights include the right to vote, the right to education, the rights of disabled persons to education, and the right to health care.

The right to a public education evolved over time. The first attempts to institute mandatory education came at the state level between 1770 and 1830 (Right to Health Care, 2005). By the early 1900s, all states had compulsory education laws. Today, all children in the United States have the right to a public primary and secondary education, regardless of legal status (citizen, resident alien, illegal alien). This right evolved over 200 years but is well established today. Similarly, the right to vote has evolved over time. When the Constitution was ratified in 1789, only property-holding white men over the age of 21 were permitted to vote.

Other barriers such as religious tests, racial restrictions, literacy tests, and poll taxes were implemented, only to be abolished over time. The religious tests faded in the early 1800s, and the property holding requirements were abolished by the mid-1800s. Former slaves and their descendants gained suffrage in 1870 (in fact, all races gained the right to vote at that time), women in 1920, and adults between the ages of 18 and 21 in 1971. Throughout the 1960s, most other barriers to voting were abolished, culminating with passage of the Voting Rights Act of 1965 (Turner Learning, 2001). Once again, the right to vote that is exercised today took almost 200 years to fully evolve.

The Constitution of the United States of America and Health Care

Interpreting the United States Constitution and determining the "constitutionality" of state and federal laws is largely the responsibility of the federal court system and, in particular, the Supreme Court of the United States. There are five generally recognized schools of thought regarding how the Constitution should be interpreted: Originalism/Original intent, Modernism/Instrumentalism, Literalism—historical, Literalism—contemporary, and Democratic/Normative reinforcement (United States Constitution.net).

Originalism/Original intent is the belief that the Constitution should be interpreted as the Framers (Founding Fathers) intended. Originalists use writings by the Framers around the time that the Constitution was drafted, such as the *Federalist Papers* (written by Alexander Hamilton, James Madison, and John Jay), correspondence, newspapers, and even notes taken during the Constitutional Convention to support their interpretation of the Framers' intent.

Modernism/Instrumentalism is the belief that the Constitution should be interpreted as it applies to today's standards and situations. Modernists believe that the "Constitution becomes stale and irrelevant to modern life if only viewed through 18th century eyes" and that the Framers intentionally left the Constitution vague so that it could evolve with society. Modernists believe that the "Constitution is flexible and dynamic, changing slowly over time as the morals and beliefs of the population shift." This thinking is often referred to as the "Living Constitution" view (http://www.USConstitution.net). This view is best illustrated by a quote from former Associate Justice William J. Brennan, Jr., who stated, "We look to the history of the time of framing and to the intervening history of interpretation. But the ultimate question must be what do the words of the text mean in our time" (http://www.BrainyQuote.com).

Literalism—historical is the belief that only the literal words of the Constitution and their meaning in the eighteenth century can be used to interpret the Constitution. Historical literalism differs from Originalism in that it does not permit reference to the writings and thoughts of the Framers. This belief is often referred to as the "strict constructionist" view. A corollary of this thinking is to define words according to a "reasonable" construction, or the meaning of a text apart from anyone's intent, sometimes called textualism.

Literalism—contemporary is the belief that only the literal words of the Constitution can be used to interpret the Constitution, but this school of thought uses modern or contemporary definitions of those words.

Democratic/Normative reinforcement is the belief that the "Constitution is not designed to be a set of specific principles and guidelines, but that it was designed to be a general principle, a basic skeleton on which contemporary vision would be built. Decisions about the meaning of the Constitution must consider the general feeling evoked by the Constitution, and then use modern realism to add flesh to the skeleton." (http://www.USConstitution.net).

The following discussion utilizes the Historical Literalism view as an illustration of the use of the Constitution to address the formulation and implementation of health policy.

Historical Literalist View

A recent comment by sitting U.S. Supreme Court Justice Antonin Scalia embodies the Historical Literalist perspective. He stated:

> The Constitution says what it says and does not say what it does not say. Text is to be given the same meaning and same application to facts as it had when it was adopted. . . . Where the original meaning or application of the text cannot be determined, it should be interpreted and applied as it is reflected in the traditional practices of the American people. (Ave Maria School of Law: Events)

The Preamble to the Constitution states:

> We the People of the United States, in Order to form a more perfect Union, establish Justice, insure domestic Tranquility, provide for the common defense, promote the general Welfare, and secure the Blessings of Liberty to ourselves and our Posterity, do ordain and establish this Constitution for the United States of America.

Several of the phrases in the preamble can be used to rationalize government programs in defense as well as health care and the development of health policy. The strongest constitutional justifications for government involvement seem to come from its mission to provide for the common defense. Programs to combat bioterrorism, although not a new mechanism of warfare, have gained more attention since September 11, 2001, and the anthrax attacks that followed. Two agencies of government, the United States Army Medical Research Institute for Infectious Diseases (USAMRIID) and the Centers for Disease Control and Prevention (CDC), have actively engaged in the search for strategies to combat bioterrorism. These agencies' missions are derived from the constitution's promise to provide for the common defense.

The United States and state and local governments use the phrase "promote the general Welfare" to rationalize their development of public health policies and interventions. State and local health departments promote the general welfare by providing sanitation (e.g., sewage treatment plants, drinking water filtration, food-handling regulations), controlling communicable diseases (including vaccinations), promoting health and education, and delivering preventive health services (screenings for certain diseases).

However, many argue that none of these phrases in the preamble justify programs such as Medicare and Medicaid—that promoting the general welfare should not be so broadly interpreted as to encompass providing health insurance for the elderly and poor.

Here, we outline the general process of making law at the federal level, often used to promote health policy agendas.

Article 1.

Section 7. All Bills for raising revenue shall originate in the House of Representatives, but the Senate may propose or concur with Amendments as on other bills.

Every bill . . . .

When government needs to raise revenue to fund its health care programs, such bills must be introduced in the House of Representatives.

Section 8. The Congress shall have power to lay and collect taxes, duties, impost, excises, to pay the debts and provide for the common defense and general welfare of the United States, but all duties, imposts and excises shall be uniform throughout the United States.

This section gives Congress the authority to raise or create taxes to pay for health care programs (e.g., FICA).

To promote the progress of Science and useful Arts, by securing for limited times to authors and inventors the exclusive right to their respective writings and discoveries (patents).

This section justifies funding NIH programs for health care and social science research and for allotting pharmaceutical and equipment companies patent protection.

To make all laws which shall be necessary and proper for carrying into execution the foregoing powers and all other powers vested by this Constitution in the Government of the United States, or in any Department or Office thereof.

This section gives Congress the power to enact laws. For example, to promote the general welfare, Congress enacted the Social Security Act of 1935 and its related amendments (among which are Medicare and Medicaid). However, many believe these programs are a modernist interpretation of promoting the general welfare.

> Article II.
>
> Section 2. He shall have power, by and with advice and consent of the Senate, to make treaties . . . . shall appoint Ambassadors, other public Ministers and Consuls, Judges of the Supreme Court, and all other Officers of the United States whose appointments are not herein otherwise provided for. . . .

This section gives the president the authority to appoint judges to the Supreme Court and lower federal courts and nominate cabinet members, such as the Secretary of the Department of Health and Human Services. This clause has had a substantial impact on health policy because of the courts' involvement in defining health policy.

> Section 3. He shall from time to time give to the Congress information on the State of the Union, and recommend to their consideration such measures as he shall judge necessary and expedient. . . .

This clause gives the president the power to set a legislative or policy agenda. Through the State of the Union speech, the president reports to Congress on the performance of the country during the previous year and discusses what the president intends to propose for the upcoming year. The president and executive branch can also prepare bills that are then submitted by a "friendly" congressman. Although Congress makes the laws, this clause gives the president authority to develop and direct policy, including health policy.

> Article III.
>
> Section 1. The judicial power of the United States shall be vested in one Supreme Court and in such inferior Courts as the Congress may from time to time ordain and establish.

This section established the judicial branch, but it does not define the power of the judicial branch. It was not until President Jefferson's term that the power of the judiciary was defined through the court case *Marbury v. Madison* (1803). *Marbury v. Madison* is credited with establishing judicial review (i.e., the court is able to deem a law unconstitutional). (For a discussion of *Marbury v. Madison*, see http://ourdocuments .gov/doc.php?flash=true&doc=19.)

> Section 2. The judicial power shall extend to all cases in law and equity, arising under this Constitution, the laws of the United States, and Treaties made, or which shall be made, under their authority; —to all cases affecting Ambassadors, other public ministers and consuls; —to all cases of Admiralty and maritime Jurisdiction; —to controversies to which the United States shall be a party; —to controversies between two or more States; —between citizens of different states; —between citizens of the same state claiming lands under grants of different states, and between a state, or the citizens thereof, and foreign States, Citizens or Subjects.

This section describes what types of cases fall under the federal judiciary. For example, if a person or organization sues the Department of Health and Human Services or its secretary, the case belongs in the federal courts. However, if a person or organization sues a company for malpractice it does not enter federal court because such litigants are not covered in this section of the Constitution.

Article V.

The Congress, whenever two thirds of both Houses shall deem it necessary, shall propose Amendments to this Constitution, or, on the Application of the Legislatures of two thirds of the several States, shall call a Convention for proposing Amendments, which in either Care, shall be valid to all Intents and Purposes, as Part of this Constitution. . . .

This article gives Congress and states the rights to amend the Constitution. The 18th Amendment (Prohibition), a form of public health policy, became part of the Constitution for 24 years. Other amendments address aspects of health policy such as: 5th, 7th, 9th, 10th, 11th, part of the 14th, 16th, 18th, and 21st.

The 10th Amendment is especially important because it states: "The powers not delegated to the United States by the Constitution, nor prohibited by it to the States, are reserved to the States respectively, or to the people.

This amendment clearly states that the powers that are attributed to the federal government in the Constitution are all that the federal government should have. The rest of the powers belong to the states, or to U.S. citizens. This amendment was intended to limit the role of the federal government. Some argue that judicial review and further amendments to the Constitution have extended the federal role and have diluted the intent of the 10th Amendment to a certain extent.

▪ Considerations Regarding National Health Insurance

The following are issues that must be considered when debating the passage of national health insurance.

▪ Who Should Be Covered?

- **The Poor:** Covering just the poor would cost less than covering everyone; the rich can draw on their own resources, but the poor may have no alternative if public funding is not available. Would this financing scheme produce two classes of health care? The British fund 5 percent of their health care bill from the wealthy, who pay directly for their health care. Are Americans comfortable with formalizing a two-class health care system where some individuals receive higher quality care based on ability to pay?

- **Employment Based:** The Social Security System in part protects individuals from poverty, but entitlements are based on what individuals have paid in taxes on earned income. Therefore, poor individuals will never receive as much Social Security as wealthier individuals. If insurance is employment based, how does the program address the self-employed and permanently disabled?

- **Voluntary versus Compulsory:** In a voluntary system, are we prepared to let those who choose not to pay into the system, become ill or die? What about those who do not fall into any predefined category—do we have coverage for them, for instance, foreign visitors, young unemployed, and both legal and illegal immigrants? From an administrative cost perspective, it might be more expedient to make the system compulsory.

- **Equity:** Universal coverage regardless of family composition, employability, or Social Security contribution not only seems most equitable but could also be more efficient and effective. For example, administrative costs would be lower than they are currently because everyone is eligible and benefits are specified.

What Services Should Be Covered?

A national health insurance plan must determine priorities for coverage of certain health care services. Important choices must be made between services that are known to be effective with demonstrable outcomes (e.g., prenatal care, immunizations) and services that can substantially avoid personal significant financial burden (e.g., hospitalizations, specialists' fees, management of chronic illness).

Priorities would need to be assigned to essential services such as cancer treatments and cardiovascular surgery. As a nation we would need to decide between acceptable lower cost substitutes for high-cost procedures (e.g., physician services versus physician assistant or nurse practitioner care; hospital services versus emergency care facility [ECF]). We would need to place special emphasis on special cases such as outreach services for the uneducated poor or those with special risks.

Vignette

HOW DO WE REDUCE COSTS DURING THE LAST SIX MONTHS OF LIFE?

Mr. Arnold Sanford, an 88-year-old retired lawyer, lived a reasonably carefree life until his retirement at age 70, when his primary care provider noticed a significant rise in his serum cholesterol level. Mr. Sanford then began a regimen of anti-cholesterol medication, and he and his wife dramatically changed their lifestyles. They became very conscious of food intake and increased their consumption of fruits and vegetables. They reduced their intake of sugary desserts and pastries, fatty sauces and dressing, and red meat. They began playing doubles tennis on a regular basis, either in the warmer Florida climate or at their home in Long Island, New York. He and his wife experienced more than a decade of healthy retirement with managed cholesterol levels.

At age 83, while traveling to Florida in November, Mr. Sanford suffered a stroke. After months of rehabilitation both in a facility in Florida and then in his home, he was able to resume some normal activities but was not strong enough to resume tennis as part of his routine. For four years, Mr. Sanford fought to regain his former health status but experienced several setbacks. He continued to lose strength as he felt weaker and shorter of breath. Some of the weight that he had lost crept back. At age 88, he was diagnosed with congestive heart failure and was prescribed the conventional drugs, including diuretics, to assist his weakened heart with removing fluids.

Mr. Sanford and his wife had completed medical advance directives and other end-of-life documents that made it clear that should they reach a certain point and were unable to make decisions, heroic life-saving procedures should *not* be considered. Among those procedures was being kept alive on a ventilator or feeding tube. They made it clear that if any uncertainties arose in interpreting the living will, a health care proxy, and no one else, was to make final decisions. A copy of the directives was given to each of their relatives as well as to their physicians.

During Mr. Sanford's hospital stay for stroke, his wife provided the facility with a copy. Mrs. Sanford and their only son were clear that Mr. Sanford preferred to die in his home without technological heroics. Such advance directives, if broadly adopted, can ease the emotional pressure on the surviving families and dramatically reduce overall health care costs to society.

One day, while watching television at home, Mr. Sanford experienced significant distress. Mrs. Sanford called her internist, who suggested that she call 911 for an ambulance and that he would meet the Sanford's at the hospital. Mr. Sanford was rushed to the ICU, and hospital cardiologists attended to him, later consulting with the family internist. The cardiologists had installed dopamine shunts and were trying to reduce the build-up of fluid in Mr. Sanford's lungs. After, several hours, the cardiologists received test results and learned that Mr. Sanford's kidney capacity was only 25 percent, and there were limited options for treatment. The cardiologists consulted with Mr. Sanford's advanced directive and, in keeping with his and his family's wishes, did not engage in any further invasive or heroic live-saving procedures. His blood pressure was sinking, and Mrs. Sanford and her son bid their good-byes to an unconscious Mr. Sanford. Just one hour later, Mrs. Sanford and her son received a call from the hospital and learned that Mr. Sanford had just died.

1. How effective are advance directives when doctors are making on-the-spot decisions with less than full information?

2. When can the family intervene to assure the advance directive wishes?

3. Although dying in the hospital is very expensive, is it avoidable through use of advanced directives?

4. Although dying in the hospital is very expensive, would you want it any other way for *your* loved one?

5. Have you had a conversation with your elderly loved ones regarding their end-of-life care preferences? Have those wishes been documented in advanced directives?

■ Should Patients Share in Costs?

A national health insurance plan must include a cost-sharing structure for patients. The questions that such a plan should address include:

- Should all patients share in costs of all services?

- Should level of charges be the same for all patients?

- If there is coinsurance and deductibles, should supplemental private coverage by private insurance companies be permitted?

- How will deductibles and copays be collected?

There are advantages to cost sharing between the patient population and providers. Cost sharing reduces inflation by reducing demand for health care. It also reduces wasteful use of resources; users are more cost conscious when they must share the cost of their care. Cost sharing reduces "tax" cost, thereby reducing federal spending and avoiding tax increases (i.e., shifts cost of the plan to people that are actually using the plan).

Cost sharing can be used as an incentive for providers and patients to use less expensive alternative forms of care. Thus, cost sharing has significant impact on the quantity and mix of health care services. In a preferred provider organization (PPO), there is little or no cost sharing. In a fee-for-service arrangement, there is a cost-sharing schedule.

There are also disadvantages and limitations of cost-sharing provisions. Cost sharing increases administrative costs because claims must be processed and determinations made regarding the amount of costs to be shared. More confusion is created for patients at the point of use as they may be unclear as to their share of costs for their services.

Cost sharing may discourage use of some needed health care services, especially elective services and preventive services. Patients can avoid cost-sharing plans by purchasing *supplementary insurance* with inflation at a set amount. But cost sharing has a different impact on each income group. For example, lower income users are more likely to delay obtaining preventive health care services when they are forced to share the costs of care.

How Should the Plan Be Financed?

A tax based on utilization seems reasonable but may be tantamount to a *regressive tax* structure, imposing cost burdens on the poorest of users. A flat tax, regardless of income, is the most regressive because lower income people will pay a higher percentage of their income in taxes, regardless of their use. A progressive income tax increases the percentage paid for taxes as income increases, placing the burden on those who can most afford to carry it. Copayments are regressive because they are set amounts that are paid by the patient when they receive care. For poor people, these copayments are a higher percentage of their income.

Many liberals argue that a method of financing is required for care if its costs represent a higher percentage of income for the low-income families than for high-income families. Health care financing is usually based on premiums, payroll tax revenues, and federal and state general revenues. Private health care premiums decrease federal budgetary outlays; however, premiums are generally regressive. A payroll tax is less regressive, but it has a limit and does not account for unearned income. Progressive personal income tax for health care would mean that wealthy families would pay a higher tax for their care than low-income families.

The effects on the supply of and demand for the national labor force must be considered when determining the financial structure of a national health insurance plan. Some employers cannot cost shift premiums to their cost of production. If increased costs are substantial, some employers will either go out of business or reduce their labor force.

On the other hand, employers may obtain windfall gains from a national health insurance plan. Currently, employers allot a significant amount of their revenue for employee health insurance. With national health insurance, the employer would not have these immediate costs.

What Role Should Private Insurance Companies and State Governments Play?

In a national health insurance plan, private health insurance plans would set plan benefits, underwrite coverage, and act as a fiscal intermediary, and/or be driven from the marketplace. A fiscal intermediary is an administrative agent of a public plan that processes claims and makes payments—but they do not set premiums nor underwrite costs. In essence, the national health insurance plan would operate as Medicare functions today but would underwrite everyone, including the elderly and poor. Thus such a plan would eliminate Medicare and Medicaid.

In a national health insurance plan, the government regulates the private insurance industry and establishes standards for providers. The government would administer and subsidize coverage for low-income families. The government would increase reimbursement levels to attract physicians to states experiencing shortages. Medicaid-rich states would offer higher levels of health care and more benefits to their citizens. The government would negotiate drug costs, which might decrease profits for pharmaceutical companies.

What Role Should Consumers Have?

In a national health insurance plan, consumers would have a direct role in policy formulation, and a grievance process to address problems, beyond their elected representatives.

How Should Hospitals, Physicians, and Other Providers Be Reimbursed?

Should reimbursements constitute the total payment for a service, or can providers bill additional amounts to patients? If physicians do not accept assignment, then we are promoting a two-class system of health care. Currently, usual and customary fees are determined by a preestablished fee schedule. If providers were paid based on a salary it might promote underutilization to increase leisure time. Reimbursement based on capitation might also stimulate underutilization.

What Provisions Should Be Made for Quality Controls?

A national health insurance plan must address the following issues: What providers can participate? What providers will be evaluated? How will providers be evaluated and for what services? Would the plan employ simply utilization review, assess the process of care, or evaluate based on outcome? What penalties would the plan institute—no payment? Regarding the trade-off between access and quality, is government going to decide how we use services?

What Types of Delivery Forms Should Be Emphasized?

A national health insurance plan must choose its delivery modes. Should those modes be group practice or solo practice? What role should there be for paraprofessionals in diagnosing, treating, prescribing, and working with patients without direct supervision?

■ Summary—The Future

Although conservative thinking and constitutional interpretation have made substantial political gains in the past two decades, a significant percentage of Americans still vote for government to play a larger role in their lives, particularly in the delivery and financing of health care.

There is no doubt that decisions about government involvement in the delivery of health care will affect access, cost, and quality. Specific issues have to be addressed in upcoming debates about national health reform. How much more are Americans willing to pay through taxes and out-of-pocket payments at time of use? Americans have traditionally not wanted to pay in full for use, yet we are demanding more services. If national health reform empowers the uninsured to seek and obtain care, who will provide such care when we are currently experiencing shortages of personnel, particularly primary care providers?

How much individual freedom are we willing to sacrifice? Care has always been rationed for the poor. The middle class is now experiencing rationing. How much more rationing will we accept for the greater good? This greater good is a "statistical" greater good, because when Americans or their families become sick, they demand "Rolls Royce–level" health care regardless of the cost. However, rising expenditures in Medicare and Medicaid are not sustainable. History demonstrates that entitlement program costs always exceed the best budget estimations.

World and national events have a great impact on health care policy. For example, immediately after the attacks of Sept. 11, 2001, bio-terrorism, such as smallpox and anthrax, became an important health issue after years of "unimportance"; at the same time the then-proposed Medicare prescription drug benefit was placed on the back burner for two years. Public health initiatives to produce anthrax and smallpox vaccinations became a high priority after several people died from anthrax attacks. The cost of the war on terror has a substantial impact on the availability of government funds that otherwise could be directed toward improving access to health care and quality of services. The health care industry is a major competitor for labor and capital resources in the economy, and as the largest industry in the United States, it has a direct impact on other parts of the economy because it provides so many jobs.

What does the future hold for us? Public sector cost containment could hasten private sector changes in the health care delivery system. Some changes could be driven by what could happen among managed care companies who finance and deliver comprehensive health services to an enrolled population for a prepaid, fixed fee. More consolidation could take place among HMOs, leaving weaker health plans with limited ability to manage poor-risk populations. This result could produce fallout from the press and the public. In addition, some believe that HMOs are detrimental to patients.

Among hospitals and physicians, practice patterns could be influenced by reimbursement cuts from third-party payers, cost-shifting constraints, further declines in hospital occupancy rates, growing overcapacity, redistribution of physician supply, the size of the uninsured and underinsured populations, and risk of hospital closure. Community hospitals, a key provider of primary and secondary care have declined in number in the last 20 years, from 6,000 to 5,000. Patients also face a narrower choice of providers, a greater threat of rationed care for all (including middle class), and a shrinking safety net for the uninsured.

The future of health care reform leaves much to be determined. Some argue that the current Patient Protection and Affordable Care Act (PPACA) violates constitutional edicts, whereas others believe that it has not gone far enough. Although there is polarization, the U.S. system of government requires serious deliberation on such policy issues and, most of all, compromise. It is certain, however, that the current rate of increase in GDP share for health care is unsustainable as is the rising costs of entitlement programs such as Medicare and Medicaid. Containing costs, as the iron triangle demonstrates, will result in fewer benefits for some, reduced access for others, and diminished quality of the care currently received. Some believe that PPACA's promise to increase access for 32 million currently uninsured cannot be accomplished while trying to contain costs, unless care is rationed. Others believe that care is already rationed and that the current system does provide care for the uninsured, called uncompensated care.

There are several key issues to consider when evaluating the health care system:

- Do we have a moral obligation versus a constitutional obligation to provide health care to our fellow citizens?

- What is the appropriate role of government in the health care industry?

- How should the roles and responsibilities in the delivery of health care be divided between the federal government and the state governments?

- What should be the government's effect on the U.S. economy?

- The health care system is a major part of the U.S. economy, so how should this component be regulated and managed?

Many of these questions have remained unanswered for decades, and many of these questions and resultant challenges will continue to confront the U.S. health care system in the future. In a free, democratic society, there will always be disagreement on government's role in the economy and in the provision of services such as health care. Yet, even if we come to compromise solutions to the problems mentioned above, other challenges will materialize. Whether you are a future health care administrator, doctor, nurse, allied health provider, or just someone interested in learning more about health care, it is important to know that there are no easy answers, but the U.S. health care delivery system will need constant attention to improve. These challenges will bring about changes that will affect providers, patients, and employees.

Not surprisingly, health care does not exist in a vacuum, but within a larger economy, and not only a U.S. economy but also a world order. Our willingness for government to spend increasing percentages of GDP on health care will be influenced by the size of our national debt and such exogenous factors as the price of oil and food. As we emerge from the most serious economic crisis since the Great Depression, our recovery is still precarious, dependent on the economies of countries such as China and Japan as well as smaller countries, including Portugal, Italy, Greece, and Spain. These factors contribute to an environment where it is almost impossible to predict with any accuracy the future of the health care industry in the United States. However, what Americans want from that industry will come head to head with what the United States can afford, with additional pressure coming from a constantly changing global economy.

■ Review Questions

1. What has been the historic role of the American Medical Association in the passage of health insurance legislation?

2. What has been the impact of the Patient Protection and Affordable Care Act (PPACA) of 2010 on the U.S. health care system?

3. What is the role of federal and state governments in paying for or actually providing health services?

4. Do the national values of the United States favor mandatory participation versus voluntarily participation in health care programs?

5. Should the United States implement a comprehensive national health insurance plan like Canada's or the United Kingdom's, where government pays for the health care for all of its citizens?

6. What was the role of the AMA during the Great Depression as it relates to enacting national health insurance?

7. What did the "New Deal program" do for the retired, disabled, and the poor?

8. Who was the first American president to propose national health insurance?

9. What are the major elements of the Patient Protection and Affordable Care Act (PPACA)?

10. What are the primary problems with the PPACA?

■ Additional Resources

AcademyHealth: http://www.academyhealth.org/Training/ResourceDetail.cfm?ItemNumber=5662

Agency for Healthcare Research and Quality: http://www.ahrq.gov/

American Enterprise Institute for Public Policy Research: http://www.aei.org/ra/43

American Medical Association (AMA) health care reform: http://www.ama-assn.org/ama/pub/advocacy/current-topics-advocacy/affordable-care-act.page

American Nurses Association (ANA) health care form resources: http://www.nursingworld.org/MainMenuCategories/HealthcareandPolicyIssuesHealthSystemReform/HealthCareReformResources.aspx/

Brookings Institution Engelberg Center for Health Care Reform: http://www.brookings.edu/topics/health-care.aspx

Congressional Budget Office (CBO): http://www.cbo.gov/

Federal Health Reform: State Legislative Tracking Database: http://www.ncsl.org/?TabId=22123

Herdon Alliance Healing America's Healthcare: http://herndonalliance.org/

Kaiser EDU.org: www.KaiserEDU.org

National Association of Community Health Centers: http://www.nachc.org/

National Association of Public Health Policy: http://www.naphp.org/

National Committee for Quality Assurance: http://www.ncqa.org/Default.aspx

National Health Reform Law and Policy Project: http://www.gwumc.edu/sphhs/departments/healthpolicy/healthReform/

National Institute for Health Care Reform: http://www.nihcr.org/index.html

Office of Rural Health Policy: http://www.hrsa.gov/ruralhealth/

State Refor(u)m: http://www.statereforum.org/

The Commonwealth Fund: http://www.commonwealthfund.org

USAID Health Policy Initiative: http://www.healthpolicyinitiative.com/index.cfm?id=index

References

Carmalt, J., & Zaidi, S. (2004). The right to health in the United States. What does it mean? Center for Economic and Social Rights. Retrieved August 8, 2005, from http://www.nhchc.org/Advocacy/RighttoHealthinAmerica.pdf.

Esmail, N., & Wrona, D. (2008). *Medical technology in Canada*. Fraser Institute.

Kaiser Family Foundation (KFF). (2004). Study estimates that the U.S. will spend nearly $41 billion for uncompensated care for the uninsured in 2004; while full-year uninsured receive about half as much care as those fully insured. Press Release. Retrieved August 8, 2005, from http://www.kff.org/uninsured/kcmu051004nr.cfm.

Kaiser Family Foundation (KFF). (2011, April 19). Focus on health reform: Summary of new health reform law. Retrieved February 3, 2012, from http://www.kff.org/healthreform/upload/8061.pdf.

Kelley, D. (n.d.). Is there a right to health care? The Objectivist Center. Retrieved August 8, 2005, from http://www.objectivistcenter.org/articles/dkelley_right-to-health-care.asp.

Right to Health Care. (2005). Philosophy and history of the right to health care. Retrieved August 8, 2005 , from http://www.righttohealthcare.org/Phil.htm.

Roosevelt, F. D. (1944). Economic Bill of Rights: Excerpt from January 11, 1944, message to Congress on the State of the Union. Retrieved August 8, 2005, from http://www.worldpolicy.org/globalrights/econrights/fdr-econbill.html.

Turner Learning, Inc. (2001). Your choice. Your voice. Lesson 1: Voter backgrounder. Retrieved August 8, 2005, from http://www.turnerlearning.com/cnn/election/l1_backgrounder.html.

Glossary of Key Terms

A

access   Potential or ability to use health care services. Access may be influenced by the ability to pay for services and the cost of services as well as ability to visit a provider.

accountable care organization (ACO)   Network of providers (physicians and hospitals) that share responsibility for providing care to patients. The purpose of an ACO is to provide seamless continuity of care between providers at lower cost, and for ACOs to work, member providers would have to seamlessly share information.

activities of daily living (ADLs)   The most basic tasks performed throughout the day. They measure dependence on others for assistance with personal care functions. Examples include bathing, dressing, eating, walking and mobility (which includes transferring from bed to wheelchair or from toilet to wheelchair), and toileting.

acute care   Short-term care provided to a patient in either a hospital or clinical setting where the need is for immediate intervention and treatment.

adult day care   May be derived from either a social model or medical model or combination of both. Social model includes social activities and custodial care provided in senior centers. Medical model provides medical care and rehabilitation.

adverse selection   The demand for health insurance is correlated with the risk of illness of the buyer of the insurance, but the seller of insurance is unable to incorporate the higher risk into the insurance price. In other words, the predisposition of sick people to purchase health insurance in order to access treatment for their condition.

alternative medicine   Uses of alternative therapies such as acupuncture and chiropractic in place of conventional medicine.

allopathic medicine   Conventional or traditional scientific medicine. Doctors trained in allopathic medicine use drugs, devices, and surgery to treat diseases to produce alterations in the paths of diseases.

ambulatory care   Also referred to as outpatient care and includes personal health or medical health care services that are provided to a patient who is not institutionalized (the person does not need an overnight stay).

ambulatory surgical center (ASC)   A facility that furnishes outpatient surgical procedures to patients who do not require an overnight stay following the procedure. Many such facilities are owned by physicians or have at least one physician-owner and may also be a joint venture between a physician group and a hospital or health system.

American Medical Association (AMA)   Founded in 1847, the professional organization for physicians that initially opposed Medicare in the 1960s, comparing it with socialized medicine. When it seemed that passage was inevitable, the AMA lobbied for the program to cover only the poor elderly.

Anderson's model of utilization of health services   A behavioral model of health services utilization that uses societal determinants, individual factors, and health industry characteristics to predict use of services.

assisted living   Type of long-term care service for patients who have limitations in some activities of daily living (ADLs) or instrumental activities of daily living (IADLs) but do not need full-time nursing care.

Avedis Donabedian   Born in 1919 and died in 2000, known as the father of quality in health care, he developed an algorithm for measuring health care quality that contained three components of the delivery of care: structure, process, and outcome. He received his medical degree from the American University of Beirut and practiced medicine in Israel before joining the New York Medical College. He next joined the faculty at the School of Public Health at the University of Michigan. He transformed the field of quality in the health care industry and successfully developed methodologies for its measurement and assessment.

average length of stay (ALOS)   Computed by dividing the number of inpatient days by the number of discharges (including deaths) during the year.

B

baby boomers   The generation of Americans who were born immediately following World War II, or from 1946 through 1964. During the time from 1946 through 1964 approximately 78 million baby boomers were born in the United States.

bad debt   Incurred from services provided by a health care provider and not reimbursed, but which are provided with the expectation of being reimbursed. May be comprised of copayments or coinsurance portions of a patient's bill that the patient subsequently cannot pay.

Balanced Budget Act of 1997   Through this act in 1997, Medicaid was expanded to cover additional children; however, it also resulted in reduced reimbursement to hospitals, physicians, and nurse practitioners. Some of these decreases were later restored by subsequent legislation.

biologically based practices   Use of natural substances such as herbs, vitamins, and supplements to improve health or prevent disease. Examples include taking Ginkgo biloba to improve memory, or zinc or vitamin C to prevent a cold.

C

capitation   A set amount of money given to physicians for each person who enrolls in their practice prior to the provision of any care (usually used with primary care physicians). In return, the physician is responsible for providing specified services for a designated period of time.

case management   Care for the patient by coordinating a combination of services that will allow for the most independent level of functioning within a supportive system. It involves joint decision making among the patient (whenever possible), the family, physicians, and social services, to determine the care plan most appropriate for the patient.

Centers for Medicare and Medicaid Services (CMS)   Created by legislation signed into law in 1965 by President Lyndon Johnson, it is a division of the Department of Health and Human Services that administers the Medicare and Medicaid service plans. The agency was previously known as the Health Care Financing Administration (HCFA). It is also responsible for working with states to implement the State Children's Health Insurance Program (SCHIP) and portability standards for health insurance.

Certificate of Need   A state-level program whereby a state board must approve applications for new health care facilities, capital improvements, or high-cost equipment.

certified nurse midwife   An advanced practice nurse who is trained to deliver relatively low-risk births and provide primary gynecological care for women. A certified nurse midwife provides care in diverse settings, including hospital labor and delivery services, physician offices, homes, and clinics.

certified registered nurse anesthetist (CRNA)   An advanced practice nurse who provides the majority of anesthetics to patients. A CRNA earns a Master's of Science in Nursing (MSN) degree and is one of the first advanced practice nurse positions created.

charity care   Hospital services provided for which a hospital does not expect to be reimbursed or services provided to patients who are uninsured and have no means to pay for their care.

Children's Health Insurance Reauthorization Act of 2009 (CHIPRA)   Signed by President Barack Obama in 2009, it increased funding by $32.8 billion to expand Children's Health Insurance Program (CHIP) to cover an additional 4 million children and pregnant women.

chiropractor   Doctoral-level clinician (Doctor of Chiropractic) who treats conditions related to the musculoskeletal system and their interconnectedness with the rest of the body as reflected in the central nervous system that travels through and emanates from the spine.

chronic illness   Medical condition lasting three months or longer; examples include many of the prevalent illnesses associated with aging, such as Alzheimer's disease and cardiac disease.

classical principles of insurance   Basic tenants that stipulate that an insurable event has a significant financial risk; the risk or the probability of event occurrence is measurable for a group; the event is infrequent; service is not desirable by the patient; and patients do not determine whether they receive care.

clinical nurse specialist   An advanced practice nurse who specializes in a field such as adult intensive care, pediatrics, gerontology, or surgical care. A clinical nurse specialist provides specialized care for physical and mental health issues in hospitals and physician offices and may have training, management, or research responsibilities.

Clinton Health Reform   Also called the 1993 Clinton Health Security Act , the health care reform plan that was proposed by President Bill Clinton in 1993 and developed by a task force headed by First Lady Hillary Clinton. The goal of the reform plan was universal health care for all Americans, and it required each United States citizen to be enrolled in a health insurance plan. All employers would be required to contribute toward the costs of insurance premiums for their employees. Americans would choose from multiple health plans that would compete for their enrollment, with the expectation that most would choose managed care plans.

closed panel   A managed care plan that contracts with physicians and other primary care clinicians on an exclusive basis for services; the clinicians do not treat any other patients other than those who are members of the plan.

coinsurance   Portion of a bill for health care services that is the responsibility of the patient, once the patient has met his or her health plan deductible requirements. For example, this amount may be approximately 20 to 40 percent of the charges for a service, and the insurance company pays the remaining 80 to 60 percent, once the patient has paid the required deductible amount.

community rating   Health care insurance coverage for different groups of people in a defined service area or community at the same cost despite widely varied health spending by those in the community. As a result, everyone pays the same premium, and healthy individuals subsidize the health care consumed by sicker individuals.

complementary medicine   Uses alternative therapies such as acupuncture and chiropractic along with conventional medicine.

compressed morbidity   To live a long and healthy life and then become acutely sick toward the end and die quickly.

continuing care retirement community (CCRC)   Single facilities that combine a range of services including independent living, assisted living, and a skilled nursing home. More facilities are offering Alzheimer's and dementia care. A large entry fee, plus monthly maintenance fees, is typically required for a residence, meals, and health care coverage. Residents receive care services depending on their level of need and health status.

continuum of care   The delivery of comprehensive health care services over time for patients with a disease, from diagnosis to the end of life.

copayment   A fixed dollar amount paid by the insured for each type of service. For example, a copayment may be $20 per physician visit, $10 per prescription, or $100 for each day in the hospital.

cost   Within the context of the health care industry, the resources required to deliver health care services. For example, from the perspective of a patient, it may be the price they are charged for care services. A health care provider may identify it as the fixed, variable, direct, and indirect requirements to deliver care. A payer for health care services may determine it as a claim or charge submitted by a provider for the delivery of care services to members of a health plan.

cost–push inflation   Higher general price levels due to higher production costs from rising input costs. May stem from new technology, increased wages of health care personnel, duplication of medical services, unionization or threat of unionization, and inappropriate use of heatlh care, such as defensive medicine and inexperienced providers using services inefficiently.

critical access hospital (CAH)   A hospital located in a rural area more than 35 miles from any other hospital or 15 miles from another hospital in mountainous terrain or areas with only secondary roads. This type of hospital must be certified by the state as a necessary provider of health care to area residents and must provide emergency services 24 hours a day. It must maintain an annual average length of stay of 96 hours or less for its acute care patients and have a maximum of 25 acute care inpatient beds.

D

deductible   The annual amount patients must pay for health care expenses before their health insurance plan covers the cost of care.

defensive medicine   When providers order additional or "unnecessary" tests to protect themselves in case of a lawsuit. Defensive medicine increases costs, but does not really help the practitioner treat the patient and may even harm the patient.

demand–pull inflation   When consumer demand for services is greater than the supply offered. It is enabled by health insurance, as it increases consumers' buying power and removes price sensitivity or cost consciousness.

democratic/normative reinforcement   The belief that the "Constitution is not designed to be a set of specific principles and guidelines, rather a general principle, a basic skeleton on which contemporary vision would be built. Decisions about the meaning of the Constitution must consider the general feeling evoked by the Constitution, and then use modern realism to add flesh to the skeleton."

dentist   Doctoral-level clinician who is responsible for the prevention, diagnosis, and treatment, both surgical and nonsurgical, of the problems in the mouth and maxillofacial area and associated structures.

Department of Veterans Affairs   A department of the U.S. federal government that provides programs to benefit veterans and their families. Among the many services it provides to veterans, it operates a health care system composed of clinics, nursing homes, and hospitals to deliver health care services to veterans who qualify for care.

diagnosis-related groups (DRGs)   A prospective payment system used by Medicare and other insurance companies to group illnesses. It is a classification of 467 illness categories where all patients in the same group are expected to display the same set of symptoms and require approximately the same amount of resources to treat. The DRG code is used to determine how much the provider will be reimbursed for providing care to the patient.

diminishing marginal returns   When each additional dollar spent produces less of a gain in output, whether it is measured by increased life expectancy, lower mortality, or better quality of life.

disability-adjusted life expectancy   Calculated by subtracting the total number of sick and disabled days and years from the average life expectancy. Used to determine the percentage of a person's or group's life that is spent in good health and to compare the disease and disability burdens of different groups.

disability rates   Rates of diseases such as diabetes, hypertension, and neurological conditions that require more assistance with ADLS and IADLS.

discounted fee-for-service   A reimbursement plan under which physicians are paid for services based on a contractual discount of the usual and customary price charged by physicians in the local region.

disjointed incrementalism   Policy making that is divided into separate stages that results in a conclusion and solution that is less than optimal as opposed to when the problem and solution are considered as a whole.

disparities   In health care, refers to population-specific differences in the health outcomes, access to health care, quality of health care, that exist across socioeconomic, racial, and ethnic groups.

diversification strategies   As it relates to hospitals and health systems, developing new sources of revenue and reimbursement through development of new service lines and products. The goal is to increase profits and reduce risk for the organization.

"docs in a box"   Free-standing urgent care centers.

Donabedian model for quality   Structure, process, outcomes—a model that explains the various stages at which quality of care can be measured; structure refers to

health care inputs; process refers to standards for delivery of care; and outcomes refers to the results of the delivery of care.

donut hole   That part of Medicare Part D reimbursement between basic services and full coverage that is the Medicare beneficiaries' responsibility to pay.

dual eligibles   Medicare Part A or Part B recipients who would qualify for either the Medicare Savings Program or for Medicaid benefits. These persons qualify for programs that are part of the state Medicaid programs that pay some of the costs of Medicare; these programs may be referred to as Medicare savings programs, effectively providing full health coverage.

E

elasticity of demand   The responsiveness of demand to changes in price.

emergency care   Services provided at the scene of an accident, en route to the hospital, or at the hospital emergency department. The main purpose is to stabilize the patient until arrival at a hospital trauma center or emergency room.

Emergency Medical Treatment and Labor Act of 1986   Also referred to as (EMTALA), it requires that if a hospital does have an emergency department, it must examine and stabilize all patients who seek care there, regardless of their willingness or ability to pay.

enabling factors   Conditions or characteristics that facilitate or inhibit the use of health care services. Examples may include family income, distance, family size, health insurance, and community resources.

endemic   The usual, sustained occurrence of a disease in a population.

energy medicine   The use of biofield therapy and electromagnetic fields (bioelectromagnetic-based therapy) to affect health.

epidemic   An unusual occurrence of disease in a population. Some have caused large numbers of deaths. Measles, cholera, and certain flu strains have become epidemic throughout the world.

epidemiology   The study of the distribution and determinants of diseases in a population.

externalities   A positive or negative result experienced by a third party due to economic activity.

F

fee-for-service Reimbursement system whereby the payer reimburses the provider based on a contractual agreement for each individual service that is provided.

Final Report of the Committee on the Costs of Medical Care Formed in 1927 and comprised of 44 members of the medical community, the committee spent five years studying the health care needs of the patient population in the United States. The committee assessed the organization, distribution, and cost of health care in the 1920s. The Committee provided five primary recommendations for the delivery, access, cost, and coordination of health care services that are still applicable to modern-day conditions.

"flat-of-the-curve" medicine The point in many health care treatments where no additional increases in health status for additional spending occur.

The Flexner Report, 1910 A groundbreaking report published in 1910, prepared for the Carnegie Foundation by Abraham Flexner (1866–1959), that severely criticized the nation's medical education institutions. It gave rise to modern medical education, as many proprietary institutions closed and the medical education system was redesigned based on the Johns Hopkins model of university-based medical education. As a result, training in biomedical sciences was combined with hands-on clinical training for new physicians.

Food and Drug Administration (FDA) Federal agency that regulates drugs and medical devices.

for-profit organizations Organizations that must pay a corporate tax on their net corporate profits.

G

gatekeeper Usually a primary care physician, physician assistant, or nurse practitioner who must authorize specialty care before any is rendered.

goal A long-range statement of an ideal or desired outcome.

Great Depression A severe economic downturn that began in the United States with the New York stock market crash in 1929 and then spread to Europe and throughout the world. It lasted approximately 10 years and caused widespread poverty and unemployment.

Great Society A phrase coined by President Lyndon Johnson during his presidential campaign in 1964. It describes the effort by President Johnson to end poverty, promote equality, improve education, rejuvenate cities, and protect the environment. These efforts lead to the passage of the Civil Rights Act of 1964 and the Economic Opportunity Act of 1964, the launching of Medicare and Medicaid, and initiatives to end racial injustice.

gross domestic product (GDP) The value of all of the goods and services produced in the United States.

group model HMO A type of HMO that contracts with an established medical group for the provision of health care services. The physicians are employed by the group practice and are permitted to provide services to non-HMO patients. The clinicians operate their own medical practices and function as separate group. The HMO also contracts with hospitals to care for patients who are part of the health plan.

group practice Organizational structure which may be a single-specialty practice or a multi-specialty practice of three or more physicians. Most group practices are single-specialty and have less than eight physicians. Physicians may own the practice jointly, or there may be a mixture of owners (partners) and employed physicians.

H

health A state of complete physical, mental, and social well-being, and not merely the absence of disease or infirmity.

health care savings accounts Created in 2003 so that persons covered by high-deductible health plans could deposit tax-deferred money for health care expenses.

health care system A complex set of arrangements in our society that mediate between the human being and our vulnerability to disease. The three goals are to treat the sick, prevent disease, and set goals for maintenance and promotion of health.

health education/prevention Delivery of information to change attitudes and behaviors to prevent or lessen the impact of disease. Examples include immunizations, hypertension control, cholesterol control, smoking cessation, exercise, stress management, and breast cancer screening.

health maintenance organization (HMO) A company that performs both a health care delivery function and health insurance function for its member enrollees.

health planning A formal process where organizations or government entities devise strategies and itemize services that promote health or prevent or treat diseases. It entails the following steps: defining a problem, formulating and evaluating alternatives, implementing the chosen alternative, and evaluating the results.

health status   The level of health of a person, group, or nation.

healthy worker effect   Health care costs are lower for an employed group of individuals because working individuals are more likely to be in good health simply because they are able to perform the requirements of their job.

Hill-Burton Act   Also called the Hospital Survey and Construction Act of 1948, it was designed to bring hospital beds to areas that were previously underserved. As a result of the legislation, two-thirds of the beds built during this time were in rural areas.

HMO Act of 1973   A major federal effort to change the traditional solo practice fee-for-service system by providing $375 million over five years in grants and loans for the establishment of HMOs. Authorized for-profit IPA-HMO models in which HMOs contract with independent practice associations that contract with individual physicians for health care services at a negotiated rate. The legislation also required employers to include an HMO as a health benefit option and defined a minimum range of services that the HMO must provide.

home health care   Services provided in a person's private residence because the person is homebound and receives a prescription from a provider for home health services. It is designed to promote, maintain, or restore health, or can be prescribed to minimize the effects of a disability and/or illness.

homeopathy   The use of "very low doses of drugs that produce patient signs or symptoms" as a means of curing them. For example, a homeopath may try to relieve nausea by administering a small amount of *Psychotria ipecacuanha*, the plant used to make ipecac, which induces vomiting.

horizontal integration   The merger or combination of similar organizations, such as hospitals with hospitals, and nursing homes with nursing homes.

hospice care   Palliative care to the terminally ill or those expected to die within six months and their families. Involves the medical relief of pain and supportive services that can be provided in an inpatient setting, such as a hospital or nursing home or in a patient's home. Additionally, these programs address the emotional, social, financial, and legal needs of patients and their families. It is frequently used for the treatment of terminal cancer and AIDS patients.

hospital   An organization that provides medical or surgical care on either an inpatient or outpatient basis.

hospital outpatient centers   Hospital-based setting where ambulatory care such as surgery is delivered.

hunter–gatherer   An expression used to describe a foraging society in which most food was obtained from hunting animals and gathering wild plants, and people lived by instinctual behaviors.

incidence   A measure of the number of new cases of a disease over a period of time.

independent living facility   A residential living facility for seniors, generally for those over 55 years of age. The type of facility may vary from apartment living to freestanding houses with services to care for building maintenance and yard care. Also may be referred to as a retirement community, retirement home, or senior housing.

independent practice association (IPA)   A group of physicians, or an organization that contracts with physicians, to provide care to HMO-enrolled members, usually on a capitated basis or a negotiated fee-for-service basis. Clinicians participating in IPAs retain their right to treat non-HMO patients on a fee-for-service basis, in an open panel HMO, as well as retain their solo practice.

Indian Health Service   Federal agency within the Department of Health and Human Services that provides health services and operates health care facilities for American Indians and Alaskan Natives.

individual determinants   Part of Andersen's behavioral model of health services utilization, unique characteristics of patients that help determine their utilization of health services. The unique characteristics can be subdivided into three categories, including predisposing factors, enabling factors, and need factors.

individual or differential rating   Health insurance rates based on the risk factors, which may include health status, age, illness, tobacco use, and other factors of the individual groups.

inertia   A law of physics that states that a body in motion, left to itself, will keep moving, or that a body at rest will stay at rest if it is left to itself.

infant mortality rate (IMR)   The rate of infant deaths (from live birth to age 1 year) per 1,000 live births.

informal caregiver   Family members and friends who provide care for a patient.

informal medicine   Practiced when family and friends influence our health and medical-seeking behavior. For example, comments such as "You don't look well. You should take some vitamin C," or "You should see a doctor."

inpatient care   Care that requires the patient to spend at least one overnight stay; it can take place in many settings such as hospitals, nursing homes, assisted living, and home health and hospice care.

instrumental activities of daily living (IADLs)   Measures ability to accomplish more independent tasks such as cleaning, shopping, managing finances, preparing meals, using the telephone, preparing meals, heavy and light housework, and shopping. The need for help with IADLs increases with age.

Institute of Medicine (IOM)   Established in 1970, the Institute of Medicine (IOM) is the health arm of the National Academy of Sciences. It is an independent nonprofit organization, separate from the federal government, and provides authoritative evidence-based analysis and policy recommendations for decision makers in government and the private sector. Work is completed by volunteer researchers, analysts, and scientists who produce peer-reviewed analysis on a broad range of health and medical issues and problems.

integrated delivery system (IDS)   An organized system of health care providers that spans a broad range of health care services by using vertical integration to contract with a variety of clinicians and health plans.

Joint Commission on Accreditation of Health Care Organizations (JCAHO)   Also referred to as The Joint Commission and founded in 1951, an umbrella organization that evaluates and accredits more than 19,000 health care organizations such as hospitals.

joint venture   A legal agreement whereby two or more organizations create a new entity by both contributing resources and then sharing the markets, intellectual property, revenues, expenses, knowledge, and control of the new endeavor. The endeavor may be ongoing or limited in time, depending on the original agreement of the two parties. It differs from a merger, as there is no transfer of ownership of assets in the agreement.

Kaiser-Permanente   Based in California and founded in 1945 by Henry Kaiser and Sidney Garfield, the health insurance company with the most HMO enrollees in the United States, as well as an operator of medical centers and offices.

leading causes of death   The prevailing determinants of premature death, such as heart disease, cancer, and stroke. These chronic diseases have been the main killers, from the last half of the twentieth century into the twenty-first century.

The Leapfrog Group   Launched in 2000 by several large United States companies with funding from the Business Roundtable, it represents major corporations and purchasers of health insurance who desire to improve regulations and standards in health care quality. They also strive to improve the value and quality of health care insurance for their employees and retirees.

life expectancy   The average number of years that people in a given population live.

lifetime cap   A limit on the insurance benefits that an individual may receive during his or her lifetime. The cap may be on overall services or services for a specific condition or disease, or a combination of the two. Once the limit has been reached, the health insurance company will no longer pay for services.

literalism—contemporary   The belief that only the literal words of the Constitution can be used to interpret the Constitution, but this school of thought uses modern or contemporary definitions of those words.

literalism—historical   The belief that only the literal words of the Constitution and their meaning in the eighteenth century can be used to interpret the Constitution. Historical literalism differs from Originalism in that it does not permit reference to the writings and thoughts of the Framers.

long-stay hospital   Also referred to as a long-term hospital, where acute care services are provided to patients who typically have an average length of stay of more than 25 days.

long-term care   The treatment of chronic illnesses and disability. It is generally less expensive and less intensive than acute hospital care; the services include nursing homes, home health care, assisted living facilities, and hospice care.

long-term care hospitals (LTCHs)   Facilities that provide care to patients with an average length of stay of more than 25 days. They specialize in patients with more than one serious condition, with the goal of returning the patient home with a measure of independence.

macro planning   Planning with a focus on the national, regional, or state level. It is often centralized, where a single entity coordinates the planning of services for a large area. As an example, Certificate of Need (CON) programs, where a state board must approve applications for new facilities, capital improvements, or high-cost equipment.

managed care   A system of health care delivery that emphasizes comprehensive health services focused on preventive care and primary care to streamline services, contain costs, improve quality, expand access, and reduce the need for more expensive specialty services. A managed care organization (MCO) performs the functions of delivery of care, health insurance, and administration.

managed indemnity plans   Managed care model that is managed like a traditional indemnity plan but with the added requirement of precertification and other utilization review tools. Some of the care members receive is subject to pre-approval by the health plan. Members choose their own physician, pay a predetermined deductible for care and then a coinsurance amount, and they are reimbursed for the remaining medical costs.

manipulative and body-based practices   Care delivered by those who believe in the laying on of hands; includes chiropractic and massage therapy. Chiropractic doctors treat problems with the musculoskeletal and nervous systems, largely using spinal manipulation or "chiropractic adjustment."

mechanistic approach to the treatment of disease   A treatment approach based on the assumption that humans operate as "machines." We can disassemble machines and repair them, so medicine should be able to apply this capability to human beings. We view many parts and organ systems as parts of a machine and use invasive techniques such as replacing valves or lenses, transplants, bypass grafts, and other techniques to treat conditions.

Medicaid   Public assistance program administered by states, with the federal government providing matching funding. Healthcare service coverage varies by state and it is provided for persons whose incomes and/or assets are insufficient to pay for their own health care services. Disabled persons who are eligible for Social Security Income are also eligible.

medical care   Diagnoses and treatment of illness or disease by a professional clinician.

medical home   A team-based primary care delivery model led by a primary care physician, where the goal is to facilitate seamless communication among patients, physicians, and families. Care is enhanced through the primary care provider coordinating all of the patient's care and being available to the patient and the family. The home is responsible for providing all of the patient's care needs and for arranging care with other providers. The overall goal of the model is to promote health and manage chronic conditions, thereby reducing hospitalization and length of stay.

medical malpractice   The improper treatment of patients by physicians and other providers.

medical savings accounts (MSAs)   Tax-deferred accounts that allow money to be saved for medical expenses.

medically underserved areas (MUAs)   A region with a shortage of health care resources such as hospitals, providers, or equipment.

Medicare   The nation's largest health insurance program—beneficiaries number more than 40 million Americans. A social insurance program, or an "entitlement" program; it is not a welfare program. To qualify for Part A (hospital insurance), beneficiaries have to pay Social Security taxes for 40 quarters, or quarter years, or for 10 years by way of a payroll tax.

Medicare Part A   The hospital insurance program covers inpatient hospital, skilled nursing facility, hospice, and home health care. It is funded through a payroll tax paid by employees and employers.

Medicare Part B   Supplementary medical insurance that covers physician and other medical services, such as outpatient hospital care, lab tests, medical supplies, and home health. The program is funded through beneficiary premiums and general revenues.

Medicare Part C   Managed care plans that provide Part A and Part B benefits, also called Medicare Advantage (MA), to enrollees. Medicare Advantage (MA) plans contract with Medicare to provide both Part A and B services to enrolled beneficiaries.

Medicare Part D   Outpatient prescription drug benefit implemented in 2006 through the Medicare Prescription Drug Improvement and Modernization Act of 2003 (MMA) and funded through beneficiary premiums and general revenues.

Medicare Prescription Drug, Improvement and Modernization Act (MMA) of 2003   Legislation that enacted the most sweeping changes to Medicare since its inception by affording Medicare beneficiaries a prescription drug benefit. Starting in 2006, individuals who are eligible for Medicare Part A or enrolled in Medicare Part B were eligible to participate in the program, which provides a voluntary drug benefit for beneficiaries through private companies.

Medicare+Choice   Plan in which enrollees can contract with other types of private health plans such as preferred provider plans (PPOs), point-of-service organizations (PSOSs), and medical savings accounts (MSAs). Plan members continue to pay monthly premiums but must obtain all Medicare-covered benefits through a private plan. Enrollees can choose among insurance products, such as an HMO, for their care delivery.

Medigap   Insurance purchased by Medicare beneficiaries to fill gaps in their health insurance coverage by enrolling in health maintenance organizations (HMOs) and purchasing private insurance. These policies pay most of Medicare coinsurance amounts and may provide coverage for Medicare's deductibles.

micro planning   Health planning targeted at the institutional or individual level. For example, a local hospital might conduct a needs assessment before deciding what types of new services to offer or which services to discontinue. Usually decentralized where no one agency or organization is in charge of planning what services can or should be delivered.

mind–body medicine   Care designed to "enhance the mind's capacity to affect bodily function and symptoms" (NCCAM, 2007). These interventions include support groups such as Alcoholics Anonymous or cancer support groups, meditation, faith medicine (healing practices, such as prayer, that appeal to a supernatural power), and creative therapies such as art.

modernism/instrumentalism   Belief that the Constitution should be interpreted as it applies to today's standards and situations.

moral hazard   A phenomenon where individuals who have health insurance tend to over-consume health services because they do not bear the full cost of consuming those services. As a result, insurance companies must use coinsurance, copayments, and deductibles to provide incentives to consumers not to over-consume health care services.

morbidity rate   The number of people in a population who have a disease at one point in time per 100,000 people.

mortality rate   The number of deaths in a population at risk during one year.

national debt   The sum of all annual federal deficits or, in other words, all outstanding federal government debt.

national deficit   The amount by which the federal government's expenditures exceed its tax revenues.

The National Practitioners' Data Bank (NPDB)   Established by Congress as part of the Health Care Quality Improvement Act of 1986, it is a repository of data regarding payments made in response to lawsuits against physicians for medical malpractice, as well as peer sanctions against clinicians' licenses, clinical privileges, and professional society membership. Regulation requires that any payments made as a result of malpractice lawsuits or adverse actions must be reported to the NPDB. The information is considered confidential to the public but may be released to eligible parties or other clinicians.

naturopathy   Care delivery that uses all-natural treatments such as herbal medicine, massage, acupuncture, manual manipulation, hydrotherapy, and aromatherapy. Naturopaths believe that natural treatments can help the human body to heal itself.

network model HMO   A model in which the HMO contracts with multiple physician groups to deliver health care to the health plan members. The physician network may be a large single multi-specialty group or it may be composed of many small groups of primary care physicians (PCPs), or a combination of both.

not-for-profit   Also called 501(c) (3) status and based on the section of the Internal Revenue Code that governs tax exemption, no profit can accrue to any shareholders. It is legal for such organizations to show excess income, a "profit" or surplus in the hospital's balance sheet of profits and losses. Any excess income must be reinvested in the organization, and the organization must provide community benefits as part of its tax-exempt status.

nurse practitioner (NP)   An advanced practice nurse who works in many types of clinical settings, including hospitals, clinics, and physician offices. He or she provides primary, specialty, and preventive care to pediatric, adult, and geriatric patients, as well as prescribes medications, orders tests, and diagnoses and treats many common injuries and illnesses.

nursing home   Facility with three or more beds that provides nursing or personal care services to the senior, infirm, or chronically ill populations. They are classified as skilled nursing facilities (SNFs), nursing facilities, sub-acute care facilities, and post-acute care facilities.

objective   A specific, measurable target that must be reached within a defined time frame.

Omnibus Budget Reconciliation Act (OBRA) of 1989   Legislation that established a new method of Medicare physician reimbursement effective in 1992, using a resource-based relative value scale (RBRVS), which replaced the former method of charge-based reimbursement. This legislation also prohibited physicians from referring Medicare patients to clinical laboratories in which they had a financial investment.

open panel   A managed care plan that contracts with private clinicians to deliver care; however, the clinicians may see other patients not in the health plan.

Organization for Economic Cooperation and Development (OECD)   Formed in 1961 and headquartered in Paris, France, it is an international organization of the most industrialized countries with market economies. Its goals are to foster economic stability and democracy in its member countries and in developing countries.

originalism/original intent   The belief that the Constitution should be interpreted as the framers of the Constitution, or the Founding Fathers, intended.

osteopathic medicine   Care delivery that believes structure influences function; if there is a problem in one part of the body's structure, function in that area, and possibly in other areas, may be affected. Many of the manipulative techniques used are aimed at reducing or eliminating the impediments to proper structure and function so the self-healing mechanism can assume its role in restoring a person to health.

overuse of care   The use of health care resources and procedures in the absence of healing evidence.

"pain and suffering"   A legal term that refers to the mental anguish and physical distress of going through treatment and recovery from an injury and avoiding activities that were customary before the injury.

palliative care   Services for patients with a chronic incurable or terminal illness with a focus on ensuring that the end of life is filled with dignity and as little pain as possible.

pandemic   An unusual occurrence of a disease that spreads around the world or in a large geographic area; for example, HIV/AIDS is now pandemic.

Patient Protection and Affordable Care Act (PPACA), 2010   Signed on March 23, 2010, by President Obama, with the goal of expanding health insurance coverage to 32 million Americans by 2019. It is intended to provide affordable health care for all Americans and to reduce the growth in health care costs. Specifically, among its provisions, it requires most United States citizens and legal residents to purchase health insurance by 2014. It bars all existing insurance plans from imposing lifetime caps on coverage. Restrictions will also be placed on annual limits on coverage. Insurers can no longer cancel insurance retroactively for reasons other than outright fraud. Funding for the legislation would come from $438 billion in new taxes and more than $500 billion in spending reductions, primarily in Medicare.

per member per month (PMPM)   A set amount of money paid or received per enrollee in a managed care plan. May also be referred to as *capitation*.

personal health care services   Services designed to provide individual treatment of sick persons, which may be performed on a per visit or a per hour basis.

physician   A doctoral-level clinician (Doctor of Medicine or Doctor of Osteopathy) responsible for the diagnoses and treatment of illness, injury, and disease. He or she refers patients to hospitals, performs tests and procedures, and coordinates the care of patients.

physician hospital organization (PHO)   A legal entity that combines physicians and hospitals together to form an integrated delivery system. They possess advantages in contracting with managed care plans, sharing financial risk, contracting directly with employers, and enhancing the quality of care for patients.

physician's assistant   A provider who works under the supervision of a physician to perform a variety of services such as triaging patients and performing physical examinations, tests, and procedures. A physician's assistant plays a key role in providing patient education, counseling, and prescribing medications and treatments.

point-of-service organization (POS)   A type of managed care plan with characteristics of both a health maintenance organization and a preferred provider organization. In this plan, a primary care physician is selected from participating providers, and all health care is coordinated by this physician or "point of service." Referrals by the primary care physician for specialist care are made to other in-network physicians. When visiting an out-of-network specialist, the patient is responsible for submitting claims for reimbursement.

post-acute care   Care similar to sub-acute care but always occurs following an acute care hospitalization and does not have to be provided in an inpatient setting. Typical settings in which this type of care is provided include nursing homes and rehabilitation and long-term care hospitals; it is also provided through outpatient physical and occupational therapy.

predisposing factors   The propensity of individuals to use health services based on their demographics, socioeconomic status, and beliefs in the benefits of the health services.

preferred provider plan (PPO)   A plan where different types of providers, physicians, hospitals, and clinics contract with a preferred provider organization to provide care to its members. Insured members pay a copayment at the time of service and a yearly deductible before the insurance begins to pay a percentage of medical fees for an in-network provider. Patients may visit out-of-network providers without a referral and pay a higher percentage of fees.

President George W. Bush   Born in 1946, served as governor of Texas (1995–2000), and was the 43rd president of the United States from 2001–2009. He supported and signed the Medicare Prescription Drug Improvement and Modernization Act (MMA) of 2003, which made the most sweeping changes to Medicare by providing Medicare beneficiaries a prescription drug benefit.

President Harry S. Truman   Born in 1884 and the 33rd president of the United States, he succeeded President Roosevelt upon the latter's death in 1945. As part of the Fair Deal in 1949, he proposed a comprehensive, prepaid medical insurance plan for all people through the Social Security system. His proposal was referred to as National Health Insurance, and although the legislation failed to pass the Congress, it provided the basis for President John F. Kennedy's promises of health insurance for the elderly.

President John F. Kennedy   Born in 1917 and the 35th president of the United States from 1961–1963. He proposed legislation calling for health insurance for the elderly. The proposed legislation became the focus of debate throughout the early 1960s. President Kennedy was unable to pass health care coverage for the elderly during his presidency, but the bill was passed during the Johnson administration and was a cornerstone of his "Great Society" program.

President Lyndon B. Johnson   Born in 1908 and became the 36th president of the United States upon the death of President John F. Kennedy. He was president of the United States from 1963–1969. He signed into law the Civil Rights Act (1964) and initiated major social service programs as part of the Great Society. He signed legislation that funded the Medicare and Medicaid programs, which, respectively, provided health benefits for the elderly and the poor.

prevalence   The number of total cases of a disease (existing and new) over a period of time. Healthier groups or nations should have fewer cases for a given standardized group (such as per 1,000 or 100,000 people).

preventive care   Services that aim to stop the onset of disease through health education and healthy changes in lifestyle to produce significant societal health benefits.

preventive public health   The most cost-effective health care interventions to date, they include immunizations, prenatal care, smoking cessation, and cholesterol control. They also include health screening programs and many disease management programs.

primary care   Often referred to as "first contact" care, care that is received from the family doctor, hospital outpatient department, community health center, or university health service. It is delivered by clinicians in general practice and the medical specialties of family practice, obstetrics and gynecology, pediatrics, and general internal medicine.

primary prevention   Precluding disease processes from ever getting started. Examples of these public health programs include immunizations, water and air purification, fluoridation of the water supply, and education, such as diet and exercise programs.

program of all-inclusive care for the elderly (PACE)   A system of managed care serving frail elderly who are eligible for nursing home care. It provides case management and an all-inclusive set of acute and long-term care services under one umbrella, thereby ensuring coordination of care.

public health   Strategy to improve the health of communities through education, promotion of healthy lifestyles, and a focus on disease and injury prevention. Efforts focus on improving the health and wellbeing of people in the local patient population.

public health problems   Diseases or issues that may be common or even increasing in incidence and prevalence in a community.

quality assessment   The process by which quality of care is measured at some point in time.

quality assurance   The process of conducting ongoing measurement activities in conjunction with the installation of feedback mechanisms designed for continuous quality improvement.

quality improvement (QI) initiatives   Strategies employed by stakeholders in the health care industry to enhance health care quality through a diverse set of strategies. Some focus on publically reporting quality measurements of providers and payers. Others may focus on clinical outcomes and improving the overall health of patients before, during, and after inpatient and outpatient care.

quality improvement organizations (QIO)   Private not-for-profit entities staffed by professionals, such as physicians and other health care professionals, who are trained to review the quality of health care and assist Medicare beneficiaries with their care issues. They also work to improve the quality of health care available to beneficiaries throughout the health care continuum.

quality of health care   The measure of the degree to which the right care was provided to the right patient at the right time, every time. There are three fundamental dimensions to quality, including structure, process, and outcomes. A high level of health care quality is consistently safe, equitable, effective, timely, efficient, and patient centered.

quality-adjusted life years   The percentage of life span that is healthy (free of significant disease or disability), it also measures both quantity and quality of a person's healthy life.

reactive planning   No specific sequence of stages or events are made in advance, but a set of conditions and a goal are identified. Decisions are made based on rules that account for conditions or contingencies and actions that should result. Or, future actions are taken as a response to past or present events or conditions.

regional variation in health   Differences in health status or health care based on location or residence of the patient(s).

regulation   Centralized planning that has the force of law behind it through the power of federal and state agencies. In the health care industry, these agencies may include the Center for Medicare and Medicaid or the Food and Drug Administration.

rehabilitation   Care provided in different settings such as inpatient facilities, outpatient facilities, or in the patient's home. May follow an acute illness such as a stroke, an injury such as a hip fracture, or total knee replacement, with the goal of optimization of function, maintenance of health, and slowed decline of the patient's health. It can also be used to treat drug and alcohol addictions.

residential care facility   A facility designed for residents who need minimal assistance with activities of daily living (ADLs) or who are in the early stages of dementia.

resource-based relative value scale (RBRVS)   Implemented in 1992, a method of standardized physician payment schedule that attempts to contain costs by instituting the same pay for similar services. Payment for services is based on the resource costs as measured by time, skill, and intensity needed to provide them.

respite care   Service designed to give informal caregivers a break by providing assistance to their family member or loved ones who require long-term care. It encompasses a wide variety of services including traditional home-based care as well as adult day care, skilled nursing, home health, and short-term institutional care.

Roemer's law   The tendency to fill hospital beds with patients when there is an excess of hospital beds; it therefore guarantees use of the beds and reimbursement for providers. This law assumes that the population is insured and that physicians influence their patients to demand more services through induced demand.

Rosenstock's model of health services   Developed in 1966, it holds that four factors predict use of health care services: the perceived susceptibility to the disease, the perceived threat of the disease and its seriousness, the belief in benefit or the efficacy of the health system in treating their condition, and the individual's cues to action through the media, friends, family, or well-known persons.

Rural Hospital Flexibility Program (Flex Program)   Begun under the Balanced Budget Act of 1997, a federally funded program that provides assistance to critical access hospitals (CAHs), encourages the development of rural health networks, assists with quality improvement efforts, and improves rural emergency medical services.

S

secondary care   An intermediate level of health care that may involve, for example, an admission to a hospital or consultation with a specialist. The services are typically delivered as part of an episode of care and focused on a specific health problem, test, or procedure.

secondary prevention   The early detection of the presence of the initial stages of diseases to avoid their developing into later stages of those diseases; examples include high blood pressure screening, cholesterol screening, pap smears, and mammograms.

senior center   Community facilities that provide social activities and custodial care for seniors.

short-stay hospital   The most common type of hospital in the United States, with a majority being voluntary, not-for-profit, community general hospitals with an average length of stay of approximately 5.5 days.

skilled nursing facility   Entity designed to deliver short-term nursing care on an inpatient basis, usually following hospitalization. They provide the most intensive care available outside of a hospital and most are in nursing homes, but many hospitals may also have skilled nursing facility (SNF) beds.

Social Security Act of 1935   Federal legislation that was part of Roosevelt's "New Deal" social program. It was enacted to provide retirement security for retired American workers. It created a pension system funded by taxes on employers and employees. Amendments to the Social Security Act in 1965 added health insurance benefits through the Medicare and Medicaid programs.

societal determinants of utilization   Norms, beliefs, and standards which influence the perceived need for health services on a societal level. These beliefs may be reflected in legislation, regulation, and trends in health care practice.

socioeconomic status (SES)   The stature in society one holds that is dependent on such diverse factors as income, profession, residence, education, or income.

solo practitioner   A physician practicing independently without any partner physicians.

space shot mentality   Belief that technology can achieve anything which leads to a concentration on acute care settings, rather than on prevention, disease management, or long-term care. Leads to medical research focused on finding medicinal or surgical cures for idiosyncratic or rare diseases.

specialty hospital   A facility that provides specialized services, such as cardiology, orthopedics, and surgery, or focuses on treatment of specific conditions, such as cancer or pediatrics. Distinguished from general acute care hospitals by its focus on providing a select core of services. May also be dedicated to a specific category of patients, such as children or women. Most are small and less likely to be teaching hospitals and to treat low-income patients.

staff model HMO   A managed care model that employs physicians to deliver care to HMO enrollees exclusively at their facilities.

State Children's Health Insurance Plan (SCHIP)   The partnership between states and the federal government that permits states either to expand Medicaid coverage or develop a proposal for a new program to be reviewed by the Centers for Medicare and Medicaid Services. In general, states are permitted to insure kids living in families whose income is up to 200 percent of the federal poverty level. Eligibility requirements are set so that uninsured children who are ineligible for Medicaid can still be covered under SCHIP. There are many benefits to enroll in SCHIP, including a full range of inpatient, outpatient, and physician services.

sub-acute care   Care that is delivered in the inpatient setting to patients who are suffering from an injury or acute illness or an exacerbation of an existing condition. It may focus on care right after a serious illness in the hospital or in place of an acute care hospital stay. The treatment is goal oriented and is designed around one or more specific conditions or complex treatments.

Supplemental Security Income (SSI)   Implemented in 1974, a federal program funded by general funds to provide eligible persons supplemental income to meet basic needs. Program provides assistance for the aged, blind, and disabled persons, and those with little or no income.

T

teaching hospital   A facility that has at least one approved residency program for medicine or dentistry.

Temporary Aid for Needy Families (TANF)   A federally funded need-based grant program that allows states to administer their own assistance programs. The goal of the program is to provide families with children under the age of 18 with both financial assistance and work opportunities. The program provides cash assistance, job preparation, and support services. Recipients are required to participate in work activities for a specified period every week and be fully employed within a specified time.

terminally ill   A patient who has a life expectancy of six or fewer months due to an incurable illness.

tertiary care   Referred to as "super" specialty care, services are often delivered at large medical centers, referral hospitals, and teaching hospitals. Tertiary care hospitals do provide almost all levels of service, including primary and secondary care. They also perform complex medical procedures such as transplants, open heart surgery, neurosurgery, and advanced cancer treatment, and are likely to have intensive care and critical care units such as neonatal intensive care, cardiac intensive care, and burn units.

tertiary prevention   The treatment of diseases once they are present, to avoid further complications; examples include cardiac rehabilitation to prevent further heart attacks, stroke rehabilitation to limit permanent disability, disease management of diabetes or congestive heart failure, and treatment and management of HIV to prevent the transition to AIDS.

underinsured   Individuals who have health insurance coverage, but do not have comprehensive coverage. As a result, they face significant cost sharing requirements or limits in their benefits that may diminish their ability to access or pay for needed health services.

underpayment   The difference between the hospital cost of care and the amount the hospital is reimbursed for providing that care.

underuse of care   Failure to use evidence-based health care practices that have proven to be beneficial to patients.

uninsured   Persons who lacked health insurance coverage at any time during a defined 12-month period.

usual source of care (USOC)   A health care clinician who provides regular and customary care to patients.

vertical integration   The combination or coordination of different stages of the delivery of health care. For example, when a hospital joins with one or more health maintenance organizations (HMOs), outpatient clinics, home health agencies, rehabilitation centers, long-term care facilities, surgi-centers, technical laboratories, or wellness clinics. Potential benefits may include economies of scale, efficiency, reduced duplication of services, and increased market share.

"way-of-life" factors   Factors that impact health status and life expectancy and are due to individual decisions and behaviors . Examples include smoking, seat-belt wearing in automobiles, and nutritional and diet decisions.

World War I   Begun in 1914 and ended in 1918; also called the Great War, it was between the Allies (including the United States and Western Europe) and the Central Powers (the German Empire, the Austro-Hungarian Empire, the Ottoman Empire, and the Kingdom of Bulgaria).

World War II   Begun in 1939 and ended in 1945, it was between the Allies (including the United States and Western Europe) and the Axis Powers (Germany, Italy, and Japan).

yearly deficit   The amount by which the federal government's annual expenditures exceed its tax revenues.

years of healthy life   Calculated by subtracting the total number of sick and disabled days and years from the average life expectancy. It is used to determine the percentage of a person's or group's life that is spent in good health and to compare the disease and disability burdens of different groups.

zero sum game   Resources are scarce, and there is a finite amount that can be spent on societal programs; therefore, resources dedicated to one need require that less money be spent on a different societal need.

Index

D